TOPICS IN CLINICAL CHIF
Robert D. Mootz,

Chiropractic Care of Special Populations

TOPICS IN CLINICAL CHIROPRACTIC Series
Robert D. Mootz, Editor

Chiropractic Care of Special Populations
Robert D. Mootz and Linda J. Bowers

Chiropractic Technologies
Robert D. Mootz and Daniel T. Hansen

Sports Chiropractic
Robert D. Mootz and Kevin A. McCarthy

Best Practices in Clinical Chiropractic
Robert D. Mootz and Howard T. Vernon

TOPICS IN CLINICAL CHIROPRACTIC Series
Robert D. Mootz, Editor

Chiropractic Care of Special Populations

Robert D. Mootz, DC
Editor
Topics in Clinical Chiropractic
Associate Medical Director for Chiropractic
State of Washington Department of Labor and Industries
Olympia, Washington

Linda J. Bowers, DC
Associate Editor
Topics in Clinical Chiropractic
Professor
Northwestern College of Chiropractic
Bloomington, Minnesota

AN ASPEN PUBLICATION®
Aspen Publishers, Inc.
Gaithersburg, Maryland
1999

The author has made every effort to ensure the accuracy of the information herein. However, appropriate information sources should be consulted, especially for new or unfamiliar procedures. It is the responsibility of every practitioner to evaluate the appropriateness of a particular opinion in the context of actual clinical situations and with due consideration to new developments. The author, editors, and the publisher cannot be held responsible for any typographical or other errors found in this book.

Library of Congress Cataloging-in-Publication Data

Chiropractic care of special populations/
[edited by] Robert D. Mootz, Linda J. Bowers.
p. cm.—(Topics in clinical chiropractic series)
Consists of updated articles from Topics in clinical chiropractic.
Includes bibliographical references and index.
ISBN 0-8342-1374-5 (pbk. : alk. paper)
1. Chiropractic Miscellanea.   I. Mootz, Robert D.   II. Series. [DNLM: 1. Chiropractic—methods—Aged.
2. Chiropractic—methods—Child.   3. Chiropractic—methods—Infant.   4. Women's Health.
WB 905 C5413 1999]
RZ242.C45 1999
615.5'34—dc21
DNLM/DLC
for Library of Congress
99-31809
CIP

Copyright © 1999 by Aspen Publishers, Inc.
All rights reserved.

Aspen Publishers, Inc., grants permission for photocopying for limited personal or internal use. This consent does not extend to other kinds of copying, such as copying for general distribution, for advertising or promotional purposes, for creating new collective works, or for resale. For information, address Aspen Publishers, Inc., Permissions Department, 200 Orchard Ridge Drive, Suite 200, Gaithersburg, Maryland 20878.

Orders: (800) 638-8437
Customer Service: (800) 234-1660

About Aspen Publishers • For more than 35 years, Aspen has been a leading professional publisher in a variety of disciplines. Aspen's vast information resources are available in both print and electronic formats. We are committed to providing the highest quality information available in the most appropriate format for our customers. Visit Aspen's Internet site for more information resources, directories, articles, and a searchable version of Aspen's full catalog, including the most recent publications: **http://www.aspenpublishers.com**
Aspen Publishers, Inc. • The hallmark of quality in publishing
Member of the worldwide Wolters Kluwer group.

Editorial Services: Stephanie Neuben
Library of Congress Catalog Card Number: 99-31809
ISBN: 0-8342-1374-5
Series ISBN: 0-8342-1710-4

Printed in the United States of America

1 2 3 4 5

*For Norbert who taught perspective, and
Helen who taught integrity and hope. (RDM)*

*For Ashley, thanks for bringing light
and love to my life. (LJB)*

Table of Contents

Contributors ix

Series Preface xi

Preface xiii

Understanding and Appropriate Use of Clinical Algorithms xv
    Robert D. Mootz and Daniel T. Hansen

PART I—INFANTS AND CHILDREN 1

    1   **Clinical Assessment of Selected Pediatric Conditions:**
           Guidelines for the Chiropractic Physician 3
        Linda J. Bowers

    2   **Childhood: A Crucial Age for Health Promotion** 16
        Jennifer R. Jamison

    3   **Periodic Health Examination of Infants and Children** 21
        Linda J. Bowers

    4   **Otitis Media: A Conservative Chiropractic Management Protocol** 30
        Lester Lamm and Lorraine Ginter

    5   **Chiropractic Management of the Special Needs Child** 41
        Tracy Barnes

    6   **Infantile Colic: Identification and Management** 50
        Dorrie M. Talmage and Diane Resnick

    7   **Understanding Childhood Cancer: Keys for the Chiropractor** 56
        Tracy Barnes

    8   **Adjusting the Pediatric Spine** 69
        Gregory Plaugher and Joel Alcantara

    APPENDIX I–A—The Periodic Health Examination 80

    APPENDIX I–B—Adolescent Health: On-line and Text Resources 85

    APPENDIX I–C—Children's Health Internet Sites 86

viii CHIROPRACTIC CARE OF SPECIAL POPULATIONS

PART II—WOMEN'S HEALTH ... 87

9 Heart Disease in Women ... 89
Jennifer R. Jamison

10 Osteoporosis: Assessment and Treatment Options ... 99
Donna M. Mannello

11 Diagnosis and Management of Premenstrual Syndrome in the Chiropractic Office ... 113
Tolu A. Oyelowo

12 Breast Cancer: A Current Summary ... 124
Leona Berestiansky Sembrat

13 Considerations in Adjusting Women ... 135
Kevin M. Bartol

14 Partner Abuse: Recognition and Intervention Strategies ... 145
Dorrie M. Talmage

APPENDIX II–A—A Guide to Women's Health Resources ... 154

PART III—GERIATRIC HEALTH ... 157

15 Normal Aging ... 159
Thomas Souza and Shahihaz Soliman

16 Clinical Assessment of Geriatric Patients: Unique Challenges ... 168
Linda J. Bowers

17 Management Considerations in the Geriatric Patient ... 184
Kevin A. McCarthy

18 Manipulative Care and Older Persons ... 195
Thomas F. Bergmann and Link Larson

19 Trauma in the Geriatric Patient: A Chiropractic Perspective with a Focus on Prevention ... 204
Lisa Zaynab Killinger

APPENDIX III–A—Internet Sites for Seniors ... 211

Index ... 213

Contributors

Joel Alcantara, DC
Palmer College of Chiropractic—West
San Jose, California
Gonstead Clinical Studies Society
Mount Horeb, Wisconsin

Tracy Barnes, DC
Kentuckiana Children's Center
Louisville, Kentucky

Kevin M. Bartol, DC
Northwestern College of Chiropractic
Bloomington, Minnesota

Thomas F. Bergmann, DC
Center for Clinical Studies
Northwestern College of Chiropractic
Bloomington, Minnesota

Linda J. Bowers, DC
Northwestern College of Chiropractic
Bloomington, Minnesota

Lorraine Ginter, DC
Western States Chiropractic College
Portland, Oregon

Jennifer R. Jamison, MBBCh, PhD, EdD
Royal Melbourne Institute of Technology
Bundoora, Victoria, Australia

Lisa Zaynab Killinger, DC
Palmer Center for Chiropractic Research
Davenport, Iowa

Lester Lamm, DC
Western States Chiropractic College
Portland, Oregon

Link Larson, DC
Northwestern College of Chiropractic
Bloomington, Minnesota
Private Practice
St. Paul, Minnesota

Kevin A. McCarthy, DC
Palmer College of Chiropractic—West
San Jose, California

Donna M. Mannello, DC
Logan College of Chiropractic
Chesterfield, Missouri

Tolu A. Oyelowo, DC
Center for Clinical Studies
Northwestern College of Chiropractic
Bloomington, Minnesota

Gregory Plaugher, DC
Life College of Chiropractic—West
San Lorenzo, California
Gonstead Clinical Studies Society
Mount Horeb, Wisconsin

Diane Resnick, DC
Los Angeles College of Chiropractic
Whittier, California

Leona Berestiansky Sembrat, DC
Private Practice
Calgary, Alberta, Canada

Shahihaz Soliman, MD
Palmer College of Chiropractic—West
San Jose, California

Thomas Souza, DC
Palmer College of Chiropractic—West
San Jose, California

Dorrie M. Talmage, DC
Los Angeles College of Chiropractic
Whittier, California

Series Preface

This book includes contributions to the first six volumes of *Topics in Clinical Chiropractic* (TICC) that have particular relevance to the health care needs of unique patient populations including children, the elderly, and women. This text is part of an initial four-volume series that collects and updates many of the most relevant works from the journal's archives. Where necessary, articles and care pathways have been updated from their initial publication to reflect current practices. The original idea for a scholarly chiropractic journal focusing on clinically relevant topics came from Martha Sasser, an Aspen Publishers, Inc., acquisitions editor at the time. Her first choice for editor was Reed Phillips who was in his ascendancy to president of Los Angeles College of Chiropractic.

Much to the profession's loss, Reed was unable fit the project on his rather full plate. Martha arranged to meet with me to discuss a "book manuscript review project" during a routine promotional visit to Palmer College of Chiropractic–West where I was professor. Little did I know, but by the time our lunch meeting rolled around, Martha had already met with the President and Dean to secure their support and my release time to take on the editorship of Aspen's new journal, TICC. With great trepidation, I agreed, provided that Aspen would support an expanded associate editor structure that allowed me to spread editorial tasks among eminently more qualified individuals in the publishing world.

Regrettably, most of the people I knew who were experienced with journal editing were also much smarter than I and turned down involvement, leaving me to turn to a cast of good friends and co-workers who knew no more than I did about operating a peer-reviewed scientific journal. And what good fortune that was. Linda Bowers, Dan Hansen, Kevin McCarthy, and Tom Souza all agreed to work on the project under the experienced tutelage of Martha who, before the ink was dry on the contracts, left Aspen for other publishing opportunities.

That left the five of us to make the project into our own, building the editorial board from scratch, developing issue topics, and twisting the arms of chiropractic practitioners, researchers, and academicians to submit their wares to our new upstart of a journal. Luckily, Martha's replacement was Jane Garwood, a bright and supportive Aspen insider who worked diligently and patiently with the five of us to get TICC off and running and assure that resources were there to make it a first class publication. Jane, too, was promoted, followed by Steve Zollo. When Tom Souza left to to write a couple of the profession's most respected textbooks, I was very lucky to have Howie Vernon join our Associate Editor staff.

My thanks go out to Martha Sasser for both her original idea and her persistence in getting it off the ground. I thank Reed Phillips for giving the "second-in-line" the opportunity to make a lasting contribution to chiropractic scholarship. I must especially thank my friends and colleagues, TICC's associate editors, Linda Bowers, Dan Hansen, Kevin McCarthy, Tom Souza, and Howie Vernon for their willingness to give up the incredible amount of time and energy it takes to maintain the quality and consistency that are the journal's hallmarks.

Steve Zollo was responsible for first approaching me to put together this series of essential reading books based on TICC's contributions, but it has been Amy Martin who brought the project through to fruition. Mary Anne Langdon and Stephanie Neuben, whose competence in creating the finished product, has assured its success. In addition, TICC's long-time production editor, Sandy Lunsford, has been an absolute joy to work with. Through three new children she has continued to put up with our publishing naiveté, our missed deadlines, forgotten permission requests, and our stressful last minute revisions. She has been supportive of us, patient, understanding, and resourceful when things just would not come together as planned. She continues to be the behind-the-scenes glue that holds the project together. For our lasting endearment to Sandy: *"Deadlines mean always having to say you're sorry!"*

My thanks also go to all of the authors who submit their work to the journal, particularly the contributors to this book. The quality of their work, and their willingness to share their knowledge is greatly appreciated. A special thanks to the college faculty members that have found value in our publication to make it required reading within their curriculum. And on behalf of the editors and contributors, we would also like to thank our readership—*our customers*—for the valuable feedback toward the improvements we've made and toward the recognition that what we've provided to our profession is meaningful and has made a difference.

I hope you will find the entire series of value for enhancing your educational opportunities, your practice, your community of health care, and mostly to the patients you serve.

—*Robert D. Mootz*
Editor

Preface

The topic of this book, "Chiropractic Care of Special Populations," is the title we have selected to capture chiropractic clinical strategies that fall outside of applicability to the "standard 70 kg man." Interestingly, the vast majority of clinical research that has been performed to date has excluded vulnerable populations such as the young and elderly, and frequently women.[1] The rationales may seem scientifically and socially justified because metabolisms vary with age and gender, and the concept of protecting vulnerable subjects from undue exposure to experimental regimens is laudable at face value.

However, as clinical knowledge rapidly accumulates for a predominantly young to middle aged male population, children, the elderly, and females have seen clinical practices, tested only on men, applied in practice to everyone. The same ethical rationale for protecting vulnerable subjects, or potentially skewing results due to fluctuating metabolisms, now subjects those very same populations to risk on a larger scale, but without the benefit of controlled scientific observation.

Recently, the National Institutes of Health (NIH) implemented research policies that require inclusion of age and gender representative populations in all research designs.[2] As a result, clinical interventions will increasingly have the benefit of knowledge regarding applicability to broader populations of patients. With chiropractic research really just beginning to outgrow its infancy, little is known about the impacts age and gender have on the specific care we deliver. Still, clinical experience and information from the greater clinical domains can offer insight into some of the most fruitful clinical strategies we might embrace.

Providing health care for children can be one of the most rewarding experiences of one's professional life. It can also be one of the most challenging and demanding. Every aspect of care, from evaluating a symptom or chasing down an observation brought forth by a concerned parent, requires attenuation of history and examination protocols, if not outright mental telepathy. Differences in risk factors, non-adult psychosocial variables, and basic alterations from adult physiology will all impact the care decisions and care planning we do.

The opportunities for early intervention, promotion of good habits that can influence long term health status, and the sheer joy on the face and in the heart of healing a child outweigh any and all of the extra work that may accrue the delivery of care in this special group of people. Most of the time, the resilience and recuperative abilities of growing bodies help facilitate recovery from disease or injury, in greater harmony with the interventions chiropractors offer. However, sometimes life deals an unfair hand. There is nothing more heart-wrenching in our clinical experience than caring for a child whose life will be cut short by cancer, or whose full human experience has been limited by disease, injury, or genetic predisposition. Partnering with these children and their families to find hope, relief, or function can be difficult, yet incredibly fulfilling. Often, insight to the dilemmas and limitations that these individuals confront allows a chiropractor to make a bit more of a difference.

Women make up the majority of chiropractic patients.[3] Their health concerns often differ substantially from those of men. The subject of women's health is an extremely broad one encompassing unique cancer risk factors, wellness and health promotion strategies, biomechanical and fitness issues, osteoporosis, particular nutritional considerations as well as reproductive health concerns. Domestic violence is a national tragedy that affects women in far greater numbers than men. All health care providers will see victims of it in their practice, and recognition, intervention tactics, and appropriately meeting legal obligations require skill and finesse from providers.

The number of individuals over the age 65 is expected to double between 1989 and 2030.[4] Currently, nearly 10 million elderly persons in the US experience difficulty engaging in basic activities of living such as walking and self care.[5] This rapid aging of industrialized populations will require greater geriatric health expertise from providers functioning in primary care roles. As life span increases, so do expectations of patients regarding the quality of their lives. Care seeking behavior, coverage benefits, and utilization data suggest that demand for chiropractic services will continue to increase.[6] As a result, DCs will likely find themselves harnessing clinical and management skills tailored to the needs of the elderly with greater regularity.

As with pediatric and female patients, caring for elderly persons offers unique circumstances that demand interventions that are optimized and focused to their needs. Although chiropractic practices provide abundant opportunities for managing geriatric patients, specific treatment protocols remain difficult to find. Living arrangements, functional abilities, concurrent pathologies, drug-related symptoms, healing times, and response to intervention represent examples of issues chiropractors must address when working with the elderly.

These three special populations of patients are addressed in this text. The material included only begins to scratch the surface of the issues these individuals present to chiropractors who care for them. However, we think you will agree that it represents a solid foundation of information that is essential for the DC's clinical toolbox. The authors of the material presented here come from an international and diverse group with vast clinical and academic experience. We hope you find that the informed clinical suggestions they provide will be invaluable to your practice.

—*Robert D. Mootz*
—*Linda J. Bowers*

REFERENCES

1. Finegan LP. The NIH women's health initiative: its evolution and expected contribution to women's health. *Am J Prev Med.* 1996;12(5): 292–293.
2. National Institutes of Health. NIH Guide for Grants and Contracts. Bethesda, MD: US Department of Health and Human Services, National Institutes of Health, 1997.
3. Phillips RB, Mootz RD, Nyiendo J. Cooperstein R, Mennon M. The descriptive profile of low back pain patients of field practicing chiropractors contrasted with those treated in the clinics of six west coast chiropractic colleges. *J Manip Physiol Therap.* 1992;15(8):512–517.
4. Miller DK, Kaiser FE. Assessment of the older woman. *Clin Geriatr Med.* 1992;9:1–31.
5. Harada N, Chiu V, Damron-Rodriguez J, Fowler E, Siu A, Reuben DB. Screening for balance and mobility requirements in elderly individuals living in residential care facilities. *Phys Ther.* 1995;75:462–469.
6. Cherkin DC, Mootz RD (eds). *Chiropractic in the United States: Training, Practice and Research.* AHCPR Pub. No. 98-N002. Rockville, MD: Agency for Health Care Policy and Research, Public Health Service, US Dept of Health and Human Services, 1997.

Understanding and Appropriate Use of Clinical Algorithms

Robert D. Mootz and Daniel T. Hansen

Among the most popular features of *Topics in Clinical Chiropractic* (TICC) are the clinical algorithms found in the appendixes of each issue of the journal. When used properly, a well-done clinical algorithm can be an important learning tool in clinical training and can help inform clinical decision making. The editors of TICC decided from the beginning to utilize this tool whenever possible as an adjunct to the presentation of the various clinical topics. Our original 1994 article[1] reviewed the nature and use of clinical algorithms. We update that piece here to allow better appreciation for the intended use and application of these graphic guidelines. In addition to informing the doctors and patients who use them, care pathways for chiropractic procedures can also provide guidance to non-DC providers when a chiropractic referral may be prudent.

RELEVANCE OF ALGORITHMS

The health care system continues to experience turbulent changes in delivery and accountability never before seen in the industry. Where other elements of manufacturing and service industries have been "assuring quality" and "lower costs" for products and services, the health care profession has lagged in its response to this change of culture. Health care providers cannot work a day now without some sort of contact with the new paradigm of health delivery and some element of managed care being applied to their practices. Preauthorization for procedures, benefit limitations, additional or standardized reporting requirements, and utilization reviews are all examples of managed care methodologies that providers must regularly cope with.

These changes are the result of a strong public mandate for the purchase of health care that is patient centered, evidence based and protocol driven. Patient outcome has become the tangible focus of care and coverage decisions. In practice, this means that the selection of diagnostic tests or a sequence of care is increasingly driven by accepted, evidence-based protocols. From a provider's perspective, one of the most useful forms that such guidelines can take are as *algorithms* or *care pathways*.

Because well-done algorithms are clear, concise, and graphically represented, they are an excellent basis for communicating and representing typical considerations in delivering optimal clinical care. They help convey the sequential and linked nature of many care decisions. Well-done algorithms can facilitate thinking through tiers of decisions and can systematically identify emergent and ambiguous clinical considerations. When viewed by other providers and health care administrators, they can offer a sense of predictability and a systematic organization to case management that provides assurance that the approach a chiropractor is using is reasonable and well founded.

Many common conditions have management sequences shown to be clinically efficient. Less variation in the use of

---

Algorithms offered in this book are presented with the intention of clarifying the relationships among various conditions. They are not intended for use as diagnostic guides for individual patients. Each patient's case has its own unique characteristics and must be addressed by someone well trained and competent to render a diagnosis and care. These guidelines are not presented as definitive but rather as examples of typical kinds of thought processes the practicing chiropractor might want to consider. Parameters such as these are designed to assist the DC by providing a framework for the evaluation of the patient in situations characterized by the algorithms. These guidelines are not intended to replace the physician's clinical judgment or to establish a protocol for diagnosis and/or treatment of patients with any particular set of symptoms.

resources can contribute to quicker and more optimal outcomes and, ultimately, to a reduction in health costs.[2] Algorithmic care pathways can be used to communicate expected ranges of care for a majority of patients presenting with those common problems. Physician discretion is then applied to those patients who may exhibit exceptions based on age, sex, comorbidities, or other health complications. Ideally, the algorithm should include insight as to when additional variables or confounding issues can come into play. In the era of highly competitive care, the better we can do in terms of outcomes and cost, compared with others, the more likely it is that we will be considered the provider of choice.

For doctors, this provides benefit, in that those issues that have been demonstrated to impact quality and efficiency (eg, when to order tests, how long to pursue a course of care, and how to sequence second opinions or additional diagnostics) are accessible from an algorithm in a readily identifiable fashion. Such "expert" evidence-based guidance may also benefit the doctor by providing protection from malpractice exposure. On the flip side, poorly written algorithms or inappropriate interpretation by payers may contribute to confusion and inept oversight in managed care settings. An understanding by doctors of algorithm processes and quality can promote the benefits and reduce possibilities of negative consequences from inappropriate use.

Health care disciplines have been developing and publishing algorithms for more than 30 years. In today's environment of accountability, there has been a virtual explosion of these kinds of guidelines, particularly in managed care settings.[1] Development of care pathways is a part of *continuous quality improvement* (CQI) programs. As we move into the twenty-first century, health care "best practice" algorithms are being embedded into sophisticated, network-based or internet-based information systems for ready access and data retrieval by health planners, providers, and even patients themselves. Those who purchase, use, and refer for health services are better informed than ever before. The need for well-done, provider-developed, evidence-based algorithms cannot be understated.

The chiropractic profession is responding to this charge and has developed and published several pertinent algorithms in the management of common presenting patient complaints. Chiropractic colleges and privately owned chiropractic managed care organizations (MCOs) are developing and implementing clinical algorithms for teaching and management purposes.[3]

With the recent surge in algorithm development and publication, there appears to be greater variation in algorithm formats. It has become necessary for some standards to be developed and implemented in the design, development, and production of algorithms. The standards adopted by the editorial board of TICC are included here.

HISTORY OF ALGORITHM USE IN HEALTH CARE

Graphic algorithms have been widely incorporated in health care literature since the mid-1960s. Algorithms have also been seen in the popular press in self-help books focused on common, uncomplicated health management, such as back pain and headache. Technical algorithms are currently being used in many diverse health delivery systems, such as hospitals and health maintenance organizations (HMOs), and among cohesive physician groups, such as IPAs and EPOs. Governmental and academic institutions, as well as both public and private sector payers, are increasingly turning to such graphical presentations to efficiently summarize key clinical thresholds and decision points.

The Hartford Foundation was the primary funding organization in a nationwide demonstration project that incorporated quality improvement principles used in major industries into health delivery systems. From this effort came projects aimed at identifying wasteful health practices and designing solutions for improvement and systems to implement the improvement processes.[4] The National Demonstration Project on Health Care Quality Improvement developed logical sequences for creating clinical algorithms using "quality improvement teams."[5] The effort sought to develop systems and procedures that assure reliability and validity of the algorithms.

The approach taken in the demonstration project was first validated at the Harvard Community Health Plan in Boston. The process incorporated systematically developed algorithms, review and feedback by providers expected to incorporate them, and measurement and follow-up on patient outcomes and quality markers.[5] Since then, the methods for constructing and implementing clinical algorithms have been distributed widely through course work and published literature. Currently, these methods are widely incorporated as essential steps for quality improvement in health care in both the private and public sectors.[6] There are examples of state level requirements that any health care that is purchased be protocol driven, to the extent possible, and based on published evidence and the consensus of recognized experts and community-based practitioners.[7]

ALGORITHM TERMINOLOGY

It is important to distinguish between some of the terms mentioned in this chapter. Whereas for the most part, there are conceptual similarities, there may indeed be subtle or specific differences.

Algorithms are a series of specifically shaped boxes connected by lines, usually with arrow tips. They can serve as pathways for clinical decision making in a step-wise fashion, identifying the more important or critical steps in the beginning and allowing for transitions into other management sequences or terminal steps. Clinical algorithms have their origins from *decision charts*, which analyze the various clinical decisions that can be made for a problem or patient complaint.

Care pathways are essentially the decision-making and process flow components that appear in algorithms. Algorithms represent one way to graphically illustrate a care pathway in a sophisticated, standardized, graphical manner. Whereas a care pathway may be represented by an algorithm, it may also be characterized in narrative fashion, by step-by-step lists or in a nonstandardized flow chart fashion.

Clinical guidelines are systematically developed statements to assist practitioner and patient decisions about appropriate health care for specific clinical circumstances. These can be in the form of rules or algorithms that reflect the best or most appropriate way to care for certain clinical conditions. Ideally, the use of the term *guideline* implies that some form of formalized review or consensus process has been applied to the content. Examples include recent publications from the Agency for Health Care Policy and Research and the Canadian Chiropractic Association.[8,9]

Practice parameters relate to the inventory of health practice in general. The recommendations found in parameters of care documents relate to the acceptance of procedures, devices, and other attributes of medical or chiropractic practice, according to the available science and opinions of recognized experts. They do not make any distinction for the management of condition-specific issues commonly found in practice.[10]

"Seed" algorithms, guidelines, or *pathways* are ideally well-thought-out first efforts at characterizing the components of clinical decision making in an informal fashion by an individual or a small group of authors. Any time the word *seed* appears as a modifier, it can be implied that minimal or no formalized processes of consensus or review were applied in their development. Peer review, local input, and revisions may or may not be inherent in seed efforts but formalized testing, implementation, and consensus methodologies are unlikely to have been incorporated.

Standards of care are legal standards, established by the trier of the fact in malpractice cases, describing the conduct that society finds acceptable. If a doctor's conduct falls below the applicable standard of care, liability may result. Standards of care are identified by evidentiary rules of discovery and expert testimony, and may vary from region to region and from case to case. The legal test of a standard of care is typically based on the trier of fact's assessment as to whether or not a "reasonable" doctor in a "similar" situation would have acted in a "similar" fashion.[11]

Clinical algorithms or clinical guidelines are not the same as standards of care. However, under common law in most states, a practice parameter or practice guideline may be introduced as evidence of a standard of care in a medical negligence case, as long as it is relevant to the clinical issues involved and is demonstrated to be reliable. Even if a practice parameter or practice guideline is introduced as evidence, it is not considered a predetermined standard of care that a court is required to apply.

WHAT ARE ALGORITHMS?

Algorithms are simply a series of "if, then" statements with dichotomous choices and action steps. For example, a paragraph of complex prose could describe how to compute capital gains tax where there are statements that *"if* you did this, that, and the other thing" with your real estate, *"then* you pay this amount." Alternatively, a series of boxes and lines could be used where the "if" questions are asked and the "then" action steps are clearly presented graphically. Obviously, there can be many different applications of algorithmic sequences, and specific situations can involve additional information that is not addressed in a given algorithm. In the chiropractic literature, we have seen numerous applications of graphical algorithms for assessment of technology;[12] development of standardized terminology;[13] diagnostic decision making;[14–16] and therapeutic management of specific clinical circumstances.[17–19]

Health educators have expressed interest in using clinical algorithms in the teaching and learning environment. Students can use algorithms in learning situations for quick graphic reference to logical clinical decision making. Additionally, applications of clinical algorithms as tools for collaborative and interactive teaching have already shown promise.[20] Generation of seed algorithms has been included as a learning tool for practicing chiropractors in some postgraduate orthopedic programs as a part of their course of study.

Seed clinical parameters for the management of industrial low back injuries have been presented as a part of a prospective clinical trial comparing chiropractic management with medical care.[21] These care pathways are not of the classic algorithm "boxology" but are chronological "if, then" statements identifying anticipated courses of care and expected outcomes. Investigators can then go back and compare the thresholds of care for the individual cases against their projected algorithmic steps.

Despite recent gains in popularity, algorithms and care pathways are still not prevalent in clinical practice at this time. However, with the advance of information systems technology, combined with the development of contemporary clinical pathways, a practitioner may gain access to computerized condition-specific databases with probabilities of successful management.[22] In the future, widespread availability of authoritative software seems likely to allow for the input of clinical characteristics or diagnoses to obtain a series of algorithms or care pathway options that can help the doctor to synthesize the latest clinical research, contemporary outcomes data, and expert opinion into the immediate needs of a given patient.

These computer-based tools will also help the doctor in matters of patient education and informed consent. During the course of treatment, the doctor could be able to track an individual patient through the various decision boxes and action steps, allowing the physician to generate an informative report for the patient in easy-to-understand language. In the meantime, algorithms such as those published thus far can serve to assist competent clinicians as decision-making tools.

It is emphasized that these algorithms are clinical *tools* and are not intended to replace clinical judgment. High-quality clinical guidelines are designed to assist clinicians by providing a framework for the evaluation and treatment of the more common patient problems confronting the physician. It is again emphasized that they are not intended either to replace the clinician's clinical judgment or to establish protocol for all patients with a particular condition. Some patients do not fit the clinical conditions contemplated by such guidelines, and a guideline will rarely establish the only appropriate approach to the problem.

ARE THEY REALLY BEING USED?

Group practices, MCOs, and hospitals have already begun to implement clinical algorithms and expect tighter compliance throughout their system of physicians and support staff. The Harvard Community Health Plan HMO in Boston has shown significant advances in quality of patient care and reduction of health care costs as a result of community-based physician development and refinement of care pathways and algorithms. Additionally, they have documented patient and physician satisfaction with these sequences.[8] Algorithms are also being used in MCOs and utilization management firms to estimate care and to preauthorize expensive diagnostic tests or resource-intensive care. Often, these algorithms are part of a complicated database program and are usually proprietary. Some HMOs have developed algorithms and provided for wide dissemination, expecting system-wide implementation. Applications of algorithms such as these are not "future shock"—this is the present state of the system.

The dynamic nature of algorithms and guidelines embodies the need for modification and attenuation to individual and regional needs. Variations in clinical approach between specialties and disciplines may also account for the compulsion to write, modify, and test a given algorithm or care pathway in different clinical settings. It becomes incumbent, therefore, that modern proactive clinicians be capable of constructing, modifying, critiquing, and implementing clinical care pathways and algorithms.

CONSTRUCTING A "SEED" ALGORITHM

To construct an algorithm, there is a sequence that should be followed. "How" the algorithm is developed is considered to be the "process," but "who" develops it determines how mature and implementable the "structure" is. Applying some purposeful meaning to placing certain clinical information or decision steps into variously shaped and numbered boxes connected by lines and arrows is part of the process of developing an algorithm. This aspect of algorithm development has been termed *medical cartography*,[4] but for the purposes of this book, we can simply refer to it as *boxology*. A mild warning is offered, in that application of adequate critical study toward identifying efficient decision options relative to a given clinical problem is more important than merely arranging boxes and arrows on a page. The development process involves reviewing the pertinent literature and discussing the clinical problem with experienced advisors.

Various authors have developed "seed" algorithms[15,18] as appendixes for a clinical review article. Such algorithms are typically the products of the author (or of an editorial architect) and likely have not had revision through quality improvement teams or consensus panels. The "seeds" are included in their articles merely as suggestions to practitioners, based on clinical experience, and they are ripe for professional discourse.

Conversely, in preparation for a clinical trial on the effectiveness of chiropractic manipulation for headache patients, Nelson and Boline[14] created algorithms using the quality improvement "team approach." Initial "seed" headache algorithms were refined, using consensus methodology with a community-based physician panel, then readied for implementation. These two components, the *seed algorithm* versus the *algorithm by consensus*, represent two distinct but complementary approaches in the *structure* or "design" of algorithm development.

This discussion offers a systematic review of an approach for the development of a "seed" algorithm. A common patient problem or one that is a source of clinical uncertainty and/or variations in practice is appropriate for algorithm development. Clinical algorithms can sometimes emphasize diagnostic pathways as distinct from treatment pathways, or they can be a combination of both. Often, space and page size available for the algorithm will influence how much text or information can be included. The shape of the boxes gives the reader an idea of the various logic sequences or steps in the care pathway, but the detail of the text gives meaning to the logic. An algorithm is "user friendly" when the decision logic makes clinical sense and the content of the text is useful to the physician and patient.

Development of an algorithm requires a scholarly review of relevant literature. For some of the more common conditions that patients present with, there is a knowledge base in the literature ranging from reliability and validity studies for diagnostic technologies to case studies, cohort trials, and, in some cases, randomized clinical trials. Synthesis of information from these studies should identify which methods and procedures have been shown to be effective and which might be ineffective or even controversial. Often, the scientific and more rigorous clinical literature provides only a small piece of the puzzle. A good place to start is to find a series of qualitative literature reviews or, where possible, metanalyses (or literature syntheses) that have systematically searched for and critically appraised the scientific and clinical investigation that has been done.[23,24] The product of this literature review will eventually be made available to consultants or consensus panelists later in the sequence of algorithm development (see Figure 1).

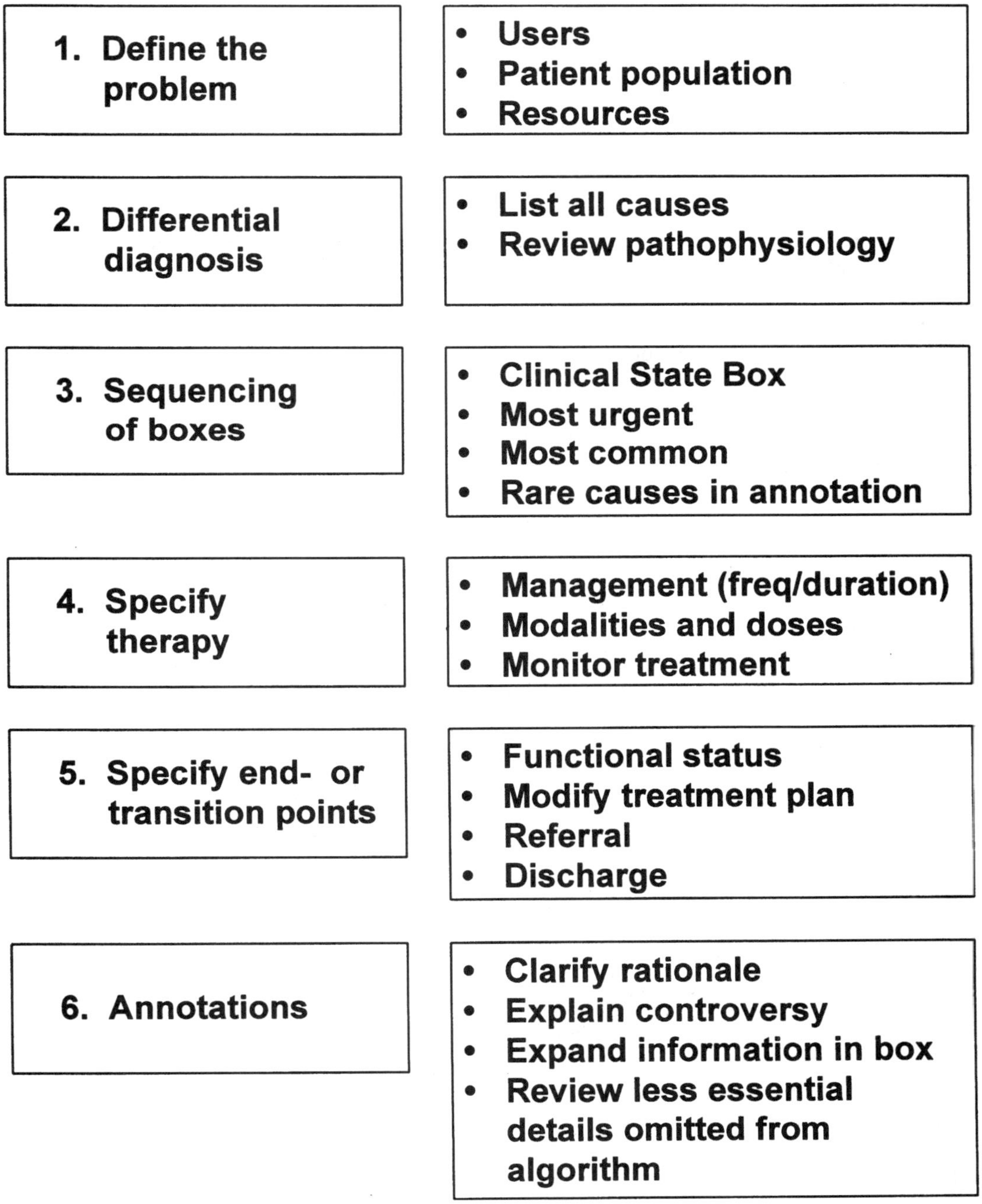

1. Define the problem	• Users • Patient population • Resources
2. Differential diagnosis	• List all causes • Review pathophysiology
3. Sequencing of boxes	• Clinical State Box • Most urgent • Most common • Rare causes in annotation
4. Specify therapy	• Management (freq/duration) • Modalities and doses • Monitor treatment
5. Specify end- or transition points	• Functional status • Modify treatment plan • Referral • Discharge
6. Annotations	• Clarify rationale • Explain controversy • Expand information in box • Review less essential details omitted from algorithm

Fig 1. How to write a clinical algorithm.

Consideration should also be given to identifying who the end-users of this algorithm will be. Practicing doctors, clinical staff, and quality assurance managers may all find utility in a given clinical algorithm. If an algorithm is geared toward a specific end-user, it may be best to include it in the algorithm's title (eg, "Efficient Hypertension Screening for the Nurse Practitioner"). Who the guideline is designed for can make a difference. Additionally, it is important to identify the patient population for which the guide is intended. Again, this may best be dealt with in the title or in the beginning statement (eg, "Hypertension Screening in the Elderly"). A clinical flow chart designed for the management of hypertension in a geriatric population cannot necessarily be generalized to the adolescent or to "twenty-something" populations. Additionally, the designer of the algorithm should be sensitive to the resources reasonably available to the end-user and the patient population.

In studying diagnostic sequences, all etiologies of the patient's presenting complaint should be identified, including pathophysiologic conditions that might be less readily apparent to the end-user. These diagnostic steps should be sequenced in a fashion designed to flush out and manage emergent and urgent conditions earlier in the algorithm. Often, the first diagnostic step is a triage-type decision and usually results in the patient exiting the algorithm. The next priority is to identify and manage the more common conditions through a series of alternating diagnostic and treatment steps. For all the common causes of the clinical condition and its treatment, details of the management should be provided. This includes treatment modalities, doses, frequency, and duration. Intermediate steps for monitoring treatment response (outcomes) should be included when indicated.

Endpoints of therapeutic cycles or phases should be noted by a discrete statement or by action steps (eg, discharge from further care, send to emergency room, etc.) Other endpoints of an algorithm may include referral for a particular diagnostic procedure, referral to a specialist, or referral to another algorithm. Typically, the algorithm will end by identifying some of the rare conditions or by determining that the patient does not fit the algorithm. Experience has shown that it is often easiest to begin by simply listing the various management considerations (etiologies, urgent situations, endpoints, etc.) and trying out various graphic sequences to identify the best way to present the first draft of the algorithm.

Once there is an appreciation for clinical decision making concerning the patient complaint and for the diagnostic or therapeutic options, it is time to start designing boxes and decision steps for the algorithm. How the boxes are shaped, sequenced, connected, and identified is now standardized through an international oversight committee.[6] Figure 2 describes the functions given to the various box shapes.

The *clinical state box* should describe the clinical problem to be addressed. Clinical state boxes that occur in the body of the algorithm are used to clarify the status of the patient or diagnosis along the path of the algorithm (ie, describe a subset of patients with a particular clinical entity).

The *decision box* contains statements that are phrased as questions and punctuated with question marks. If two assessments are to be determined, specify whether both ("and") or one ("or") must be positive for a "yes" response. Multiple questions can be asked in one box, with criteria specified for a "yes" response to the entire box (ie, are two of three present, are all present, are any present?) An example would be a multiple-choice decision box that asks whether the patient has a fever greater than 102° F, history of cancer, sudden weight loss, *or* diabetes. If any of these findings are present, it begs a "yes" response and the appropriate action step. If none are present, it receives a "no" response and the appropriate action.

The *action box* contains a single phrase, indicating a therapeutic or diagnostic action within a box. This box prompts the end-user or patient to "do" something. For clarity's sake, multiple actions that do not need to be sequenced in time may be listed in one box. When multiple actions are presented in one box, each action should be listed on a separate line (preceded with an optional number, dash, or bullet). Typically, the action phrase is not punctuated by a period.

The *link box* can be either a five-sided box or an oval shape. It is a transition step to another box sequence or page of the algorithm. The message in the box may simply read "Go to Page___" or "Go to Box___."

Figure 3 lists the standards for sequencing, connecting, and numbering the algorithm boxes. Lines and arrows should connect boxes closely, such that no lines are unduly long or angled. Boxes are numbered according to the listed guidelines. Numbers should appear outside the upper right-hand corner of the box and should be large enough to be easily read. Numbering provides ease in communication between users of the algorithm and is very convenient during consensus exercises. Algorithms should ideally be on one page but can be on multiple pages, according to the recommended guidelines.

Table 1 provides guidance on titling and use of annotations. The *title* of the algorithm is located at the top right of the page. The title should be crafted carefully because it sets the tone of the algorithm. A title of "Chiropractic Management of Pediatric Headaches" is short and succinct, and it identifies the clinical topic, the patient population, and the intended users. Identification of the author(s) and publication dates is appropriate. It is also advised that there be some designation of the explicit process used in the development of the algorithm; this can be designated as a footnote. *Annotations* are like expanded footnotes that are found at the end of the algorithm, often on a separate page. They are used to clarify rationale or to explain a controversy, with citations to references in the literature used to support the

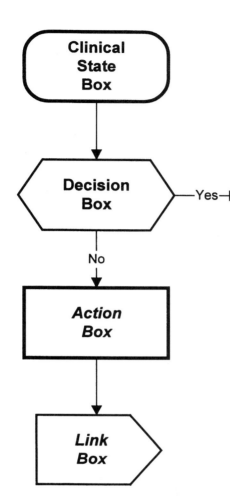

Clinical State Box
Rounded rectangle. This box defines the clinical state or problem. It has only one exit path and may or may not have an entry path. This box always appears at the beginning of an algorithm.

Decision Box
Hexagon in shape. This box requires a branching decision, whose response will lead to one of two alternative paths. It always has one entry path and two exit paths. The text is phrased in the form of a question leading to a "yes" or "no" response.

Action Box
Rectangle. This box indicates instruction for a specific action, usually therapeutic or diagnostic. Oftentimes it serves as an end-point and may suggest transfer to another place on the algorithm.

Link Box
Five-sided (can be oval). This box can be used in place of an arrow, to link boxes for graphic clarity (at page breaks or between separated nodes to maintain path continuity).

Annotations:
(A) Make annotations here...

Fig 2. Algorithm box shapes and functions.

recommendation(s) of the algorithm. They can expand on a statement in an algorithm box (ie, how to perform a procedure, possible side effects, or recommended therapy and when to monitor). Alternatively, they can explain clinical details not essential to the clinical algorithm (ie, a relatively rare etiology).

With this overview of algorithm construction and the established standards for content and clarity, the care pathway can be developed as a "seed" algorithm. Once a seed algorithm is developed, multiple attempts should be made to run through various types of patient presentations to see how well the algorithm can be applied. It is a good idea to ask

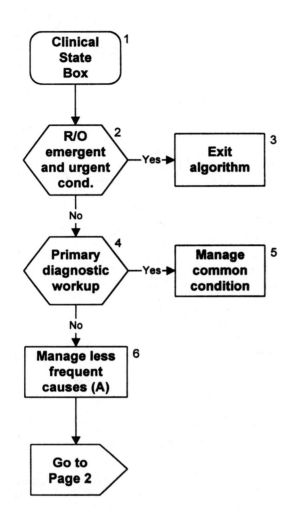

Sequencing Boxes
Present the diagnostic steps in order to rule out emergent and urgent conditions or conditions where the algorithm doesn't apply; alternate diagnostic and therapeutic steps in sequence to then rule out common to frequent to rare causes of the patient complaint.

Connecting Boxes - Arrows
Lines and arrows flow from top to bottom, and in general flow from left to right (exception: where side branch rejoins main stem).
Arrows should never intersect - link boxes can be used to avoid crossing paths.
Arrows originating from decision boxes should be labelled "yes" or "no".
No other text should be used over the arrow. Whenever possible, "yes" arrows should point right, and "no" arrows down.

Numbering Boxes
Clinical state boxes, decision boxes, and action boxes should be numbered sequentially, left to right and top to bottom. Link boxes should not be numbered.

Paging
Whenever possible, consolidation should be sought so an algorithm can be presented on one page.
When page breaks are needed, they should be inserted where clinically logical.
A single box should never be isolated on a page.
For complex algorithms, the first page could best serve as a directory to clinical subsets of patients, identified as clinical state boxes.

(A) *Annotation* regarding rare causes, controversies or clarification of clinical issues.

R/O, rule out; cond., conditions

Fig 3. Algorithm box sequencing, connecting and numbering standards.

---

other potential end-users to try it out, offer their input, and make any further refinements that may be needed. The next step is to seek broader dissemination for testing. In-house algorithms may be tried for a period of time, then evaluated; or seed algorithms can be submitted for peer review and publication. Once it is published as a seed, it can be explicitly reviewed in a number of ways to refine, edit, and improve its content, flow, logic, appearance, and applicability to the intended users. Just getting this far is often a challenge to many clinicians and educators but is usually characterized as a fun and rewarding scholarly accomplishment.

Algorithms can be generated using computer graphic programs such as *Harvard Graphics*™, *Corel Draw*™, *ABC Flowcharter*™, or *Visio*™ (preferred by editors of TICC). It is advisable to utilize a program that features "click and drag" and ample templates of box shapes and line/arrow configura-

Table 1. Algorithm title and annotations

Title
- ❑ Title should define clinical topics and intended users.
- ❑ Authors should be listed under the title, including degree and institutional affiliation.
- ❑ Date of publication and revisions (if applicable) should be specified.
- ❑ A footnote to the title should state the explicit process by which algorithm logic was decided (ie, group consensus after literature review, individual recommendation based on clinical experience, and so forth).

Annotations
- ❑ Annotations are an intrinsic part of the algorithm, and they are used to clarify the rationale of the decisions and cite the supporting literature, or expand on less essential details of the clinical information contained in the box.
- ❑ Annotations following a single phrase should be cited by a capital letter (A) at the end of the phrase.
- ❑ When multiple statements are contained in a single box, annotation(s) should appear at the end of the phrase(s) to which applicable.
- ❑ If an annotation is applicable to the entire box with multiple statements, the annotation should be cited by a capital letter (A) centered on a separate line at the bottom of the box.
- ❑ Annotations should be written in text format, appearing on the bottom of the algorithm page or on a separate page.

---

tions. It is also helpful to have diversity in text formatting and merge capabilities with other supportable software. The value of these desired features will become very apparent once the algorithm is edited or reworked.

FORMAL PROCESSES FOR IMPROVING, CRITIQUING, AND TESTING ALGORITHMS

For a detailed description of the formal processes employed in refining algorithms through consensus methods, critiquing algorithmic guidelines, and testing these pathways and guidelines for reliability and validity, refer to the full text of the article offered in TICC Volume 4, Number 1, 1994.[1] This article has been used extensively as a basis of training in college teaching situations, as well as in practice environments.

The article also offers an explanation of how these development and improvement tools find their way into practice applications in a socially meaningful way. This response by delivery and reimbursement systems has been due to the changes in social tolerances for variations in practice and quality of care. Unfortunately, not all applications of clinical or system-based algorithms are done correctly, or their implementation has occurred without critical input from the respective end-users. Practitioners must be wary of clinical algorithms and guideline systems that do not employ those formal development and implementation processes.

CONCLUSIONS

As mentioned previously, algorithms and care pathways are intended to clarify relationships among clinical conditions and possible decisions—not as diagnostic or treatment guides for individual patients. They just synthesize graphically or in an organized narrative fashion a reasonable hierarchy of clinical decision making. This is especially important to understand when attempting to apply or test a seed algorithm. The thought processes illustrated in guidelines and algorithms are not definitive, but rather examples of typical and supportable thought processes that a clinician might want to consider when addressing a similar clinical situation. They neither replace a clinician's judgment nor establish a protocol, standard for diagnosis, and/or treatment of patients with any particular set of symptoms.

As sometimes happens with medical, chiropractic, and clinical information, a flawed care pathway may be used, or inappropriate interpretation or application of an algorithm may occur, as the result of a well-intentioned attempt by an overseer to standardize adjudication processes or to contain costs. The best defense against such misuse is to have a good working knowledge of the basis of a guideline, the process by which it was developed, and the unique circumstances of any given case. Overall, the utility of condition-specific synthesis of literature and expert opinion through the vehicle of clinical algorithms has been demonstrated to improve quality of care for patients and to improve efficiency of application of clinical resources.[1,24]

Algorithms are dynamic tools and are subject to continuous revision, based on new knowledge, new technology, and, most importantly, new experience gained through implementation, evaluation, and revision.[25] Critical debate and scholarly discourse in the letters to editors sections of journals—in which both seed and refined algorithms have been published—are fertile grounds for important new input for the ongoing revision of clinical guidelines and algorithms.

Development of a useful clinical algorithm is best accomplished by following these steps (refer to Algorithm 1):

1. Review quality clinical and scientific literature on a given clinical situation. This may most easily be accomplished by searching for any published qualitative literature reviews or metanalyses on the topic.
2. Using this review and an algorithm architect's clinical experience, draft a list of key clinical issues, decisions, and options to address in constructing the algorithm.

3. Next, use the tools described in the "boxology" section of this paper to construct a seed algorithm. Attempt to identify a direct strategic endpoint to work toward in the lower portion of the page, identifying key yes or no decisions that can branch off to other clinical options horizontally.
4. Follow through the algorithm using a variety of different clinical situations to see whether it flows adequately.
5. Ask peers to also review and critique it, offering their suggestions and revisions. Incorporate them and repeat steps 4 and 5 until the flow is smooth and limitations have been dealt with.
6. A seed algorithm should now be ready for publication and dissemination. Peer scrutiny is an important step in development and refinement of workable algorithms. TICC requests authors of clinical protocol articles to develop seed algorithms for publications as an appendix.[15-19] Seed algorithms and care pathways are quite common in medical literature[24] because they can be useful references for practicing clinicians.
7. Next, algorithms should be subjected to expert consensus, implementation, testing, and further revision. After testing and refinement, algorithms should again be disseminated through publication, with a full report of the methodology and revisions that resulted from the process. These kinds of algorithms are likely to be the most reliable and useful form of this clinical aid. It should be pointed out that as new technologies are developed and validated, and other new knowledge arises, all clinical algorithms are likely to need revisiting for further upgrading.

Seed algorithms and care pathways can be useful clinical aids for chiropractors in documenting clinical thought processes. This profession has often been misunderstood by other providers, policy makers, and payers. Much of this lack of understanding of chiropractic procedures can be attributed to inadequate information from chiropractors themselves in documenting and refining their methodologies and clinical decision-making practices. There are no clinicians better prepared to describe and refine chiropractic protocols than DCs.

When well designed, not only can these tools be useful clinical adjuncts to practicing chiropractic physicians, but an abundance of such protocols available for peer review, scrutiny, and refinement can help position chiropractic as a responsible and viable health care resource. Perhaps the biggest complaints about chiropractic from policy makers and purchasers center around the disunity, unpredictability, and practice variation that often characterize chiropractic care. An evidence-based process of algorithm development can be axiomatic in both providing clinicians with important clinical insight and improving the credibility of and comfort with chiropractic services. Rather than limiting the decision-making capabilities of individual physicians, condition-specific algorithms can actually stimulate more appropriate patient referrals to chiropractors from other providers, as well as help to assure quality and consistency for the most important constituent—the patient.

REFERENCES

1. Hansen DT, Mootz RD. Understanding, developing and utilizing clinical algorithms. *Top Clin Chiro.* 1994;1(4):44–57.
2. Gottlieb LK, Margolis CA, Schoenbaum SC. Clinical practice guidelines at an HMO: Development and implementation in a quality improvement model. *Quality Rev Bull.* 16(2):80–86, 1990.
3. Hansen DT. Development and use of clinical algorithms in chiropractic. *J Manipulative Physiol Ther.* 1991;14(8):478–482.
4. Berwick DM, Godfrey AB, Roessner J. *Curing Health Care: New Strategies for Quality Improvement.* San Francisco, CA: Jossey-Bass, Publishers; 1990:23–28.
5. Berwick D, Gottlieb L. *Clinical Quality Improvement: Designing Care.* Brookline, MA: National Demonstration Project on Quality Improvement in Health Care; 1990.
6. Margolis CZ. Proposal for clinical algorithm standards. Society for Medical Decision Making Committee on Standardization of Clinical Algorithms. *Medical Decision Making.* 1992;12(2):149–154.
7. Cheadle A, Franklin G, Wolfhagen C, et al: Factors influencing the duration of work-related disability: A population-based study of Washington state Workers' Compensation. *Am J Publ Health.* 1994;84(2):190–196.
8. Vibbert S, Reichard J, eds. *The 1993–4 Medical Outcomes and Guidelines Source Book.* Washington, DC: Faulkner & Gray; 1993:169–318.
9. Henderson D, Chapman-Smith D, Mior S, Vernon H. Clinical guidelines for chiropractic practice in Canada. *J Can Chiro Assoc Suppl.* 1994;38(1):1–203.
10. Haldeman S, Chapman-Smith D, Petersen DM. *Guidelines for Chiropractic Quality Assurance and Practice Parameters.* Gaithersburg, MD: Aspen Publishers; 1993.
11. Adler RH, Giersch EP, Ennis ML, Heermans H. *Survival Guide: Chiropractic Practice Guidelines.* Seattle, WA: self-published; 1993.
12. Kaminski M, Boal R, Gillete RG, Peterson DH, Villnave TJ. A model for the evaluation of chiropractic methods. *J Manipulative Physiol Ther.* 1987;10:61–64.
13. Gatterman MI, Hansen DT. Development of chiropractic nomenclature through consensus. *J Manipulative Physiol Ther.* 1994;17(5):351–359.
14. Nelson C, Boline P. A consensus on the assessment and treatment of headache. *J Chiro Technique.* 1991;3(4):151–168.
15. Souza TA. Back to basics: Differentiating mechanical pain from visceral pain. *Top Clin Chiro.* 1994;1(1):67–69.

16. Henninger R. Back to basics: Evaluation of soft tissue pain. *Top Clin Chiro.* 1994;1(2):77.
17. Cook RD, Mootz RD. Determining appropriateness of exercise and rehabilitation for chiropractic patients. *Top Clin Chiro.* 1994;1(1):75–77.
18. Mullen D, Bowers LJ. Myofascial pain syndromes: A look at the lower extremity. *Top Clin Chiro.* 1994;1(2):81.
19. Souza TA. Conservative management of orthopedic conditions of the lower leg, foot, and ankle. *Top Clin Chiro.* 1994;1(2):82–83.
20. Hansen DT. Construction of "seed" algorithms in chiropractic postgraduate interactive learning opportunities. In: Hansen DT. ed. *Proceedings of 1993 Conference on Research and Education, Consortium for Chiropractic Research.* San Jose, CA: 1993;182–183.
21. Mootz RD, Waldorf VT. Chiropractic care parameters for common industrial low back conditions. *J Chiro Technique.* 1993;5(3):119–125.
22. Office of Quality Assurance and Medical Review. *Directory of Practice Parameters: Titles, Sources and Updates.* Chicago, IL: American Medical Association; 1993.
23. Goertz C, Mootz R. A review of chiropractic management strategies in the care of hypertensive patients. *J Neuromusculoskel System.* 1993;1(3):91–108.
24. Hadorn DC, McCormack K, Diokno A. An annotated algorithm approach to clinical guideline development. *JAMA.* 1992;267(24):3311–3314.
25. Hansen DT. Prospect for the future of chiropractic guidelines. In: Lawrence D, ed. *Advances in Chiropractic.* Vol. 1. St. Louis, MO: Mosby-Year Book; 1994:372–409.

Algorithm 1

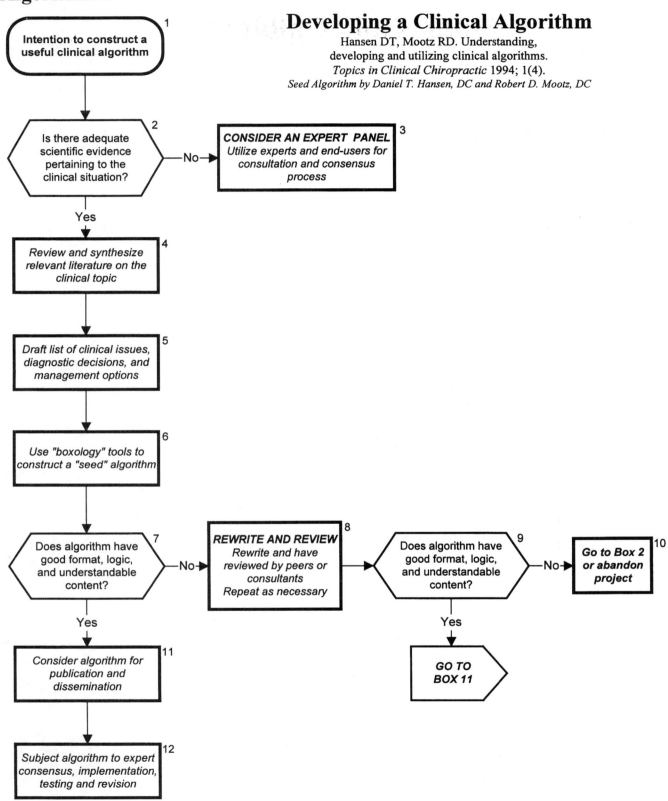

Developing a Clinical Algorithm
Hansen DT, Mootz RD. Understanding,
developing and utilizing clinical algorithms.
Topics in Clinical Chiropractic 1994; 1(4).
Seed Algorithm by Daniel T. Hansen, DC and Robert D. Mootz, DC

Part I

Infants and Children

1

Clinical Assessment of Selected Pediatric Conditions: Guidelines for the Chiropractic Physician

Linda J. Bowers

This chapter reviews the assessment of several relatively common pediatric conditions: sudden infant death syndrome (SIDS), otitis media, lead toxicity, hypercholesterolemia, growing pains, gait disturbances, and scoliosis screening. It also lists some of the guidelines available for the practicing clinician interested in providing care to infants and children.

COMMON PEDIATRIC CONDITIONS

Sudden infant death syndrome

The history of a newborn provides an ideal time for clinicians to counsel parents on SIDS. SIDS is defined as the unexpected death of an infant younger than 1 year of age that remains unexplained after a complete autopsy, death scene investigation, and review of the family history.[1,2] SIDS remains the number one cause of infant mortality between 1 month and 1 year of age in the US.[1,2] Approximately 6,000 infants die each year from SIDS, with an incidence of 1.5 per thousand live births.[2] Fifty-two percent to 60% of SIDS cases are males.[3] Although there has been a significant reduction in infant mortality in the United States over the past 10 years, the SIDS rate has varied little.

Though the pathophysiology of SIDS is still not well understood, several risk factors for SIDS have been delineated. Maternal smoking and prematurity have both been identified as risk factors; breastfeeding has been associated with decreased risk.[4] SIDS is rare in the first month of life, with peak occurrence in infants between 2 and 4 months of life.[3] Several international studies have identified a new risk factor for increased SIDS: prone sleeping position.[1] The most common position currently used in the United States is the prone position.[4] The American Academy of Pediatrics (AAP) recommended in April 1992 that healthy term infants be put to sleep on their side or back.[4] Since 1992, substantially more information regarding SIDS and sleeping position has become available. In countries that have advocated side or back sleeping for infants, there have been large, sustained decreases in the incidence of SIDS concomitant with similar declines in the proportion of infants sleeping prone.[2] The National Institute of Child Health and Development, with the support of the US Surgeon General, recently announced a "Back to Sleep" campaign aimed at changing infant sleep position practices in the United States.[1] It seems clear that SIDS rates do decrease significantly after public campaigns aimed at reducing the incidence of prone sleeping.[5]

There are still good reasons for placing certain infants prone. For premature infants with respiratory distress, for infants with symptoms of gastroesophageal reflux or with certain upper airway anomalies, and perhaps for some other infants, prone may well be the position of choice.[4] For healthy infants, there appears to be little hazard associated with the lateral or supine positions.[4] Algorithm 1 summarizes strategies for the prevention of SIDS.

Otitis media

Otitis media is one of the most common conditions encountered in primary care settings and is the most frequent primary diagnosis in children under 15 years of age.[6,7] Otitis media particularly affects infants and preschoolers: almost all children experience one or more episodes before age 6.[6] Annual direct and indirect costs of otitis media in the United States may exceed $3.5 billion.[7] Two types of otitis media are seen most: acute otitis media (AOM) and otitis media with effusion (OME). AOM is characterized by (1) fluid in

Adapted from *Top Clin Chiro* 1997; 4(4): 1–8
© 1997 Aspen Publishers, Inc.

the middle ear accompanied by signs or symptoms of ear infection, such as a bulging eardrum, usually accompanied by pain, or (2) a perforated eardrum, often with drainage of purulent material. OME is characterized by fluid in the middle ear without signs or symptoms of ear infection.[8]

It has been shown that physicians can generally detect AOM when it is present, about 90% of the time.[7] The frequency of overdiagnosis, which has been reported to be as high as 40%, is of major concern, because treatment with antibiotics may have adverse effects, cause undesired drug interactions, and induce drug resistance.[7] Further, recent meta-analysis showed a significant rate of spontaneous resolution of AOM in children who were not treated with antibiotics.[9]

There appears to be no agreement on the precise definition of AOM. However, a useful case definition is as follows: bulging or opacification of the tympanic membrane with abnormal tympanic membrane mobility, with or without erythema, accompanied by at least one of the following signs and symptoms of acute infection—fever, otalgia, irritability, otorrhea, lethargy, anorexia, vomiting, or diarrhea.[9] Two of the "classic" symptoms of ear infection, earache and fever, are often absent in children with AOM. Fever occurs in 22% to 69% of cases of AOM, but, even when it is present, fever is usually low grade (less than 38.3°C [101.0°F]) and not persistent, often lasting less than 24 hours.[7] Earache has a reported frequency of between 47% and 83%.[7] In contrast, 94% of children with AOM have either cough or rhinitis, which suggests that caution should be used when making this diagnosis in the absence of concurrent upper respiratory infection. While many children with AOM do not have ear pain, it is also true that many children with ear pain do not have an ear infection. Less than one-half of children complaining of otalgia in one study were found to have AOM.[7]

Appropriate equipment is essential for the accurate diagnosis of otitis media. The amount of light necessary for optimal visualization of the landmarks and the color of the tympanic membrane is 100 foot-candles.[7] Interestingly, most office otoscopes emit less than 100 ft-c because of weak power or bulbs, most often a worn-out bulb.[7] The life span of a typical otoscope bulb is about 20 hours. The pneumatic otoscope head was first described in 1864, and most standard textbooks and journal articles strongly support the use of pneumatic otoscopy for making the diagnosis of AOM. It is generally accepted that pneumatic otoscopy provides more accuracy than regular otoscopy because absent or decreased movement of the tympanic membrane is detectable with the pneumatic otoscope when positive and negative pressures are applied.

Congenital or early onset hearing impairment is widely accepted as a risk factor for impaired speech and language development. Because OME is often associated with a mild to moderate hearing loss, most clinicians have been eager to treat the condition to restore hearing to normal and thus prevent any long-term problems. However, no reliable evidence that OME has such long-term effects on language or learning exists.[6] Specific recommendations by an expert panel have been published for the management of otitis media with effusion in young children aged 1 through 3 years who have no craniofacial or neurologic abnormalities or sensory deficits (Table 1).[6,8] Use of these recommendations needs to be tempered by the fact that rigorous, methodologically sound research to support the relationship between OME and speech/language delays or deficits is lacking. The expert panel also advised that a number of treatments are not recommended for OME in the otherwise healthy child aged 1 through 3 years, such as steroid medications, antihistamine/decongestant therapy, adenoidectomy, and tonsillectomy. The association between allergy and OME was not clear from available evidence.[8] Evidence regarding other therapies for the treatment of OME was sought, but no reports of chiropractic, holistic, naturopathic, traditional/indigenous, homeopathic, or other treatments cited data obtained in randomized controlled studies. Therefore, no recommendation was made regarding such other therapies for the treatment of OME in children.[8] Algorithms 2 and 3 provide a care pathway for otitis media.

Table 1. Managing otitis media with effusion in young children

1. Suspect OME in young children.
2. Use pneumatic otoscopy to assess middle ear status.
3. Tympanometry may be performed to confirm suspected OME.
4. A child who has had fluid in both middle ears for a total of 3 months should undergo hearing evaluation.
5. Before 3 months of effusion, hearing evaluation is an option.
6. Observation or antibiotic therapy are treatment options for children with effusion that has been present <4–6 months and any time in children without a 20-decibel hearing threshold level or worse in the better-hearing ear.
7. For the child who has had bilateral effusion for a total of 3 months and who has a bilateral hearing deficiency, bilateral myringotomy with tube insertion becomes an additional treatment option.
8. Placement of tympanotomy tubes is recommended after a total of 4–6 months of bilateral effusion with a bilateral hearing deficit.

Source: Stool SE, Berg AO, Berman S, et al. *Managing Otitis Media with Effusion in Young Children.* Rockville, Md: US Department of Health and Human Services, Public Health Service, Agency for Health Care Policy and Research; July 1994. AHCPR publication 94-0623.

Lead toxicity

Lead intoxication has been a problem throughout history.[10] Children are at increased risk because of incomplete development of the blood-brain barrier before age 3 years, allowing more lead into the central nervous system; ingested lead has 40% bioavailability in children compared with 10% in adults.[3] Fortunately, blood lead levels in children in the United States, on average have decreased, and rarely are children seen with levels greater than 70 µg/dL.[10] However, 17% of preschool children in the United States have a level greater than 15 µg/dL.[3] Blood lead screening should be a part of routine health care for all children.[11] Because lead is ubiquitous in the environment, screening should occur at about 9 through 12 months of age and, if possible, again at about 24 months of age.[11] A history of possible lead exposure should be assessed at health care visits when children are between the ages of 6 months and 6 years. Lead poisoning should be considered in the evaluation of children with developmental delay, learning disabilities, behavior disorder, autism, convulsions, iron deficiency anemia, intestinal parasitic infections, speech and hearing deficits, encephalopathy, recurrent vomiting, and recurrent abdominal pain.[11]

Knowledge about the extent and seriousness of childhood lead poisoning has greatly increased since the 1987 AAP statement on lead poisoning. In 1990, an estimated 3 million children under 6 years of age had blood lead levels greater than 10 µg/dL.[12] These levels are associated with decreased intellectual performance and other adverse health effects, such as behavior disorders, slowed growth, and impaired hearing. In 1991, the Centers for Disease Control and Prevention (CDC) revised its childhood lead poisoning prevention policy statement to include lowering the blood lead level of concern from 25 µg/dL to 10 µg/dL.[12] The CDC also recommended a venous blood sample as a means of screening for lead poisoning. Although a fingerstick sample can be used, it is easily contaminated by environmental lead, increasing the false-positive rate. The Committee on Environmental Health of the AAP has issued a new policy statement on the treatment and prevention of lead poisoning.[11] The statement covers background, epidemiology, toxicity, environmental sources, prevention, and treatment recommendations for children with blood lead levels over 10 µg/dL and over 20 µg/dL.

The two primary ways to prevent lead poisoning in children are to remove environmental lead and to screen for elevated blood lead levels.[11] Removal of environmental lead is the most effective preventive measure. Almost all children are considered at risk for lead poisoning. Physicians should routinely ask parents about the possibility of lead exposure, as most children with elevated blood lead levels are asymptomatic.

Because the erythrocyte protoporphyrin (EP) test that had been previously recommended for screening is not sufficiently sensitive for blood lead levels less than 25 µg/dL, measurement of blood lead was identified as the screening test of choice.[12] Abdominal radiographs are helpful only in cases of acute lead ingestion or unusual persistence of high blood lead levels. As testing of hair and fingernails is subject to external environmental contamination, it is not recommended for the diagnosis of lead poisoning.[11] Children in the same household of a child with a blood lead level exceeding 20 µg/dL should also be tested if the exposure is believed to have occurred in the home.

The CDC has summarized treatment and follow-up procedures for children with blood lead levels of 10 µg/dL and higher.[11] The mainstay in the management of lead toxicity is removal of the source of exposure. Table 2 lists steps that can be used to prevent lead poisoning. Education about nutritional sources of calcium, iron, zinc, and ascorbate is important for the parents of all children but particularly so for the parents of children with blood lead levels of 10 µg/dL and above. Children deficient in these nutrients more readily absorb and/or retain dietary lead. Chelation is not recommended for blood lead levels under 25 µg/dL.[10,11,13] In these patients, environmental intervention is necessary. Chelation therapy is not a substitute for removing a child from environmental exposure. Patients with blood lead levels of 25–45 µg/dL need aggressive environmental intervention but should not routinely receive chelation therapy, because no evidence exists that chelation avoids or reverses neurotoxicity.[10] Chelation therapy is indicated in patients with blood

Table 2. Prevention of lead poisoning

1. Remove lead-based paint from the home.
2. Control dust and paint chip debris; wet mop frequently.
3. Prevent children from eating dirt or other foreign substances.
4. Change work clothes and clean up before going home from a lead-related job.
5. Avoid the use of lead around the home for hobbies and other purposes.
6. Wash hands frequently.
7. Use cold tap water for drinking and especially for formula mixing.
8. Let the water run for 1–2 minutes to rinse lead from pipes.
9. Take shoes off before entering the home.
10. Wash toys frequently in hot, soapy water.
11. Ensure adequate amounts of iron, calcium, zinc, and ascorbate.
12. Do not store food in inverted plastic bread bags printed with colored ink.
13. Do not use lead-glazed ceramics, especially with acidic food or drink.

lead levels of 45–70 µg/dL.[10,13] Patients with blood lead levels of greater than 70 µg/dL or with clinical symptoms suggesting encephalopathy require inpatient chelation therapy.[10] Algorithm 4 reviews clinical lead toxicity.

Hypercholesterolemia

Atherosclerosis has its origins in childhood, when fatty streaks begin to appear in the coronary arteries at about 10 years of age and in the abdominal aorta at 2 years of age.[14] Based on pathologic, epidemiologic, and genetic data, the National Cholesterol Education Program's Expert Panel on Blood Cholesterol Levels in Children and Adolescents recommends a dual approach to prevent atherosclerosis: (1) a population approach for all healthy American children older than 2 years of age, which includes a Step 1 diet moderately reduced in total and saturated fat and cholesterol but increased in complex carbohydrates, along with general attention to other risk factors; and (2) an individual approach in which children and adolescents from families with premature (55 years of age or younger) coronary artery disease (CAD) and /or a high blood cholesterol in a parent (240 mg/dL or higher) and children and adolescents with two or more other CAD risk factors undergo cholesterol and/or lipoprotein screening.[15]

The population approach recommendations for preventing CAD are as follows: (1) nutritional adequacy should be achieved by eating a wide variety of foods; (2) energy (calories) should be adequate to support growth and development and allow attainment and maintenance of desirable body weight; and (3) saturated fatty acids should account for less than 10% of total calories, total fat should account for an average of no more than 30% of total calories, and dietary cholesterol should be less than 300 mg/day. The individual approach recommendations for targeted selective screening include these:

1. Screen children and adolescents whose parents or grandparents, at 55 years of age or younger, underwent diagnostic coronary arteriography and were found to have coronary atherosclerosis. This includes parents or grandparents who have undergone balloon angioplasty or coronary artery bypass surgery.
2. Screen children and adolescents whose parents or grandparents, at 55 years of age or younger, suffered a documented myocardial infarction, angina pectoris, peripheral vascular disease, cerebrovascular disease, or sudden cardiac death.
3. Screen the offspring of a parent who has been found to have high blood cholesterol (240 mg/dL or higher).
4. For children and adolescents whose parental or grandparental history is unobtainable, physicians may choose to measure cholesterol levels to identify those in need of individual nutritional and medical advice, particularly those with other risk factors.

The panel's recommendations are not intended for infants from birth to 2 years of age, whose fast growth requires a higher percentage of calories from fat. Toddlers 2 and 3 years of age may safely make the transition to the recommended eating pattern as they begin to eat with the family.[15] Screening strategies are found in Algorithm 5.

Musculoskeletal conditions

In the clinic or outpatient setting, 1 of every 6 to 10 children presents with a musculoskeletal complaint,[16] although most such complaints are benign or functional in character. Nevertheless, each child must be professionally attended to and the complaint resolved. Among the more common or serious conditions are septic arthritis, intervertebral disc space infection, osteomyelitis, leukemia, aseptic necrosis, osteochondritis dissecans, rheumatic fever, juvenile rheumatoid arthritis, and Lyme disease.

Growing pains

A common benign pediatric complaint, inaccurately referred to as "growing pains," is controversial because of its vagueness, its lack of etiologic significance, and its potential for obscuring known disorders. These pains are often associated with complaints of tension headaches and psychogenic stomachaches.[17] The current concept of growing pains describes a very specific symptom complex, consisting of deep pain, usually in the lower limbs, that is severe enough to waken the child from sleep.[18] The pains occur intermittently, are always bilateral, and are completely gone in the morning. However, some children do complain of heaviness in the limbs the next day. The pains are exacerbated by excessive exercise during the day and improved by heat, massage, and occasionally by aspirin.[19] The persistent complaint is of pain in one or both legs, usually between the knee and ankle. The pain usually occurs during first hours of the night, but neither swelling, tenderness, nor stiffness are found the following morning.[16]

The incidence of growing pains among 6- to 19-year-olds is 15%, making this, along with headache (20%) and abdominal pain (12%), among the more frequent childhood complaints. Height, weight, and rate of growth seem to have no influence on the incidence of the pains.[19] Many otherwise normal children, despite recurrent episodes of severe extremity pain, have no objective changes on physical exam and do not progress to develop serious organic illness. These pains have been the subject of extensive debate for nearly 100 years.[19] Information about growing pains in the literature is sparse, in marked contrast to the frequency of the complaint.

Between 25% and 50% of children report extremity pain that is severe enough to interrupt normal daily activities.[17]

Girls report growing pains more often than boys. Although complaints of growing pains may be elicited from children of any age, there exists a bimodal distribution that peaks at 3–9 years of age and again in early adolescence.[17]

The differential diagnosis of growing pains is extensive, and the diagnosis should be one of exclusion. A working definition includes pain persisting for at least three months that is severe enough to interrupt normal daily activity; absence of a history of trauma, fever, and structural damage; and normal complete blood count (CBC), erythrocyte sedimentation rate (ESR), and electrocardiogram (ECG) results. Physical examination reveals normal vital signs and joints that are not hot, red, tender, or swollen. Radiographs are normal. These findings provide a reasonable checklist for a screening examination.[17] An ESR is an excellent test to separate organic illness from benign limb pains.[19]

Whatever the true origin of growing pains turns out to be, it is now accepted that growing pains do exist, do not progress to serious organic disease, and usually resolve with time.[19] The greatest diagnostic error is to make a diagnosis of growing pains while overlooking some serious underlying condition.[20]

Gait disturbance

Gait disturbances in children usually result from weakness or pain and in early childhood are frequently trauma related. The pain or limp may be greater in the evening or after exercise, with improvement after rest. An antalgic gait is usually present. However, examination rarely shows tender, swollen areas or pain with limitation of motion of the joints. When the physical examination is otherwise normal, an observation period of 7–10 days is reasonable, during which time most soft tissue injuries will resolve.[16] If symptoms persist, reevaluation is indicated, including a CBC, an ESR, and radiographs. Prolonged limping may be due to a stress fracture, particularly if the child participates in sports and exercise. A bone scan may be useful if a definitive diagnosis cannot be made. Hip evaluation is indicated if signs and symptoms referable to the knee occur. Likewise, lumbosacral evaluation should be performed if signs or symptoms referable to the hip are present. Patients with a knee problem often walk with the knee flexed, whereas a hip problem may cause internal rotation of the thigh.

Scoliosis

The Scoliosis Research Society defines scoliosis as a lateral spinal curve of 11° or greater.[21] An estimated 500,000 adults in the US have scoliosis.[22] Idiopathic scoliosis accounts for about 65% of cases of structural scoliosis, and a large proportion of these cases develop during adolescence.[21] A lateral curve of 11° or greater is present in about 2% to 3% of adolescents at the end of their growth period.[23] Curves greater than 20 degrees occur in less than 0.5% of adolescents.[22] There is little firm evidence from epidemiological studies that persons with idiopathic scoliosis are at significantly greater risk for experiencing back complaints than the general population.[21]

The principal screening test for scoliosis, the physical examination of the back, has variable sensitivity (74% to 100%) and specificity (78% to 91%), depending on the skills of the examiner and the degree of spinal curve.[24] A large proportion of children screened in schools for scoliosis are found to be "positive" on initial examination, but only some of these cases are ultimately found to have scoliosis.[21] At least one-half of patients diagnosed with scoliosis based on physical examination do not in fact have the condition.[23] There is limited information about the value of repeated screening of children who have previously tested negative for scoliosis.[21]

Only a subset of curves detected through screening are destined to progress to the point of potential clinical significance. The natural history of idiopathic scoliosis is such that most cases detected at screening will not require treatment because they will not progress significantly. Indications for preventive treatment are therefore uncertain and can result in unnecessary treatment. Only a small proportion of adolescents with idiopathic scoliosis are currently thought to be candidates for treatment (eg, those who have progressive curves greater than 30°).[24] Depending on the patient population, between 25% and 75% of curves detected on screening may remain unchanged and 3% to 12% may improve.[21]

Screening of adolescents for scoliosis has been advocated for its early detection and for prevention of its potential adverse effects.[21] The Scoliosis Research Society has recommended annual screening of all children between the ages of 10 and 14 years. The American Academy of Orthopaedic Surgeons has recommended screening girls at the ages of 11 and 13 and screening boys once at the age of 13 or 14. The AAP has recommended scoliosis screening at routine health supervision visits at age 10, 12, 14, and 16.[24]

However, several other groups do not recommend routine screening. The reasonableness of scoliosis screening requires evidence that scoliosis leads to important health problems, screening tests are accurate and reliable in detecting curves, effective treatments are available for cases detected by screening, early detection of idiopathic scoliosis improves health outcomes more than later interventions, and the benefits of screening and treatment outweigh their adverse effects.[23] In 1979 and again in 1984, the Canadian Task Force on the Periodic Health Examination gave a "C" recommendation (poor evidence regarding the inclusion of the condition in a periodic health examination but recommendations may be made on other grounds) to physical inspection for scoliosis by school nurses based on grade III evidence. The British Orthopaedic Association and the British Scoliosis Society issued a statement in 1983 advising against a national policy of screening for scoliosis in the United Kingdom. Individual authors have reached similar conclusions.[24]

The policy statement from the US Preventive Services Task Force states,

> There is insufficient evidence to recommend for or against routine screening of asymptomatic adolescents for idiopathic scoliosis ("C" recommendation). The evidence does not support routine visits to clinicians for the specific purpose of scoliosis screening or for performing the examination at specific ages during adolescence. It is prudent for clinicians to include visual inspection of the back of adolescents when it is examined for other reasons. Additional specific inspection maneuvers to screen for scoliosis, such as the forward-bending test, are of unproven benefit.[22(p525)]

This recommendation is based on grade II-3 evidence (multiple time series, dramatic uncontrolled experiments) for the effectiveness of early detection and treatment and on grade III evidence (opinions of respected authorities, descriptive epidemiology) for potential adverse effects.[24] The Scoliosis Research Society disagrees strongly with this policy statement.[25]

In conclusion, the available evidence in support of scoliosis screening is generally weak. Screening has a PPV (positive predictive value) that ranges between 4% and 78% (depending on the curve magnitude); the benefits of early detection are supported by uncontrolled community studies; and the efficacy, adverse effects, and cost-effectiveness of available treatments are uncertain.[21] There have been no controlled studies to demonstrate that adolescents who are screened routinely for idiopathic scoliosis have better outcomes than those who are not screened.[24] Limitations in the design of existing studies, however, also make it difficult to conclude that screening is ineffective or harmful. Clinicians should bear in mind the limited current evidence regarding the effectiveness of scoliosis screening and treatment and the uncertainties about the natural history of the disease. There is a pressing need for clinical research to demonstrate the effectiveness or ineffectiveness of routine screening for adolescent idiopathic scoliosis. It may be prudent for clinicians to include visual inspection of the back in adolescents when the back is examined for other reasons.[23] Time spent on thorough back examinations to detect scoliosis may be better spent addressing health problems of greater consequence to adolescents, such as tobacco use, unwanted pregnancy, and drinking and driving.

PRACTICE GUIDELINES

A Medline search using the key words *practice guidelines* revealed no articles from 1966 through 1990, while only two could be identified for 1991. However, nearly 3000 articles can be found between the years 1992 and 1997, illustrating the profusion of efforts in this area. No evidence-based guidelines regarding chiropractic care of children exist. However, several medical guidelines pertinent to pediatrics are available.

The AAP recently revised and updated its guidelines on preventive health care in children. These recommendations are for children who are receiving competent parenting, have no manifestations of any important health problems, and are growing and developing satisfactorily.[26] Other AAP guidelines cover febrile seizures,[27] informed consent,[28] gastroenteritis,[29] vision screening,[30] congenital hypothyroidism,[31] and pediatric AIDS.[32] The AAP has also issued policy statements regarding child-related health concerns such as aluminum toxicity,[33] lead toxicity,[34] attentional disorders,[35] and cow's milk.[36] The National Institutes of Health Consensus Development Panels have reports on cochlear implants in children,[37] optimal calcium intake,[38] physical activity and health,[39] and early identification of hearing impairment in infants and young children[40] and guidelines on the diagnosis and management of asthma.[41] The Agency for Health Care Policy and Research has clinical practice guidelines for otitis media with effusion,[8] pain management in children,[42] sickle cell disease,[43] smoking cessation,[44] and human immunodeficiency virus.[45] The US Preventive Services Task Force has recommendations concerning immunizations[46,47] and hepatitis B screening.[48] The World Health Organization has a policy statement on polio vaccines.[49] The American Association of Family Practitioners has a position paper on fluoridation of public water supplies.[50] The National Cholesterol Education Program has an expert panel report regarding blood cholesterol levels in children and adolescents.[15]

Clinicians interested in providing preventive services to children may find the following books helpful: *Healthy Children 2000: National Health Promotion and Disease Prevention Objectives Related to Mothers, Infants, Children, and Youth*[51]; *Healthy People 2000: National Health Promotion and Disease Prevention Objectives*[52]; and the *Report of the US Preventive Services Task Force: Guide to Clinical Preventive Services.*[22]

CONCLUSION

Because children cannot always speak for themselves or clearly understand their choices or options regarding their own health, it is of paramount importance that chiropractic clinicians become well informed regarding children's health care issues. They should also keep informed about new procedures, technologies, and research regarding children. Chiropractors have the opportunity to identify important health considerations and to participate with other health care providers in identifying health risks and managing common conditions. It is essential, particularly with children, to maintain the highest degrees of respect, integrity, and honesty when providing care.

REFERENCES

1. Gibson E, Cullen JA, Spinner S, Rankin K, Spitzer AR. Infant sleep position following new AAP guidelines. *Pediatrics.* 1995;96:69–72.
2. Willinger M, Hoffman HJ, Harford RB. Infant sleep position and risk for sudden death syndrome: report of meeting held January 13 and 14, 1994, National Institutes of Health, Bethesda, Md. *Pediatrics.* 1994;93(5):814–819.
3. Griffith HW, Dambro MR. *The 5-Minute Clinical Consult.* Baltimore, Md: Lea & Febiger; 1994.
4. Kattwinkel J, Brooks J, Myerberg D. American Academy of Pediatrics Task Force on Infant Positioning and SIDS: positioning and SIDS. *Pediatrics.* 1992;89(6):1120–1126.
5. Kattwinkel J, Brooks J, Keenan ME, Malloy M. Infant sleep position and sudden death syndrome (SIDS) in the United States: joint commentary from the American Academy of Pediatrics and selected agencies of the federal government. *Pediatrics.* 1994;93(5):820.
6. American Academy of Pediatrics, Otitis Media Guideline Panel. Managing otitis media with effusion in young children. *Pediatrics.* 1994;94(5):766–773.
7. Weiss JC, Yates GR, Quinn LD. Acute otitis media: making an accurate diagnosis. *Am Fam Physician.* 1996;53(4):1200–1206.
8. Stool SE, Berg AO, Berman S, et al. *Managing Otitis Media with Effusion in Young Children. Quick Reference Guide for Clinicians.* Rockville, Md: US Department of Health and Human Services, Public Health Service, Agency for Health Care Policy and Research; July 1994. Quick reference guide for clinicians no. 12 AHCPR publication 94-0623.
9. Rosenfeld RM, Vertrees JE, Carr J, et al. Clinical efficacy of antimicrobial drugs for acute otitis media: metaanalysis of 5,400 children from 33 randomized trials. *J Pediatrics.* 1994;124:355–367.
10. American Academy of Pediatrics Committee on Drugs. Treatment guidelines for lead exposure in children. *Pediatrics.* 1995;96(1 Pt 1):155–160.
11. AAP Policy Statement on Screening, Treatment and Prevention of Lead Poisoning. *Am Fam Physician.* 1993;48(6):1161–1164.
12. State activities for prevention of lead poisoning among children—United States, 1992. *MMWR.* 1993;42(9):165–172.
13. American Academy of Pediatrics issues treatment guidelines for lead exposure in children. *Am Fam Physician.* 1995;52(3):1022–1023.
14. Kwiterovich PO. The role of fiber in the treatment of hypercholesterolemia in children and adolescents. *Pediatrics.* 1995;96(5 Pt 2):1005–1009.
15. American Academy of Pediatrics. National Cholesterol Education Program: Report of the Expert Panel on Blood Cholesterol Levels in Children and Adolescents. *Pediatrics.* 1992;89(3 Pt 2):525–584.
16. Bass JC. Clinical and diagnostic overview of the child with a musculoskeletal complaint. In: Gershwin ME, Robbins DL, eds. *Musculoskeletal Diseases of Children.* New York: Grune & Stratton; 1983; 3–23.
17. Weiner SR. Growing pains. *Am Fam Physician.* 1983;27(1):189–191.
18. Atar D, Lehman WB, Grant AD. Growing pains. *Orthop Rev.* 1991;20(2):133–136.
19. Bowyer SL, Hollister JR. Limb pain in childhood. *Pediatr Clin North Am.* 1984;31(5):1053–1081.
20. Peterson H. Growing pains. *Pediatr Clin North Am.* 1986;33(6):1365–1372.
21. US Preventive Services Task Force. Review article. Screening for adolescent idiopathic scoliosis. *JAMA.* 1993;269(2):2667–2672.
22. US Preventive Services Task Force. *Guide to Clinical Preventive Services.* 2nd ed. Baltimore, Md: Williams & Wilkins; 1996.
23. DiGuiseppi CG, Woolf SH. The family physician's role in adolescent idiopathic scoliosis. *Am Fam Physician.* 1996;53(7):2268–2272.
24. US Preventive Services Task Force. Policy statement. Screening for adolescent idiopathic scoliosis. *JAMA.* 1993;269(20):2664–2666.
25. Winter RB, Banta JV, Engler G. Screening for scoliosis. *JAMA.* 1995;273(3):185–186.
26. American Academy of Pediatrics. Recommendations for preventive pediatric health care. *Pediatrics.* 1995;96:373–374.
27. American Academy of Pediatrics, Provisional Committee on Quality Improvement, Subcommittee on Febrile Seizures. Practice parameter: the neurodiagnostic evaluation of the child with a first simple febrile seizure. *Pediatrics.* 1996;97(5):769–775.
28. American Academy of Pediatrics, Committee on Bioethics. Informed consent, parental permission, and assent in pediatric practice. *Pediatrics.* 1995;95(2):314–317.
29. American Academy of Pediatrics develops guidelines for acute gastroenteritis in young children. *Am Fam Physician.* 1996;54(5): 1796–1799.
30. AAP releases pediatric vision screening guidelines. *Am Fam Physician.* 1995;51(4):972.
31. American Academy of Pediatrics, Section on Endocrinology and Committee on Genetics; American Thyroid Association, Committee on Public Health. Newborn screening for congenital hypothyroidism: recommended guidelines. *Pediatrics.* 1993;91(6):1203–1209.
32. American Academy of Pediatrics, Task Force on Pediatric AIDS. Guidelines for human immunodeficiency virus (HIV)–infected children and their foster families. *Pediatrics.* 1992;89(4 Pt 1):681–683.
33. American Academy of Pediatrics, Committee on Nutrition. Aluminum toxicity in infants and children. *Pediatrics.* 1996;97(3):413–416.
34. American Academy of Pediatrics issues treatment guidelines for lead exposure in children. *Am Fam Physician.* 1995;52(3):1022–1023.
35. American Academy of Pediatrics, Committee on Children with Disabilities and Committee on Drugs. Medication for children with attentional disorders. *Pediatrics.* 1996;98(2 Pt 1):301–304.
36. American Academy of Pediatrics, Committee on Nutrition. The use of whole cow's milk in infancy. *Pediatrics.* 1992;89(6 Pt 1):1105–1109.
37. NIH Consensus Development Panel on Cochlear Implants in Adults and Children. Cochlear implants in adults and children. *JAMA.* 1995;274(24):1955–1961.
38. NIH releases consensus statement on optimal calcium intake. *Am Fam Physician.* 1994;50(6):1385–1387.
39. NIH Consensus Development Panel on Physical Activity and Cardiovascular Health. Physical activity and cardiovascular health. *JAMA.* 1996;276(3):241–246.
40. Summary of the NIH consensus statement of early identification of hearing impairment in infants and young children. *Md Med J.* 1994;443(2):171–172.
41. National Asthma Education Program Expert Panel Report. *Guidelines for the Diagnosis and Management of Asthma.* Bethesda, Md: National Institutes of Health; August 1991. Publication 91-3042.
42. Acute Pain Management Guideline Panel. *Acute Pain Management in Infants, Children, and Adolescents: Operative and Medical Procedures.* Rockville, Md: US Department of Health and Human Services, Public Health Service, Agency for Health Care Policy and Research.

1992. Quick reference guide for clinicians no 1. AHCPR publication 92-0020.
43. Sickle Cell Disease Guideline Panel. *Sickle Cell Disease: Comprehensive Screening and Management in Newborns and Infants.* Rockville, Md: US Department of Health and Human Services, Public Health Service, Agency for Health Care Policy and Research; April 1993. Quick reference guide for clinicians no 6. AHCPR publication 93-0563.
44. The Smoking Cessation Clinical Practice Guideline Panel and Staff. *Smoking Cessation.* Rockville, Md: US Department of Health and Human Services, Public Health Service, Agency for Health Care Policy and Research; April 1996. Clinical practice guideline no 18. AHCPR publication 96-0693.
45. El-Sadr W, Oleske JM, Agins BD, et al. *Managing Early HIV Infection.* Rockville, Md: US Department of Health and Human Services, Public Health Service, Agency for Health Care Policy and Research; January 1994. Quick reference guide for clinicians no 7. AHCPR publication 94-0573.
46. LaForce FM. Immunizations, immunoprophylaxis, and chemoprophylaxis to prevent selected infections. *JAMA.* 1987;257(18):2464–2470.
47. US Preventive Services Task Force. Childhood immunizations. *Am Fam Physician.* 1989:40(4):115–118.
48. US Preventive Services Task Force. Screening for hepatitis B. *Am Fam Physician.* 1989;40(1):131–133.
49. WHO policy statement on polio vaccines. *Wkly Epidemiol Rec.* 1995;70(49):346–347.
50. American Association of Family Practitioners, Commission on Public Health. AAFP position paper. Fluoridation of public water supplies. *Am Fam Physician.* 1996;53(7):2372–2377.
51. US Department of Health and Human Services. *Healthy Children 2000: National Health Promotion and Disease Prevention Objectives Related to Mothers, Infants, Children, Adolescents, and Youth.* Boston, Mass: Jones & Bartlett; 1991.
52. *Healthy People 2000: National Health Promotion and Disease Prevention Objectives.* Washington, DC: US Department of Health and Human Services, Public Health Service; 1990.

Algorithm 1

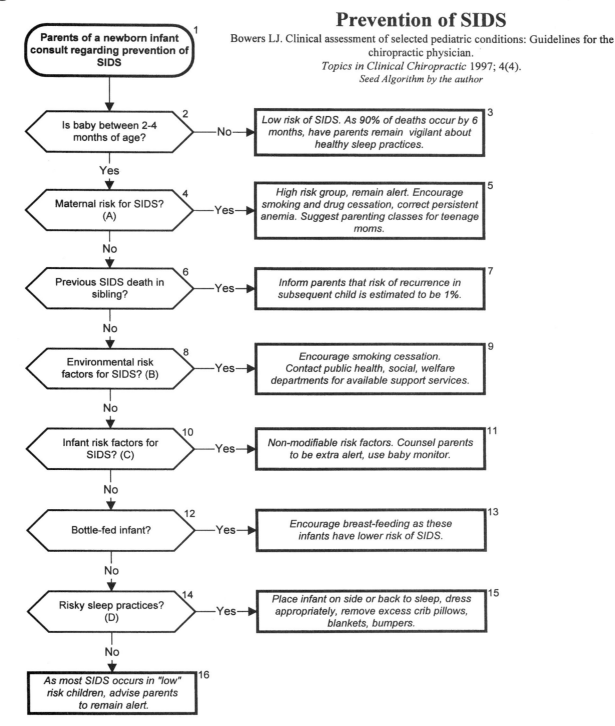

Prevention of SIDS

Bowers LJ. Clinical assessment of selected pediatric conditions: Guidelines for the chiropractic physician.
Topics in Clinical Chiropractic 1997; 4(4).
Seed Algorithm by the author

Annotations:
(A) e.g., maternal smoking, anemia, and drug use (Cocaine, opiates) during pregnancy, teenage mother, higher parity.
(B) e.g., passive cigarette smoke exposure after birth, late fall/winter season, poverty.
(C) e.g., low birth weight, Native American, African American race, recent upper respiratory or gastrointestinal infection, premature birth, male sex, intrauterine growth retardation.
(D) e.g., prone sleeping position, excessive clothing and bedding.

Algorithm 2

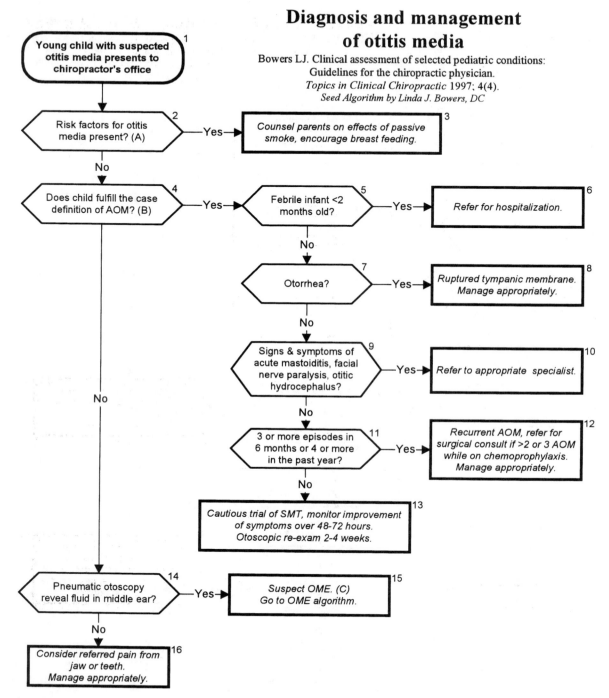

Diagnosis and management of otitis media

Bowers LJ. Clinical assessment of selected pediatric conditions: Guidelines for the chiropractic physician. *Topics in Clinical Chiropractic* 1997; 4(4).
Seed Algorithm by Linda J. Bowers, DC

Annotations:
(A) Day care, formula feeding, smoking in household, family history of middle ear disease, AOM in first year of life risk for recurrent AOM.
(B) Bulging or opacification of the tympanic membrane with abnormal tympanic membrane mobility, with or without erythema, accompanied by at least one of the following signs and symptoms of acute infection: fever, otalgia, irritability, otorrhea, lethargy, anorexia, vomiting, or diarrhea.
(C) OME = persistent inflammation manifested as asymptomatic middle ear fluid that follows AOM or arises without prior AOM.

Algorithm 3

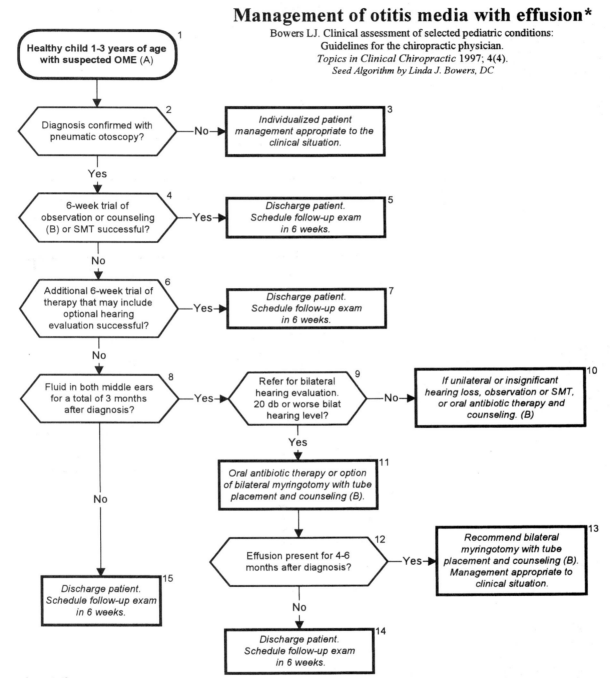

Management of otitis media with effusion*

Bowers LJ. Clinical assessment of selected pediatric conditions:
Guidelines for the chiropractic physician.
Topics in Clinical Chiropractic 1997; 4(4).
Seed Algorithm by Linda J. Bowers, DC

Annotations:
(A) Healthy = no craniofacial (e.g., cleft palate) or neurologic abnormalities (e.g., mental retardation), no sensory deficits (e.g., decreased visual acuity or pre-existing hearing deficit).
  OME = asymptomatic patient with fluid in the ear and no signs or symptoms of ear infections.
(B) Environmental risk factor control counseling, e.g., avoid exposure to cigarette smoke (passive smoke).

* Based in part on: Stool SE, Berg AO, Berman S, Carney CJ, Coley JR, Culpepper L, Eavey RD, Feagans LV, Finitzo T, Friedman E, et al. Managing Otitis Media with Effusion in Young Children. Quick Reference Guide for Clinicians. AHCPR Publication No.94-0623. Rockville, MD: Agency for Health Care Policy & Research, Public Health Service, US Dept of Health and Human Services. July 1994.

Algorithm 4

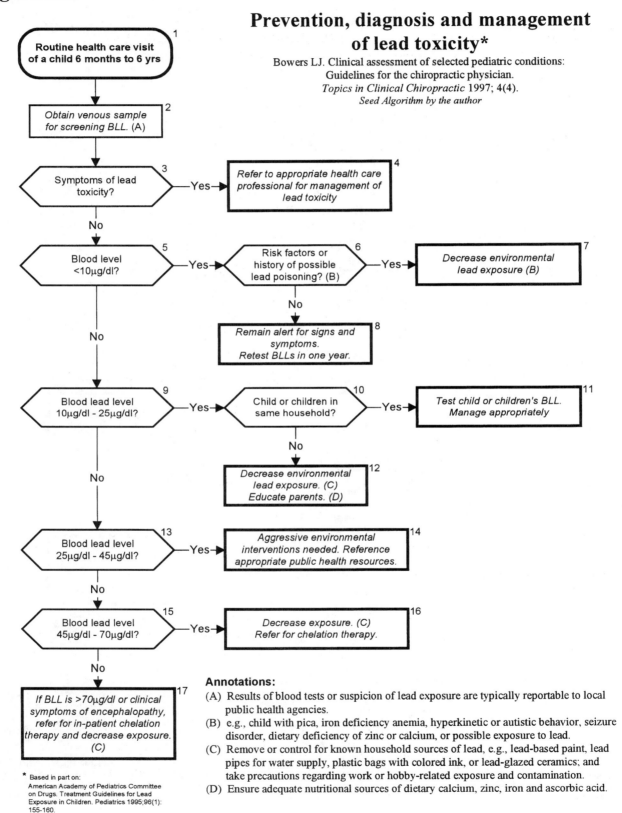

Prevention, diagnosis and management of lead toxicity*

Bowers LJ. Clinical assessment of selected pediatric conditions: Guidelines for the chiropractic physician. *Topics in Clinical Chiropractic* 1997; 4(4). *Seed Algorithm by the author*

Annotations:

(A) Results of blood tests or suspicion of lead exposure are typically reportable to local public health agencies.
(B) e.g., child with pica, iron deficiency anemia, hyperkinetic or autistic behavior, seizure disorder, dietary deficiency of zinc or calcium, or possible exposure to lead.
(C) Remove or control for known household sources of lead, e.g., lead-based paint, lead pipes for water supply, plastic bags with colored ink, or lead-glazed ceramics; and take precautions regarding work or hobby-related exposure and contamination.
(D) Ensure adequate nutritional sources of dietary calcium, zinc, iron and ascorbic acid.

* Based in part on:
American Academy of Pediatrics Committee on Drugs. Treatment Guidelines for Lead Exposure in Children. Pediatrics 1995;96(1): 155-160.

Algorithm 5

Screening and prevention of hypercholesterolemia in children*

Bowers LJ. Clinical assessment of selected pediatric conditions: Guidelines for the chiropractic physician. *Topics in Clinical Chiropractic* 1997; 4(4). *Seed Algorithm by the author*

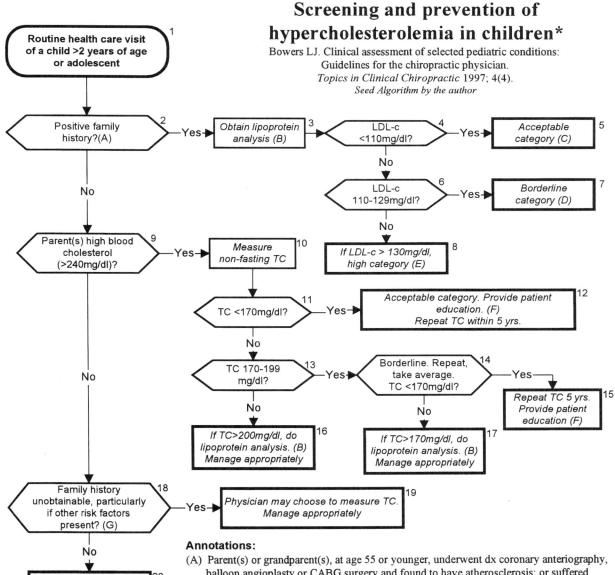

Annotations:

(A) Parent(s) or grandparent(s), at age 55 or younger, underwent dx coronary anteriography, balloon angioplasty or CABG surgery and found to have atherosclerosis; or suffered MI, angina pectoris, periph vasc disease, cerebrovasc disease, or sudden cardiac death.
(B) 12-hour fasting triglyceride (TG), total cholesterol (TC), and HDL-c, estimate LDL-c levels, measure twice and average results.
(C) Repeat lipoprotein analysis w/in 5 yrs, provide education on recommended eating pattern and risk factor reduction.
(D) Provide risk factor advice, initiate *Step-One* diet and other risk factor interventions, re-evaluate status in one year, set goal for LDL-c at <110mg/dl.
(E) Perform clinical evaluation, evaluate patient for secondary causes of hypercholesterolemia and familial disorders, screen all family members, intensive clinical intervention, set goal for LDL-c (*minimal* - <130mg/dl; *ideal* - <110mg/dl), initiate *Step-One* diet, followed (if necessary) by *Step-Two* diet, and in extreme cases, drug therapy.
(F) e.g., nutritional adequacy achieved by eating a variety of foods; energy should be adequate to support growth/development and reach/maintain desirable body weight; saturated fatty acids <10% of total calories; total fat an average of <30% of total calories; and dietary cholesterol <300mg/day, attain and maintain normal weight, exercise.
(G) e.g., smoke, high blood pressure, consume excessive amounts of saturated fatty acids and/or total fat and cholesterol, overfat, sedentary.

* Based in part on:
The National Cholesterol Education Program (NCEP): Report of the Expert Panel on Blood Cholesterol Levels in Children and Adolescents. Pediatrics 1992;89(3):525-584.

2

Childhood: A Crucial Age for Health Promotion

Jennifer R. Jamison

It is increasingly being recognized that the role and responsibilities of primary care practitioners extend beyond diagnosis and therapy. As the goal of primary care practice encompasses health promotion and disease prevention, the chiropractor is inevitably called upon to undertake the role of counselor and educator. The US Preventive Services Task Force seeks to emphasize prevention and tailor the content of the clinical examination to the particular needs of the patient.[1] Its general recommendations for the 7–12 age group include using body mass and blood pressure as screening measures. It also recommends counseling about diet (saturated fat, cholesterol, sweets, sodium, and snacks between meals); exercise; injury prevention; dental health; and, in high-risk groups, skin protection from ultraviolet light. In the 13–18 age group, history taking should include dietary intake; physical activity; sexual practices; and tobacco, alcohol, and drug use. A number of the areas in which counseling is recommended are concerned with behavioral choices. Imprudent behavioral choices made in childhood may adversely affect adult health. The adverse impact of childhood choices may be expressed as habitual behaviors that resist modification or as a failure to maximize growth during crucial phases of the life cycle. In either event, the choices made in childhood can promote or impede the realization of optimal health in adulthood. Three areas of behavioral choice in childhood that can have lifelong repercussions are "social" drug use, dietary selection, and sexual conduct.

SOCIAL DRUG USE

The regular use of alcohol and tobacco is widely accepted in many communities. Although widespread recognition of the potentially adverse social and physical impact of these substances has tempered their use, drinking and smoking remain common pastimes in modern society.

Cigarette smoking persists as a popular, albeit diminishing, habit. In 1989, the surgeon general reported that one in every six American deaths is the result of smoking.[2] Smoking is implicated in 30% of all cancer deaths and in 87% of deaths attributed to lung cancer. Smoking is also causally linked to 21% of deaths from coronary artery disease, 18% of stroke deaths, and 82% of deaths from chronic obstructive airways disease. It furthermore appears that the long-term risks of smoking may have been substantially underestimated and that about half of all regular cigarette smokers will ultimately die of a smoking-related disease.[3]

Smoking remains the most important preventable cause of death in many developed countries, and while more adults are giving up smoking, the age of initiation is falling. In America, every day more than 3,000 children and adolescents initiate tobacco use.[4] In a 1987 Australian study, 35% of 15-year-old girls were found to consider themselves regular smokers, and by the age of 17 years 40% had smoked more than 10 cigarettes.[5] Equally disturbing is the suggestion from studies in the United Kingdom that 94% of teenagers who smoke more than 2–3 cigarettes go on to become regular smokers as adults.[6] As the duration of exposure is a critical determinant of lung cancer risk, the age at which this habit is initiated is highly relevant. Ross and coworkers[7] have found that lung cancer rates rise as the number of cigarettes smoked increases and that for a fixed number of cigarettes smoked the risk of lung cancer increases with age. Furthermore, persons who stop smoking reduce their risk compared with those who continue smoking, but their risk does not revert to the nonsmoker baseline level. It is possible that the effects of smoking show a similar trend in the case of ischemic heart disease.[8]

Reprinted from *Top Clin Chiro* 1997; 4(4): 19–24
© 1997 Aspen Publishers, Inc.

The desirability of selectively providing drug-related health information during childhood is also apparent with respect to alcohol consumption. In Australia, by the age of 9, some 16% of girls and 26% of boys drink alcohol, and by the age of 15, more than 50% of children do.[5] A New Zealand study reports that children who have consumed alcohol before the age of 6 years are 1.9–2.4 times more likely to report frequent, heavy, or problem drinking at age 15 than those who did not drink alcohol before the age of 13 years.[9] This increase was found after controlling for such variables as early childhood behavior, parental alcohol use, and family sociodemographic background. As alcohol moderation may contribute to health status, awareness of the potential prudence of delaying the initiation of alcohol consumption and awareness of "safe" consumption levels should be encouraged.

In contrast to tobacco smoking, where no health benefit has been documented and no safe limits have been identified, the considered use of alcohol deserves some discussion. Although no safe level has been established for adolescents, for middle-aged or older men the mortality among regular drinkers from all causes increases above 21 units per week (three standard drinks a day) and below 1 or 2 units per day.[10] The beneficial effects of one to two drinks per day on the cardiovascular system may be related to an antioxidant effect (particularly in the case of red wine)[11,12] or to the triggering of endogenous type plasminogen activators, which reduces the risk of thrombosis.[13] In addition to the cardiovascular health advantage of moderate drinking, men who drink 30.0–49.9 g of alcohol per day also reduce their risk of non-insulin-dependent diabetes.[14] The health benefits of alcohol consumption are undisputedly dose related. Health authorities are promoting the following guidelines as consistent with responsible drinking[15]:

- Consumption of alcohol by males should not exceed 4 units or 40 g of absolute alcohol per day on a regular basis, or 28 units per week. Drinking is considered hazardous when 4–6 units are consumed per day or 28–42 units are consumed per week. Harmful drinking is defined as 6 or more units per day or 42 or more units per week. At these levels the risk of liver cirrhosis; esophageal, oral, and pharyngeal cancer; and coronary artery disease is increased. One unit is taken to be a half pint of beer, one measure of spirits, or one glass of sherry or wine.
- Consumption of alcohol by females should not exceed 2 units of alcohol per day on a regular basis, or 14 units per week. Drinking is considered hazardous when 2–4 units are consumed per day or 14–28 units are consumed per week. Harmful drinking is defined as 4 or more units per day or 28 or more units per week.
- Abstinence during pregnancy is highly desirable.
- People who undertake hazardous activities or drive should not drink.

Although a safe level of alcohol consumption has not been reported for children, delaying the initiation of alcohol consumption until the late teens would seem desirable. The guidelines for responsible drinking in social situations should also be implemented. These include

- planning drinking behavior (when, where, and how much);
- limiting consumption to one unit, that is, one standard (8–10 g), per hour or perhaps per day;
- alternating alcoholic and nonalcoholic drinks;
- diluting drinks and choosing low or very low alcohol varieties;
- eating while drinking but avoiding salty foods, which will increase thirst;
- making the first drink a soft drink and drinking only one type of alcoholic beverage; and
- avoiding drinking rounds or "shots."[15]

DIETARY BEHAVIORS

Dietary behaviors in childhood may have repercussions in adulthood, particularly for skeletal and cardiovascular health.

Prepuberty is a crucial stage of development with respect to peak bone mass. Peak bone mass, achieved between the late teens and 30 years of age, is the best safeguard against osteoporosis in later life. A high calcium intake facilitates achievement of optimal peak bone mass.[16] Milk consumption during childhood up to the age of 25 years is a significant independent predictor of bone mineral density.[17–19] A twin study found that calcium supplementation over a 3-year period resulted in a significant increase in bone density in prepubertal but not pubertal or postpubertal children.[20] This study found that calcium supplementation with a mean intake of 1612 mg per day of calcium (compared with a control group intake of 908 mg per day) resulted in a significant increase in bone density in prepubertal children. Calcium balance studies demonstrate that the threshold intake for children aged 2–8 years (1390 mg per day) and 9–17 years (1480 mg per day) is higher than for 18- to 30-year-olds (957 mg per day).[21] It is interesting to note that in the 1980s the recommended daily allowance (RDA) for calcium was 800 mg for 1- to 10-year-olds and 1200 mg for 11- to 24-year-olds. In 1994 the RDA for calcium was increased to 1200 mg for 1- to 10-year-olds and to 1500 mg for 11- to 24-year-olds.[22] It is on the basis of such information that health authorities advocate that children and adolescents select calcium rich foods. While plant sources of calcium are available,[23] the best calcium sources are milk and dairy products. As dairy products are rich in cholesterol and myristic acid, the most atherosclerotic saturated fatty acid, only low-fat varieties should be selected. Bone mass can also be protected by avoiding a high-protein, high-salt diet; by undertaking regular exercise; and by not smoking.[24] There are no data available to show whether schoolgirls are aware of these healthy behaviors, nor whether they know that the decreased bone mineral density that will result from a lifetime of two cups per day of caffeinated coffee can be neutralized by a daily glass of milk.[25]

Research over the last four decades shows that during childhood dietary and lifestyle patterns that have long-term implications for the risk of coronary heart disease in later life are initiated.[26] In Northern Ireland, a country with a high death rate attributable to coronary artery disease, a randomly selected sample of 12- to 15-year-olds found that 15% to 23% displayed increased blood pressure, 12% to 25% had unfavorable lipid profiles, and 18% to 34% were overfat.[27] Smoking, high habitual dietary intake of total and saturated fat, a low exercise level, and excessive alcohol consumption correlate with elevated serum cholesterol, obesity, and hypertension in children. Dietary measures are regarded as an important population control measure to control and lower obesity, serum cholesterol, and hypertension in childhood. Intervention studies involving children and adolescents have shown that these lifestyle risk factors can be controlled through education.

Observations from autopsies, echocardiographic studies, and long-term blood pressure studies of children also clearly indicate that primary hypertension begins in early childhood.[28] A population strategy for lowering blood pressure (or keep it from rising) involves (1) educating children to be active participants in changing their dietary and exercise behaviors and (2) instituting environmental changes, such as using less sodium in food processing.[29] Critical behavior changes include selection of a diet that is lower in sodium and fat and higher in potassium and calcium than the current diet.[30] The improved diet can be based on a high intake of vegetables, fruits, and whole grains rather than a high intake of fat derived from meat and dairy products. The dietary changes proposed for prevention of hypertension would simultaneously improve serum cholesterol levels. It is regarded as desirable that children over the age of 2 years consume less than 30% of their energy as fat, that the contribution from polyunsaturated fat should not exceed 10%, and that the contribution from saturated fat should be less than 10%.[31] In the Northern Ireland study, dietary analysis found relatively low polyunsaturated to saturated fatty acid ratios and a mean fat intake of around 40% of total daily energy.[27] In addition to alleviating hypertension and reducing serum cholesterol levels, the dietary changes proposed would reduce the prevalence of childhood obesity. Epidemiological studies of American children confirm that both obesity and high blood cholesterol levels are higher than optimal and that reducing the prevalence of these conditions in childhood will have an impact on adult health.[32]

At present, there is no consensus on how to define obesity in children and adolescents objectively.[33] A review of the literature published between 1970 and July 1992 found that, despite difficulties due to differences in definitions, study design, and analytical methods, obesity in childhood was positively associated with adult obesity.[34] For all studies and across all ages, the risk of adult obesity was at least twice as high for obese children as for nonobese children. The risk of adult obesity was greatest for children who were more overweight or obese and for older children who were obese. In a study of 5-year-olds, major risk factors were overweight parents, snacking, excessive television viewing, and short sleep duration.[35] Despite awareness of the prevalence of and risk factors for childhood obesity, the Canadian Task Force found insufficient evidence of short-term or long-term benefits from screening for treatment of childhood obesity to either recommend such screening or to recommend against it.[36] On the contrary, it concluded there is fair evidence to recommend against very low kilojoule diets for preadolescents. Nonetheless, while population-based screening cannot be recommended, primary practitioners should be aware that[37]:

- childhood obesity persists into adulthood in 30% of cases and
- the effects of adolescent obesity on adult morbidity and mortality appear to be independent of the effects of adolescent obesity on adult weight status.

SEXUAL BEHAVIORS

In our culture sexual expression is regarded as an important part of maturation. Adolescent sexual behaviors may also have enormous implications for adult health. Although since 1980 there has been some shift away from casual sex toward committed partnerships, most children have not adopted careful sexual practices, either with respect to number of partners or the use of condoms.[38] The age at which sexual activity is initiated seems to impact on the number of sexual partners encountered. Adolescents who are sexually active before the age of 13 years are nine times more likely to report three or more sex partners than those whose first sexual intercourse is at age 15 or 16.[39] Condom use is also somewhat erratic, as demonstrated by the prevalence of teenage pregnancies.[40] In a predominantly African-American sample of 69 adolescent females between 13 and 19 years, it was found that 64% used condoms half of the time or less when they had sex and that use appeared to be primarily for contraception even though 98% were aware that condoms may prevent acquired immunodeficiency syndrome (AIDS).[41]

Failure to use a condom entails potential exposure to AIDS, genital herpes, and hepatitis B. While not all of these conditions are fatal, none are curable. While genital herpes carries the potential for lifelong dyspareunia; hepatitis B carries the risk of chronic liver disease; and AIDS, owing to immune system impairment, is well recognized to shorten one's lifespan. Other sexually transmitted diseases such as gonorrhea and chlamydia can impair fertility. While oral contraceptives may have liberated young females, failure to use condoms may condemn the adolescent to serious problems in later life.

Other behavior choices also impact adolescent pregnancy. Pregnancy should be a nonsmoking, alcohol-free period.[42] Cigarette smoking has been found to substantially increase the risk of low birthweight for gestational age and is dose related. It has been reported that, although up to 39% of instances of low birthweight may be attributed to smoking, one in four pregnant women continue to smoke.[43] While some studies suggest that low to moderate alcohol use is unrelated to birthweight,[44] others report that alcohol (>100 g per week) enhances the fetal growth–retarding effects of smoking.[45–47] Wine has a slightly smaller adverse effect than beer or spirits. Low birthweight correlates with hypertension, impaired glucose tolerance, and hypercholesterolemia in adulthood.[48–50] The smoking and drinking behavior of pregnant adolescents has implications for the next generation.

AFFECTING BEHAVIORAL CHOICES

It is becoming increasingly apparent that a coordinated community approach is required to support the preventive efforts of health professionals if an environment is to be achieved in which an informed population can maximize health.[51] Social influence factors are pivotal in the initiation of smoking behavior, while perceived smoking norms, along with intrapersonal factors, appear to play an important role in maintaining the smoking habit in black adolescents.[52] The development of health promotion programs in elementary school is one way of modifying social perceptions and creating healthy norms.[53] Another is to increase the use of one-on-one clinical consultations.

As perceived self-efficacy has been identified as a strong predictor of a health-promoting lifestyle in adolescents,[54] primary practitioners should focus on providing them with the knowledge and skills to implement health-promoting behaviors.[55] While information may provide the cognitive and emotional stimulus necessary for behavioral change, it is ultimately the ability of the individual to confidently implement a strategy of personal behavior change that will raise the probability of a success. Efforts to increase condom use should, for example, focus on enhancing the adolescents' perceptions of their ability to negotiate aspects of condom use rather than merely provide them with information about the risk associated with unprotected sex.[56]

CONCLUSION

Childhood is a crucial time for making prudent behavioral choices. As we approach the turn of the century, there is increased awareness of the necessity to create a supportive environment that includes community action, family commitment, and professional leadership. Chiropractors who incorporate health promotion strategies with children may enhance their long-term impact on health in a meaningful way. It is through such interaction that our youth will be empowered to develop the personal skills necessary for adopting a healthy lifestyle.

REFERENCES

1. US Preventive Services Task Force. The periodic health examination: age-specific charts. *Am Fam Physician*. 1990;41:189–204.
2. Report of the Surgeon General. Reducing the health consequences of smoking: 25 years of progress. Executive summary. Rockville, Md: US Department of Health and Human Services; 1989.
3. Doll R, Peto R, Whetley K, Gray R, Sutherland I. Mortality in relation to smoking: 40 years' observation on male British doctors. *Br Med J*. 1994;309:901–911.
4. Shelton GE. Smoking cessation modalities: a comparison for healthcare professionals. *Cancer Pract*. 1993;1(1):49–55.
5. Australian Council for Health, Physical Education and Recreation. *Australian Health and Fitness Survey 1985*. Parkside, Australia: Australian Council for Health, Physical Education and Recreation; 1985.
6. Russell MHA. The nicotine addiction trap: a 40-year life sentence for four cigarettes. *Br J Addict*. 1990;85:293–300.
7. Ross RK, Bernstein L, Garabrandt D, Henderson BE. Avoidable nondietary risk factors for cancer. *Am Fam Physician*. 1988;38:153–160.
8. Cook DG, Shaper AG, Pocock SJ, Kussick SJ. Giving up smoking and the risk of heart attacks. *Lancet*. 1986;2:1376–1379.
9. Fergusson DM, Lynskey MT, Horwood LJ. Childhood exposure to alcohol and adolescent drinking patterns. *Addiction*. 1994;89:1007–1016.
10. Doll R, Peto R, Hall E, Wheatley K, Gray R. Mortality in relation to consumption of alcohol: 13 years' observation on male British doctors. *Br Med J*. 1994;309:911–918.
11. Fuhrman B, Lavy A, Aviram M. Consumption of red wine with meals reduces the susceptibility of human plasma and low-density lipoprotein to lipid peroxidation. *Am J Clin Nutr*. 1995;61:549–554.
12. Criqui MH, Ringel BL. Does diet or alcohol explain the French paradox? *Lancet*. 1994;344:1719–1723.
13. Ridker PM, Vaughan DE, Stampfer MJ, Glynn RJ, Hennekas CH. Association of moderate alcohol consumption with plasma concentration of endogenous tissue type plasminogen activators. *JAMA*. 1994;272:929–933.
14. Perry IJ, Wannamethe SG, Walker MK, Thompson AG, Whincup PH, Sharpe AG. Prospective study of risk factors for the development of non-insulin dependent diabetes in middle aged British men. *Br Med J*. 1995;310:560–564.

15. National Health and Medical Research Council. Is there a safe level of daily consumption of alcohol for men and women? Canberra, Australia: Australian Government Publishing Services; 1987.
16. Hu J, Zhao X, Jia J, Parpia B, Campbell TC. Dietary calcium and bone density among middle-aged and elderly women in China. *Am J Clin Nutr.* 1993;58:219–227.
17. Murphy S, Khaw K, May H, Compston JE. Milk consumption and bone mineral density in middle aged and elderly women. *Br Med J.* 1994;308:930–931.
18. Stracke H, Renner E, Knie G, Leidig G, Minne H, Federlin K. Osteoporosis and bone metabolic parameters in dependence upon calcium intake through milk and milk products. *Eur J Clin Nutr.* 1993;47:617–622.
19. Soroko S, Holbrook TL, Edelstein S, Barrett-Connor E. Lifetime milk consumption and bone mineral density in older women. *Am J Public Health.* 1994;84:1319–1322.
20. Johnston CO, Miller JZ, Selmenda CW, et al. Calcium supplementation and increases in bone mineral density in children. *N Eng J Med.* 1992;327:82–87.
21. Matkovic V, Heaney RP. Calcium balance during human growth: evidence for threshold behavior. *Am J Clin Nutr.* 1992;55:992–996.
22. New US recommendations on calcium intake. *Lancet.* 1994;343:1559.
23. Weaver CM, Plawecki KL. Dietary calcium: adequacy of a vegetarian diet. *Am J Clin Nutr.* 1994;59(suppl):1238S–1241S.
24. Hopper JL, Seeman E. The bone density of female twins discordant for tobacco use. *N Eng J Med.* 1994;330:387–392.
25. Barrett-Connor E, Chang JC, Edelstein SL. Coffee-associated osteoporosis offset by daily milk consumption. *JAMA.* 1994;271:280–283.
26. Cunnane SC. Childhood origins of lifestyle-related risk factors for coronary heart disease in adulthood. *Nutritional Health.* 1993;9(2):107–115.
27. Boreham C, Savage JM, Primrose D, Cran G, Strain J. Coronary risk factors in schoolchildren. *Arch Dis Child.* 1993;68(2):182–186.
28. Berenson GS, Wattigney WA, Bao W, Nicklas TA, Jiang X, Rush JA. Epidemiology of early primary hypertension and implications for prevention: the Bogalusa Heart Study. *J Hum Hypertens.* 1994;8(5):303–311.
29. Gillman MW, Ellison RC. Childhood prevention of essential hypertension. *Pediatr Clin North Am.* 1993;40(1):179–194.
30. Ellison RC. Should physicians intervene during childhood to prevent adult hypertension? *Schweiz Med Wochenschr.* 1995;125(7):264–269.
31. Williams CL, Bollella M, Wynder E. Preventive cardiology in primary care. *Atherosclerosis.* 1994;108(suppl):S117–126.
32. Ernst ND, Obarzanek E. Child health and nutrition: obesity and high blood cholesterol. *Prev Med.* 1994;23(4):427–436.
33. Flegal KM. Defining obesity in children and adolescents: epidemiologic approaches. *Crit Rev Food Sci Nutr.* 1993;33(4–5):307–312.
34. Serdula MK, Ivery D, Coates RJ, Freedman DS, Williamson DF, Byers T. Do obese children become obese adults? A review of the literature. *Prev Med.* 1993;22(2):167–177.
35. Locard E, Mamelle N, Billette A, Miginiac M, Munoz F, Rey S. Risk factors of obesity in a five year old population: parental versus environmental factors. *Int J Obes Relat Metab Disord.* 1992;16(10):721–729.
36. Canadian Task Force on the Periodic Health Examination. Periodic health examination, 1994 update, 1. obesity in childhood. *Can Med Assoc J.* 1994;150(6):871–879.
37. Dietz WH. Therapeutic strategies in childhood obesity. *Horm Res.* 1993;39(suppl 3):86–90.
38. Netting NS. Sexuality in youth culture: identity and change. *Adolescence.* 1992;27:961–976.
39. Durbin M, DiClemente RJ, Siegel D, Krasnovsky F, Lazarus N, Camacho T. Factors associated with multiple sex partners among junior high school students. *J Adolesc Health.* 1993;14:202–207.
40. Adelson PL, Frommer MS, Pym MA, Rubin GL. Teenage pregnancy and fertility in New South Wales: an examination of fertility trends, abortion and birth outcomes. *Aust J Public Health.* 1992;16:238–244.
41. Overby KJ, Kegeles SM. The impact of AIDS on an urban population of high-risk female minority adolescents: implications for intervention. *J Adolesc Health.* 1994;15:216–227.
42. McDonald AD, Armstrong BG, Sloan M. Cigarette, alcohol, and coffee consumption and prematurity. *Am J Public Health.* 1992;82:87–90.
43. Floyd RL, Zahniser C, Gunter EP, Kendrick JS. Smoking during pregnancy: prevalence, effects, and intervention strategies. *Birth.* 1991;18:48–53.
44. Walpole I. Is there a fetal effect with low to moderate alcohol use before or during pregnancy? *J Epidemiol Community Health.* 1990;44:297–301.
45. Haste FM, Anderson HR, Brooke OG, et al. The effect of smoking and drinking on the anthropometric measurements of neonates. *Paediatr Perinat Epidemiol.* 1991;5:83–92.
46. Peacock JL, Bland J, Anderson HR. Effects on birthweight of alcohol and caffeine consumption in smoking women. *J Epidemiol Community Health.* 1991;45:159–163.
47. Olsen J, Pereira A, Olsen SF. Does maternal tobacco smoking modify the effect of alcohol on fetal growth? *Am J Public Health.* 1991;81:69–73.
48. Hales CN, Barker DJP, Clark PMS, et al. Fetal and infant growth and impaired glucose tolerance at age 62. *Br Med J.* 1993;303:1019–1022.
49. Barker DJP, Martyn CN, Osmond C, et al. Growth in utero and serum cholesterol concentrations in adult life. *Br Med J.* 1993;307:1524–1527.
50. Barker DJP, Bull AR, Osmond C, Simmonds SJ. Fetal and placental size and risk of hypertension in adult life. *Br Med J.* 1990;301:259–262.
51. Luepker RV. Community trials. *Prev Med.* 1994;23:602–605.
52. Botvin GJ, Baker E, Botvin EM, Dusenbury L, Cardwell J, Diaz T. Factors promoting cigarette smoking among black youth: a causal modeling approach. *Addict Behav.* 1993;18:397–405.
53. Arbeit ML, Johnson CC, Mott DS, et al. The Heart Smart cardiovascular school health promotion: behavior correlates of risk factor change. *Prev Med.* 1992;21:18–32.
54. Gillis AJ. Determinants of health promoting lifestyles in adolescent females. *Can J Nurs Res.* 1994;26:13–27.
55. Robinson SM, Walsh J. Cognitive factors affecting abstinence among adolescent polysubstance abusers. *Psychol Rep.* 1994;75:579–589.
56. Joffe A, Radius SM. Self-efficacy and intent to use condoms among entering college freshmen. *J Adolesc Health.* 1993;14:262–268.

3

Periodic Health Examination of Infants and Children

Linda J. Bowers

The periodic health visit is an important opportunity for the delivery of clinical preventive services.[1] In 1984 the assistant secretary for health formed the US Preventive Services Task Force (USPSTF) and asked the members to develop age-, sex-, and other risk factor–specific recommendations concerning the appropriate use of preventive interventions in the clinical setting.[2] The guide's principal audience consists of primary care providers. The report of the USPSTF offers evidence-based recommendations for the periodic health examination of specific age groups.[3] This report is the "gold standard" for authoritative, evidence-based recommendations for clinical preventive services.[4] The major theme of the report is "talk more and test less" (ie, clinicians should use counseling and other interventions to change behaviors more often than previously). The task force divides the periodic health examination into screening, parent or patient counseling, and immunizations and chemoprophylaxis. High-risk groups as well as the leading causes of death for each age group are identified.

Recommended activities when examining infants and children include height, weight, and blood pressure measurement; neonatal screening for hemoglobinopathies; and counseling about injury prevention, diet and exercise, sexual behavior, substance abuse, and dental health. Lead screening is recommended in communities with a high prevalence of elevated lead levels. The task force did not recommend routine visual acuity screening in children, routine urinalysis, scoliosis screening, anemia testing, and routine screening for serum cholesterol levels in children.[4] Cholesterol screening may be indicated in adolescents at high risk for future coronary heart disease (eg, a family history of very high cholesterol, premature heart disease in a first-degree relative, or other major risk factors).[4]

Preventive measures targeted at conditions most likely to significantly influence the health and well-being of the patient being examined should be prioritized. The two most important factors to consider are the leading causes of morbidity and mortality in the patient and the potential effectiveness of clinical interventions in altering the natural history of those diseases.[1] Consider the fact that an estimated 350 men died from testicular cancer in the United States in 1989 and that early detection is believed to be an important means of improving survival. However, of the 39,929 deaths among young persons in the United States during 1986, 19,975 were due to injuries (15,227 from motor vehicle crashes).[1] Therefore, on the basis of mortality data alone, it appears likely that a few minutes with an adolescent male might be more productively spent discussing ways of preventing unintentional and intentional injuries, such as seat belt use and not driving drunk, rather than how to perform a testicular self-exam.

It is important to note that the task force report focuses on efficacy issues (does the procedure "work"?) and does not address issues of cost or effectiveness (does a public health strategy reach sufficient persons to significantly improve morbidity and mortality?). Any clinician interested in providing primary care will find this report a valuable reference because it delineates the scientific base for specific preventive interventions, allowing clinicians to develop rational, cost-effective preventive protocols tailored to their particular situation. The complete *Guide to Clinical Preventive Services* is now available on the Internet at the following location: http://text.nlm.nih.gov.

The author wishes to thank Drs. Tim Mick and Jeff Rich for their advice regarding radiography in children.

Schedules for ages birth to 18 months, 2–6 years, 7–12 years, and 13–18 years can be found in Appendix I–A.

ADAPTING THE HEALTH HISTORY FOR INFANTS AND CHILDREN

Because children are not merely miniature adults, pediatric health histories differ in style from histories obtained from adults and also vary depending on the particular developmental stage of childhood.[5] However, there are many similarities between pediatric and adult health interviews. For example, the basic organization of a clinical history is the same for patients of all ages: chief complaint, history of present illness, past health history, family health history, current health status, and review of systems.[6] Empathy, respect, privacy, and confidentiality—attitudes and values that facilitate good adult doctor-patient interactions—are equally important in pediatric interactions. Table 1 outlines the data that need to be acquired during pediatric health interviews.

The two most important distinctions between adult and pediatric patient interviews involve who participates in the conversation and the topics that are emphasized at a particular stage of development.[5] For example, parents, caregivers, or other family members often provide information instead of or in addition to the child. This introduces potential problems in gathering information, and the precise point at which a verbal child has the skill to contribute to his or her own health history is not always easy to determine. With regard to topics that are emphasized, the prenatal history is vitally important in the case of a newborn but not in the case of an adolescent, and the achievement of developmental milestones, while critical in the assessment of a 6-month-old infant, is of minimal significance in the evaluation of a 7-year-old child with a sore throat.

The infant or child should be comfortable and quiet so that the parents will be relaxed enough to provide detailed information. A good relationship with a child begins by making friends with him or her. One of the best ways to make a child comfortable is through praise.[7] In the case of a preschool child, offering the child a toy to occupy his or her attention may well improve the efficiency of the interview. It also may be useful to admire something the child has—a toy or a pair of new shoes—instead of uttering an overly enthusiastic greeting. White clinic jackets may contribute to a child's fear. It can be helpful to spend a few moments talking to the parents or caregiver in order to give the child time to size you up.[5]

The infant and toddler

A very young patient, while the focus of the interview, will not usually be a participant.[5] Ideally, the clinician should conduct the interview with the infant or toddler present, as both parents and child are likely to be more comfortable. In the case of a preschool child, it may be easier for the child to trust the doctor if the child sees the doctor interact with the parents.[5]

Although most of the history is provided by the parents or caregiver, some questions may be asked of the child. Two

---

Table 1. Pediatric history elements

Identifying data
  Date and place of birth, nickname, first names of parents (and last of each, if different).
Chief complaint
  Determine if they are the concerns of the child, the parent(s), a schoolteacher, or some other person.
Present illness
  Determine how each member of the family responds to the child's symptoms, why he or she is concerned, and the secondary gain the child may get from the illness.
Birth history
  Important when neurologic or developmental problems are present.
  - Prenatal: maternal health, medications, drug and alcohol use, vaginal bleeding, weight gain
  - Natal: nature of labor and delivery, birth weight
  - Neonatal: resuscitation efforts, cyanosis, jaundice, infections, nature of bonding
Feeding history
  Important with under- and overnutrition.
  - Breast feeding: frequency and duration of feeds, difficulties encountered, timing and method of weaning
  - Artificial feeding: type, amount, frequency, vomiting, colic, diarrhea, vitamin, iron, and fluoride supplements, introduction of solid foods
  - Eating habits: likes and dislikes, types and amounts of food eaten, parental attitudes and response to feeding problems
Growth/development
  Important with delayed growth, psychomotor and intellectual retardation, and behavioral disturbances.
  - Physical growth: weight and height at birth and 1, 2, 5, and 10 years; periods of slow or rapid growth
  - Milestones: ages child held head up, rolled over, sat, stood, walked, and talked
  - Social: day and night sleeping patterns; toilet training; speech problems; habitual behaviors; discipline problems; school performance; relationships with parents, siblings, and peers
Current health status
  - Allergies: eczema, urticaria, perennial allergic rhinitis, insect hypersensitivity, foods, penicillin
  - Immunizations: dates given, untoward reactions
  - Screening tests: inborn errors of metabolism, sickle cell disease, blood lead, vision, hearing, scoliosis

Source: Bates B. *A Pocket Guide to Physical Examination and History Taking.* Philadelphia, Pa: Lippincott Williams & Wilkins; 1991.

useful rules in questioning children are as follows: (1) do not ask too many questions too quickly and (2) use simple language.[7] Observing the child at play while interviewing the parents may provide useful information. Allowing a toddler to play with a stethoscope or penlight may increase familiarity and comfort with equipment that will be used later in the physical examination.

Information concerning the perinatal period should be obtained: complications and problems during the pregnancy, duration and complications of labor, and problems during the infant's first days of life. Crying, sleeping, and bowel and bladder function should also be discussed. A careful review of developmental stages must be obtained. It should focus on different milestones depending on the age of the child. The doctor should ascertain the child's immunization status, including any reactions to vaccines.

Age-appropriate questions related to nutrition can help identify potential consequences of malnutrition, including defective neurologic development, stunting of growth, and decreased immunocompetence.[5,7] Three screening questions often suffice: (1) "How many ounces of formula (or, for older children, milk) does your baby take each day?" For breastfed babies, "How many times does the baby nurse in 24 hours?" and "What's the longest he or she goes between feedings?" (2) For older infants and toddlers, "Are there any foods your child refuses to eat?" (3) "Does your child eat much in the way of sweets and junk food?"[5]

The pediatric family history and review of systems are basically the same as in the adult history. However, there should be increased emphasis on symptoms related to the respiratory, gastrointestinal, and genitourinary systems.[7] The high incidence of symptoms and diseases related to these systems obligates the interviewer to be very methodical. The clinician should obtain enough information to be able to later discuss accident prevention, feeding, toilet training, and developmental issues such as teething and the acquisition of normal speech patterns.

The symptoms of pediatric illness, particularly in the preverbal child, are often nonspecific and may indicate more about how sick the child is than precisely what the illness is. A 13-month-old toddler cannot say that an ear hurts; rather crying, irritability, fever, and possible a loss of appetite or even vomiting and diarrhea may be present. With luck, the child may tug at an ear, but many children with healthy ears do that as well. If the child is preverbal, physical examination is necessary to arrive at the diagnosis of otitis media.

The school-aged child

When a child reaches the age of 5 or 6 years, the interactive balance in the interview begins to shift. The child will now be more able to contribute substantially to the collection of data, but his or her reports will usually be broad and sometimes difficult to interpret. Thus, the clinician, while seeking to elicit information from the child, must turn to the parents to provide accuracy and precision. An enormous variation in maturation is found in elementary school-aged children, and taking cues from observing the child can help guide the interview process.

In general, the school-aged child is a healthy child. In addition to obtaining historical information concerning immunizations, development, and nutrition, the psychosocial aspects of the child's history become gradually more important. Knowledge of the child's school performance and friends is necessary for an understanding of the child's general well-being. Anticipatory guidance at this age emphasizes accident prevention, both in the home and at school, and good nutrition.

PHYSICAL EXAMINATION

Most techniques used to examine adults are applicable to infants and children; however, there are specific methods for examination during infancy (first year of life), early childhood (1–4 years), and late childhood (5–12 years). Some portions of the physical examination can be conducted with the infant or child supine or sitting on the parent's lap. However, the supine position on the examining table is essential for examination of the abdomen, hips, genitalia, and rectum, and of the mouth and the ears when the infant is resisting.[6] No special sequence of examination techniques is required in infancy and early childhood, except that the mouth and ear examinations, abduction of the hips, and the rectal examination, if needed, should be saved until last, as these can cause the infant to cry. It is important to listen to the heart and lungs and palpate the abdomen when the infant is quiet. Tables 2 and 3 list musculoskeletal and neurological system examination techniques that can be used for patients in infancy, early childhood, and late childhood.

Attainment of developmental milestones should be determined using the Denver Developmental Screening Test (DDST). This test detects developmental delays in the first 6 years of a child's life, with special emphasis upon the first 2 years.[7] It should be emphasized that the DDST is a screening device for developmental delays and not an intelligence test. It assesses the four main areas of development: gross motor, fine motor, language, and personal development. Failure to perform an item passed by 90% of children is significant. Two failures in any of the four main areas indicate a developmental delay.[7]

Musculoskeletal and nervous system examination of the newborn

A physical examination of a newborn child will detect gross abnormalities. Appearance of extremities at birth usually reflect the positioning of the child within the uterus, a condition

Table 2. Physical examination of the musculoskeletal system of infants and children

Test	Significance
Palpate clavicle	Fracture
Observe child with feet together	Foot deformities, bow legs, knock-knees, scoliosis
Observe walking and running	Limp, gait abnormalities due to weakness or spasticity
Observe stooping to pick up an object	Eye-hand coordination and muscle balance
Observe rising from a supine position	General neurologic integrity and the proximal leg muscle weakness of muscular dystrophy
Palpate spine for defects	Defects associated with an underlying spinal cord anomaly
Check spine for pigmented spots, hairy patches, or deep pits that might overlie external openings of sinus tracts that extend to the spinal canal	Sinus tract provides potential entry to the spinal canal for organisms that can cause meningitis
Ortolani test	Click heard or felt as the femoral head enters the acetabulum near the end of abduction signifies congenitally dislocated hip
Trendelenburg test	Positive sign is present in diseases of the hip associated with gluteus medius muscle weakness
Decreased cervical range of motion	Torticollis

known as intrauterine packing. Palpate the clavicle. An area of crepitus over the distal third is suggestive of a fractured clavicle. Decreased motion in the upper extremity may also be associated with a clavicular fracture. Inspect for brachial palsy.

The most important musculoskeletal assessment in infants is evaluation of the lower extremities. Examine the hips for the possibility of dislocation. Inspect the contour of the legs while the child is lying supine. The presence of asymmetric skin folds on the medial aspect of the thigh is suggestive of a proximally dislocated femur. The perineum should not be visible with the child in this position, because the normal position of the thighs should cover most of the perineum. If the perineum is visible, suspect bilateral hip dislocation. After inspection, gently perform the Ortolani test. Flex the newborn's legs at the hips. Hold the legs by placing your thumbs over the lesser trochanters and your index fingers over the greater trochanters and press downward toward the examination table (Barlow variation). Simultaneously abduct the hips to almost 90°. The presence of an audible "click" suggests a dislocated hip as the femoral head snaps back into the acetabulum. After the newborn period, the Ortolani test may be falsely negative.[7]

Musculoskeletal and nervous system examination of infants and children

The infant of 1 week to 6 months can be examined on the examination table, with the parent standing nearby. It may be easier to perform part of the examination while the infant is in a parent's arms or lap. Between the ages of 6 months and 1 year, infants may be best examined entirely on the parent's lap. This strategy is useful for many parts of the examination up to age 3. Again, the more difficult portions of the examination, such as the evaluation of the pharynx and the otoscopic examination, should be performed last. Take advantage of any time when the infant is quiet to listen to the lungs and heart. Palpate the clavicle. At 1 month of age, the presence of a callus formation suggests a healed clavicular fracture. The hips must be reexamined for dislocation at every routine visit for the first year of life.[7] By the 4th month, when the supine infant is pulled into a sitting position, no head lag should be present. By the 8th month, the infant should be able to sit without support. Coordination of the hands begins at about 5 months, when the infant can reach and grasp objects; by 7 months, the infant can transfer objects from hand to hand. At 8–9 months, the infant should be able to use a pincer grip to pick up small objects.

The child of 1–5 years needs to be relaxed in order for an adequate examination to be performed. It is very important to speak softly to the child and to demonstrate parts of the examination prior to performing them. Conversation with the parents during the examination can be reassuring to the child.[7] Observe the gait by telling the child to walk back and forth. Watch for in-toeing or out-toeing, which are very common in children. Inspect for genu varum and genu valgum. The normal gait of a child 2–4 years of age is wide based, with a prominent lumbar lordosis. The child with a limp should be examined for evidence of trauma or localized bone tenderness. The presence of a limp and knee pain in a child, especially a boy, 3–8 years of age suggests Legg-Calve-Perthes disease. Inspect the child's shoes for evidence of abnormal wear. The development of speech, reading ability, and the ability to manipulate small objects, throw a ball, and understand simple directions are the best indicators of a nor-

Table 3. Physical examination of the nervous system of infants and children

Test	Significance
Triceps reflex	Not present until after 6 months
Abdominal reflexes	Absent at birth, appears within 6 months
Ankle reflex	Unsustained means ankle clonus normal (8–10 beats); sustained suggests severe CNS disease
Plantar reflex	Babinski present in normal newborns (<10%) and may remain for as long as 2 years
Palmar grasp reflex	Disappears at 3–4 months
Rooting reflex	Disappears at 3–4 months; may be present longer during sleep
Truck incurvation (Galant's) reflex	Disappears at 2 months
Ventral suspension positioning	Disappears after 4 months; fixed extension and crossed adduction of the legs (scissoring) indicate spastic paraplegia or diplegia
Placing response	Best after 4 days; disappearance time variable
Rotation test	Disappearance time variable
Tonic neck reflex	Usually appears at 2 months and disappears at 6 months, considered abnormal when it occurs every time it is evoked
Perez reflex	Disappears after 3 months
Moro response/startle reflex	Disappears by 4 months

mally developing neurologic system. Deep tendon reflexes are generally not tested unless there is reason to suspect there is a developmental abnormality.

The child of 6–12 years is usually a pleasure to examine. He or she understands the purpose of the examination and rarely presents any problems. It is often very helpful to engage the child in conversation regarding school, friends, and hobbies to aid in relaxation. Allow the child to wear a gown or drape. The order of the examination is essentially the same as for the adult. Brief explanations about each part of the examination should be given. Observe for scoliosis. A limp and knee pain in a child 9–16 years of age must be considered to be a result of a slipped epiphysis of the hip until proved otherwise. The pathognomonic sign of a slipped epiphysis is a hip that goes into external rotation as it is flexed.[7] The neurologic examination is essentially the same as for an adult. However, a complete neurologic examination is indicated only when there is evidence of developmental abnormalities.[7]

Somatic growth is one of the most important focuses of the pediatric examination. Deviations from the standard curves are often early sensitive indicators of a pathologic process. Children with a discrepancy between length and weight by more than two percentage lines also require further evaluation.[7] The American Academy of Pediatrics (AAP) recommends that children's height and weight be measured throughout infancy, annually from 1 to 6 years of age and biennially thereafter.[8] The USPSTF recommends that height and weight be measured regularly and plotted on a growth chart throughout infancy and childhood.[3] The Canadian Task Force on the Periodic Health Examination recommendations are similarly designed to identify children who are failing to thrive.[8] This task force also believes there is insufficient evidence of short- or long-term benefits from screening for or treatment of childhood obesity to recommend for or against it. There is fair evidence to recommend against a very low kilojoule diet for preadolescents, and there is insufficient evidence to recommend for or against exercise programs or intensive family-based programs for most obese children.[8]

DIAGNOSTIC IMAGING

Guidelines concerning clinical indicators for radiological imaging of children are generally the same as for adults. However, special emphasis is often placed on minimizing or eliminating the exposure of developing tissues to radiation. Roentgenographic joint surveys in search of subclinical joint disease are usually not performed in children because of the radiation dose and low diagnostic yield.[9] The process of evaluating the joint or bone in question begins with plain roentgenograms taken in two projections and includes for comparison the joint of the opposite side.[9] Knowledge of the normal variants and changing appearance of the growing skeleton is vital in interpretation of pediatric roentgenograms. Table 4 lists clinical indications for imaging in children.

NUTRITION ASSESSMENT

Infancy

The first 2 years of life, characterized by rapid physical and social growth and development, is a period in which many changes that affect feeding and nutrient intake occur.[10]

Table 4. Indications for imaging in children

Arthritis (eg, septic arthritis, juvenile rheumatoid arthritis)
Back pain (Scheuermann's disease, spondylolisthesis)
Failure to respond to conservative therapy within 2 weeks
Painful scoliosis
Upper respiratory infection with torticollis
Osteomyelitis
Osteoid osteoma
Significant trauma
Stress fracture

Healthy, well-nourished infants have the energy to respond to and learn from the stimuli in their environment and to interact with their parents or caregivers in a manner that encourages bonding and attachment. Nutrient needs of infants reflect rates of growth, energy expended in activity, basal metabolic needs, and the interaction of nutrients consumed.[10]

Normal infants who are breastfed to satiety and infants fed a standard 20-kcal/oz formula whose mothers are sensitive to their cues of hunger and satiety generally adjust their intake to meet their energy needs. The best method to determine the adequacy of an infant's energy intake is to carefully monitor his or her gain in height and weight. Protein is needed for tissue replacement as well as for growth. Requirements during the rapid growth of infancy are higher on a per kilogram basis than those for the adult or older child. Essential amino acid needs are the same for infants as for adults. It is recommended that infants consume a minimum of 3.8 g and a maximum of 6 g per 100 kcal of fat. Carbohydrates should supply 30% to 60% of the energy intake during infancy.[10]

Some nutritional concerns in infancy are baby bottle tooth decay, over- and undernutrition, botulism (honey and corn syrup are sources of Clostridium botulinum spores), water imbalance, vitamin K (hemorrhagic disease of the newborn), and cow's milk allergy.

Childhood

The rate of growth slows considerably after the first year of life. Although physical growth may be less remarkable and steadier than during infancy, preschool and middle school years are a time of significant growth in the social, cognitive, and emotional areas.[11] In general, growth is steady and slow during the preschool and school-aged years, but it may be erratic in individual children. Some children may be in an apparent "holding pattern" for several months or even years and then have a spurt in height and weight. This pattern of growth usually parallels changes in appetite and food intake.[11] Periods of slow growth and poor appetite can cause anxiety on the parent's part, which may lead to mealtime struggles.

The complete assessment of nutritional status includes the collection of anthropometric data, including height, weight, weight for height, upper arm circumference, and triceps or subscapular fatfolds.[12] Growth measurements must be recorded at regular intervals to show the growth pattern. Regular monitoring of growth enables trends to be identified early and treatment begun so that long-term growth is not compromised.

Because children are growing and developing bones, teeth, muscles, and blood, they need more nutritious food in proportion to their weight than do adults.[11] The suggested proportion of energy for children is 50% to 60% as carbohydrate, 25% to 35% as fat, and 10% to 15% as protein.[11]

Nutritional concerns in this age group are iron deficiency anemia, obesity, underweight (failure to thrive), dental caries, and food allergies. As any parent can attest, from the child's viewpoint an important nutritional concern is that foods do not touch each other. There are unique nutritional concerns for child athletes[13] and children who are vegetarian.[14]

ASSESSMENT OF PHYSICAL FITNESS

Although growing evidence suggests that regular physical activity and exercise leads to good health,[15] physical activity levels of children have declined.[16] The national objectives for health promotion, *Healthy People 2000 National Health Promotion and Disease Prevention Objectives*, include the relatively modest goal of increasing the proportion of people "aged 6 or older who engage regularly, preferably daily, in light to moderate physical activity for at least 30 minutes per day."[17(p97)] The National Institutes of Health consensus statement on physical activity and cardiovascular health concurs.[18] Although studies have not shown conclusively that exercise in childhood reduces coronary risk, many experts agree that it is desirable for children and adolescents to establish regular exercise habits that may continue through life.[19] Any physical activity is better than none at all. All children should be asked about the frequency, type, and duration of their physical activities. Television watching and parental activity patterns are factors that affect a child's exercise habits.[19] The more time children spent watching television, the poorer their mile walk/run performance and the greater their skinfold thickness. The more active the parents, the more active their children.[19]

The terms *physical activity, exercise,* and *physical fitness* are often confused and sometimes used interchangeably. Physical activity is defined as any body movement produced by skeletal muscle that results in energy expenditure.[19,20] Exercise is planned, repetitive physical activity designed to improve physical fitness. Physical fitness encompasses a set of attributes that are health related, skill related, or both.[20] Physical fitness is difficult to address without discussing its components. The five components of health-related physical fitness are cardiorespiratory endurance, muscular strength, muscular endurance, flexibility, and body composition.[20] A variety of tests are available that can be administered in the office setting to assess these components of fitness.

Body composition

Body composition is an important health-related component of fitness. Clinical measurement of body composition can assist in educating patients about its importance, identify patients who are becoming obese, and monitor the progress of weight-loss efforts. Body composition can be assessed using methods such as BMI, skinfold measurements, bioelectrical impedance, infrared reactance, or hydrostatic weighing. Skinfold measurement is the most practical method in an office setting. It requires a skilled examiner, but the methodology is well described. Physicians should be cognizant that reporting a percentage body fat to an adolescent may be very upsetting, as adolescents are very conscious of body image. The predictive accuracy of BMI is less than that for estimates based on skinfold thickness and often overestimate body fatness because the measurement reflects muscle and bone content as well as fatness.

Cardiorespiratory fitness

Cardiorespiratory endurance (aerobic power) may be assessed by utilizing a cycle ergometer, an arm ergometer, a step test, or a motor-driven treadmill. The most accurate method is to use a motor-driven treadmill, but the cost of the equipment and the personnel required make this method impractical for most settings. A cycle ergometer is less expensive than a treadmill.

Protocols performed according to body height are well suited to children.[19] Because direct measurement of oxygen uptake is not feasible in most offices, indirect measurement of oxygen uptake can be made using the performance of the child and the Borg scale rating of perceived exertion.[21] Recent studies[19] of step tests for children are promising because such tests are easier to perform in most offices than other tests of aerobic power.

Flexibility

Flexibility is specific to each joint, and there are no standardized flexibility tests available. The sit and reach test (SRT) is commonly used to assess flexibility of the lower back and length of the posterior thigh muscles, and it is the only test for which norms are available for children 5–17 years of age.[19] This simple field test can easily be performed in the office with a wooden box and a yardstick. It is an important test to do because decreased flexibility, particularly in the hamstring muscles and the back, is thought to contribute to development of low back pain. Data confirming this supposition are still lacking, however.

The child sits on the floor with knees fully extended and ankles in neutral dorsiflexion against a standardized box. The child places one hand on top of the other and slowly reaches forward as far as possible while keeping knees extended. The child's fingertips are extended slowly along the surface of the box and the placement of the fingertips on the ruler (on top of the box) is recorded. The minimum acceptable score to pass as determined by the American Alliance for Health, Physical Education, Recreation, and Dance (AAHPERD) is 25 cm, or 2 cm beyond the toes, for all ages and both genders without consideration of anthropometric variables.

Strength and endurance

Although muscle strength and endurance are probably less related to health than body composition and cardiorespiratory fitness, some physicians may want to assess these components in the office. There are no simple strength tests that do not use equipment such as a grip dynamometer or an isokinetic machine. Push-ups, sit-ups, or pull-ups can be performed to test muscular strength, but these activities also test endurance.[19] Norms for school-aged children are available.[19]

Factors that influence physical activity among children include perceptions of physical or sports competence; perceived benefits; enjoyment (the major reason young people engage in physical activity); favorable attitudes toward physical education; parental activity; physical activity of friends and siblings; parental encouragement; direct help from parents, such as organizing exercise activities or providing transportation; access to play spaces and facilities; and time spent outdoors.[22] Competition motivates boys more than girls, whereas weight management motivates girls more than boys.[22] The clinician can use knowledge of these factors to support and encourage physical activity in his or her pediatric patients. Though school-based interventions to promote physical activity among children have been consistently effective, health care professionals also have a potential role to play.[22]

There are standardized, commonly used tests of physical fitness in children. Studies of both children and adults have shown that increased levels of regular physical activity are associated with improved scores on tests of physical fitness.[15] The President's Council on Physical Fitness and Sports reports that only 36% of US schoolchildren in grades 1–12 are enrolled in daily physical education classes.[16] The Youth Fitness Test was developed in the early 1960s under the auspices of the President's Council of Physical Fitness and Sports.[15] It has been standardized and used to test more than 23 million US schoolchildren.[15] It consists of the following six subtests: 45-m (50-yd) dash, standing broad jump, sit-ups (maximum number), pull-ups (maximum number), shuttle run, and 548.6-m (600-yd) run. The individual subtests, particularly the 548.6-m run, have been shown to have a strong correlation with cardiorespiratory fitness (maximal oxygen consumption determined by treadmill or bicycle ergometry testing).[15] The childhood 548.6-m run has been shown to be the fitness test most predictive of physical inactivity in young men.[15]

Because many lifestyle habits are established during childhood and adolescence, physical activity and exercise habits may also be established during these formative years. Identification of children at high risk of becoming physically inactive adults might allow intervention programs to be targeted toward these children. The best primary strategy for improving the long-term health of children and adolescents through exercise may be to create a lifestyle pattern of regular physical activity that will carry over to the adult years rather than promote childhood physical fitness.[20] The AAP has published recommendations regarding physical fitness and children.[19]

INJURY PREVENTION COUNSELING

Observers of national health trends have predicted that the next great increase in life expectancy will result, not from major medical breakthroughs, but rather from changes in lifestyle.[23] In recent years, physicians have become more concerned about the prevention of childhood accidents. Unintentional injuries are the leading cause of death in childhood and adolescence in the United States.[24-26] More children die from injuries than from all other diseases combined.[25] The most common causes of injury in children are motor vehicle accidents, bicycle accidents, falls, penetrating injuries, and gunshot wounds.[26] Because most injuries from accidents are preventable, health care providers should address safety issues with young patients and their parents. Increased knowledge, safer behavior, and reduced injury rates have been demonstrated in primary care settings.[27]

In April 1983 the AAP officially launched the first nationwide drive to prevent injuries: The Injury Prevention Program (TIPP).[27] TIPP was developed to help physicians teach parents how to avoid unintentional injury. Anticipatory guidance has now been recognized as an essential part of routine health supervision.[23] TIPP consists of three major elements: (1) a policy statement on injury prevention by the AAP Committee on Injury and Poison Prevention; (2) a childhood safety counseling schedule; and (3) a packet of materials, including safety information sheets and safety surveys, for use in providing anticipatory guidance to parents. TIPP has evolved over the years to become a comprehensive program for children from birth through age 12 years. It is based on the principle that injury prevention counseling should emphasize strategies that have proven effective (eg, car seats), should reinforce these strategies at age-appropriate visits, and should be individualized.

The AAP believes that health education through office-based counseling can contribute to childhood injury prevention.[28] A literature review supports the AAP's recommendation to include injury prevention counseling as part of routine health supervision.[24] The 1991 edition of *Healthy Children 2000* suggests increasing to at least 50% the proportion of primary care providers who routinely provide age-appropriate counseling aimed at preventing unintentional injury.[29]

Injury is the leading cause of childhood medical spending,[28] and thus injury prevention counseling has the potential for significant health cost savings.[28] Current pressure by payers, however, is forcing pediatricians to offer less counseling. A cost-benefit comparison of injury prevention counseling concluded that it is a cost-effective method of preventing childhood injuries and should be more widely adopted.[28] Each dollar spent on TIPP childhood injury prevention targeting children aged 0–4 years returns nearly $13 in medical savings.[28] Each visit at which TIPP counseling occurs saves an estimated $5.50 in future medical spending and preserves future earnings and quality of life valued at $74.50.[28] TIPP materials are available from American Academy of Pediatrics Publications, PO Box 927, Elk Grove Village, IL 60009-0927 (or call 1 800 433-9016).

Clinicians interested in providing preventive services to children may find the following books useful: *Healthy Children 2000: National Health Promotion and Disease Prevention Objectives Related to Mothers, Infants, Children, and Youth*[29]; *Healthy People 2000: National Health Promotion and Disease Prevention Objectives*[17]; and *Report of the US Preventive Services Task Force: Guide to Clinical Preventive Services*.[3]

CONCLUSION

The periodic health examination provides the chiropractic clinician an opportunity to discuss many key health measures, including preventive measures. Familiarity with recommendations from various health organizations can enhance the clinician's ability to best use time during office visits as well as contribute to improving the health of pediatric patients. The evidence-based recommendations of the US Preventive Services Task Force exemplify the kinds of strategies that maximize effectiveness and facilitate optimal use of health care dollars.[3]

Because it is impractical to cover all areas during one office visit, clinicians should focus on a few key areas, individualizing health care and advice and progressively adding components of the periodic health examination on successive encounters. Key areas chiropractors can address include high-risk behaviors, diet, exercise, physical fitness, and injury prevention. Performance of baseline and progress measurements (eg, height, weight, and blood pressure measurements) is essential. Selected screening tests (eg, blood lead and cholesterol tests) may also be appropriate for chiropractic clinicians to consider. Such tests, if within the clinician's area of competency and jurisdictional scope of practice, can be performed by the clinician; other tests can be referred out.

REFERENCES

1. US Preventive Services Task Force. The periodic health examination: age-specific charts. *Am Fam Physician.* 1990:41(1):189–204.
2. Report of the US Preventive Services Task Force. *JAMA.* 1990:263(3):436–437.
3. *Report of the US Preventive Services Task Force: Guide to Clinical Preventive Services.* Baltimore, Md: Williams and Wilkins; 1989.
4. Frame PS, Berg AO, Woolf S. US Preventive Services Task Force: highlights of the 1996 report. *Am Fam Physician.* 1997:55(2):567–576.
5. Coulehan JL, Block MR. *The Medical Interview: A Primer for Students of the Art.* 2nd ed. Philadelphia, Pa: FA Davis; 1992.
6. Bates B. *A Pocket Guide to Physical Examination and History Taking.* Philadelphia, Pa: JB Lippincott; 1991.
7. Swartz MH. *Textbook of Physical Diagnosis. History and Examination.* Philadelphia, Pa: WB Saunders Company; 1989.
8. Canadian Task Force on the Periodic Health Examination. Periodic health examination, 1994 update, 1: obesity in childhood. *Can Med Assoc J.* 1994;150(6):871–879.
9. Winchester P, Brill PW. A guide to the radiographic analysis of pediatric arthropathies. In: Gershwin ME, Robbins DL, eds. *Musculoskeletal Diseases of Children.* New York: Grune & Stratton; 1983: 641–647.
10. Pipes PL. Nutrition in infancy. In: Mahan KL, Escott-Stump S, eds. *Krause's Food, Nutrition, and Diet Therapy.* 9th ed. Philadelphia, Pa: WB Saunders; 1996.
11. Lucas B. Nutrition in childhood. In: Mahan KL, Escott-Stump S, eds. *Krauses's Food, Nutrition, and Diet Therapy.* 9th ed. Philadelphia, Pa: WB Saunders; 1996.
12. Bowers LB. Back to basics: assessment of nutritional status. *Top Clin Chiro.* 1995;2(4):1–12.
13. Bowers LB. The child athlete. *Top Clin Chiro.* 1997;4(2):27–39.
14. Berestiansky L. Vegetarianism at each stage of the life cycle. *Top Clin Chiro.* 1996;3(4):14–24.
15. Dennison BA, Straus JH, Millits ED, Charney E. Childhood physical fitness tests: predictor of adult physical activity levels? *Pediatrics.* 1988;82:324–330.
16. Schlicker SA, Borra ST, Regan C. The weight and fitness status of United States children. *Nutr Rev.* 1994;52(1):11–17.
17. *Healthy People 2000: National Health Promotion and Disease Prevention Objectives.* Washington, DC: US Department of Health and Human Services, Public Health Service; 1990.
18. *Physical Activity and Cardiovascular Health.* NIH consensus statement. Washington, DC: National Institutes of Health, Office of the Director; 1995.
19. American Academy of Pediatrics, Committee on Sports Medicine and Fitness. Assessing physical activity and fitness in the office setting. *Pediatrics.* 1994;93:686–689.
20. Rowland TW, Freedson PS. Physical activity, fitness, and health in children: a close look. *Pediatrics.* 1994;93(4):669–672.
21. Borg GA. Psychophysical bases of perceived exertion. *Med Sci Sports Exercise.* 1982;14(5):377–381.
22. Physical activity and health: a report of the surgeon general. Atlanta, Ga: US Department of Health and Human Services, Centers for Disease Control and Prevention, National Center for Disease Prevention and Health Promotion; 1996.
23. Krassner L. TIPP usage. *Pediatrics.* 1984;74(suppl):976–980.
24. Bass JL, Christoffel KK, Widome M, et al. Childhood injury prevention counseling in primary care settings: a critical review of the literature. *Pediatrics.* 1993;92(4):544–550.
25. Hobbie C. The Injury Prevention Program (TIPP). *J Pediatr Health Care.* 1991;5(5):279–280.
26. Moront ML, Williams JA, Eichelberer MR, Wilkinson JD. The injured child: an approach to care. *Pediatr Clin North Am.* 1994; 41(6):1201–1226.
27. Bass JL. TIPP: the first ten years. *Pediatrics.* 1995;95(2):274–275.
28. Miller TR, Galbraith M. Injury prevention counseling by pediatricians: a benefit-cost comparison. *Pediatrics.* 1995;96(1):1–4.
29. US Department of Health and Human Services. *Healthy Children 2000: National Health Promotion and Disease Prevention Objectives Related to Mothers, Infants, Children, Adolescents, and Youth.* Boston, Mass: Jones & Bartlett; 1991.

4

Otitis Media: A Conservative Chiropractic Management Protocol

Lester Lamm and Lorraine Ginter

Otitis media is the clinical term used to describe a spectrum of inflammatory middle ear diseases in which fluid is present in the middle ear space.[1,2] Anatomic and functional qualities of the eustachian tube as well as the relative inadequacy of the maturing immune system in infants and children are believed by many experts to be important causative factors.[1,3–6] Although the sequence of events leading to otitis media is incompletely understood, eustachian tube dysfunction, chronic upper respiratory infections, food sensitivities, and environmental and social risk factors have been implicated as contributing significantly to the prevalence of this disorder.[1,7] Children under the age of 6 are most frequently afflicted,[8] and many clinical researchers attribute the high rate of occurrence to the smaller, shorter, and/or less rigid orientation of the pediatric eustachian tube.[5,8–11] While the risk factors involved in middle ear disease are well understood,[1,2,12,13] it is difficult to predict which cases of middle ear disease will resolve without complication and the need for intervention and which will culminate in suppurative infection.

The presence of infection can be definitively diagnosed only when aspirated fluid (tympanocentesis) from the middle ear has been analyzed by clinical lab procedures.[2] Because of the invasive nature of tympanocentesis, most patients with ear complaints are not subjected to this procedure. Despite the lack of a definitive diagnosis, it has become a common practice for physicians to administer antibiotics for most presentations of otitis.[7,8,14,15] A debate now centers around the use of antibiotics in the management of middle ear disorders.[2,15–19] Many of the cases diagnosed as frank infections are, in fact, acute cases of serous otitis media or mild, self-limiting infections that spontaneously resolve or can be managed conservatively without antibiotic therapy.[2,16–19]

Acute otitis media is an acute bacterial infection of the middle ear. It is most common in children and is frequently preceded by an upper respiratory infection.[1,12,20] It has been suggested that the combination of immature immune system, dysfunctional eustachian tube, and frequent bouts of upper respiratory infections lead to the inadvertent viral and/or bacterial inoculation of the middle ear and subsequent suppurative infection.[1,3–6,12,20] *Strep pneumonia* and *S pyrogenes* and *Haemophilus* influenza are the most common pathogens associated with this disorder.[20]

Serous otitis media, otitis media with effusion, or "glue ear," may be the sequela of acute otitis media.[6,8] This disorder is believed to be caused by a number of factors, including recurrent acute otitis media, dysfunctional eustachian tubes, allergic manifestations, hypertrophic adenoids, and tumors.[7,8] Serous otitis media is characterized by the accumulation of fluid in the middle ear, which, in turn, causes discomfort and behavior changes in the patient.[2]

This condition can spontaneously resolve within a matter of days to weeks or it can persist for months.[21] Because so many of these cases initially appear with many of the same signs and symptoms as bacteria-related otitis, they have been misdiagnosed as ear infections and managed as infections.[2,11,15,19]

The "Antibiotic Therapy" section was reviewed by Thomas Harris, DO, and Patricia Canfield, DO. The content of this chapter was derived from review work of the Western States Chiropractic College Clinical Standards, Protocols, and Education Committee. The authors acknowledge the contributions of Laura Baffes, DC, CCSP; Daniel DeLapp, DC, DABCO; Tom Dobson, DC; Kathleen Galligan, DC; Ronald LeFebvre, DC; Owen Lynch, DC; Bruce Marks, DC, DABCO; Charles Novak, DC; Steve Oliver, DC; Karen Petzing, DC; Ravid Raphael, DC, DABCO; Lisa Revell, DC; and Anita Roberts, DC.

Reprinted from *Top Clin Chiro* 1998; 5(1): 18–28
© 1998 Aspen Publishers, Inc.

EPIDEMIOLOGY

Middle ear infections are one of the most common childhood illnesses.[11,12,15,22,23] Although the vast majority of otitis media cases occur in infants and children, the adult population is not immune to this affliction.[20] It is most common in children under the age of 6.[1,6,12] The incidence rate has been reported to be as high as 62% by the first birthday and 83% by the third. Forty-six percent of 3-year-old children have experienced three or more episodes.[1,8,12] Acute otitis media is very much age dependent. In one study it was reported that 84% of infants and younger children (0–3 years) are afflicted with this disorder whereas only 46% of children aged 8–11 are afflicted.[6]

Natural history: untreated acute versus untreated serous otitis media

Acute, suppurative, or bacteria-related otitis media is most frequently heralded by otalgia; fever, irritability, sleep disturbances, nausea, vomiting, and diarrhea may also be present.[12] Temporary hearing loss can occur during the infection.[1,2] Ear infections tend to recur, and fluid can accumulate in the middle ear and cause hearing impairment.[1,2,12,24] No epidemiologic study has addressed the true incidence and prevalence of the complications of otitis media. However, the available literature does document the marked decrease in complications that has occurred since the advent of antimicrobial usage, and it puts the complication rate at approximately 6.5%.[8]

An untreated infection can lead to spontaneous rupture of the tympanic membrane.[5] After an acute perforation of the tympanic membrane, the middle ear will drain for up to 2 weeks after which the repair process begins. Over 90% of otitic perforations heal spontaneously within 2 months.[5] When ear infections are treated promptly, serious complications such as mastoiditis rarely manifest.[12] Chronic or recurrent infections can lead to the need for myringotomy with or without insertion of tympanostomy tubes.[1,8,12]

Serous otitis media, otitis media with effusion, or chronic otitis media does not always present with the signs and symptoms of an acute infection.[6] Otitis media with effusion is often noted at a well-child check-up or at follow-up examinations after an episode of acute otitis media. It may be acute (lasting less than 3 weeks), subacute (lasting 3 weeks to 3 months), or chronic (lasting longer than 3 months). Effusions can be serous, mucoid, or purulent.[8] Otitis media with effusion commonly has milder symptoms than the symptoms caused by the acute infectious form of this disorder and can present in an asymptomatic patient.[8] Patients may experience ear pain and conductive hearing loss.[8]

In most instances, this condition is self-limiting; most cases of nonsuppurative otitis media with effusion spontaneously resolve within a month and 80% of cases of effusion clear within 2 months.[6,8] It is suspected that the eustachian tube normalizes and becomes patent, the fluid drains from the middle ear, the air pressure equalizes, and the patient becomes asymptomatic. However, if otitis media with effusion goes undetected or is allowed to persist for months or years, chronic hearing loss develops.[6] There is a concern that withholding treatment for these chronic cases may have an adverse effect on hearing, speech, language development, learning, and behavior.[2,25]

Risk factors

A number of risk factors for infant and childhood otitis media have been identified.[1,13,24,26–38] Most important appear to be climate, dietary habits, and exposure to various environmental factors. Table 1 lists key risk factors. Although the factors identified are based on infant and childhood population studies, they may also be of consequence for otitis media in adult populations.

EVALUATION STRATEGY FOR OTITIS MEDIA

In order to accurately diagnose an earache or hearing loss disorder, it is important to determine whether the problem is related to the middle ear and/or the eustachian tube, is related to the external ear and/or the auditory canal, or involves pain referred from other sources. The types of disorders and subsequent management protocols for external ear complaints differ significantly from disorders of the middle ear. General evaluation procedures for infants and young children with suspected otitis media should include assessment of growth and development. For the general population, assessment for possible infectious diseases and examination of the head and neck are important (see Tables 2 and 3).

Take appropriate history

It is through the history that the physician is able to identify those factors most frequently associated with the various types of otitis media. Look specifically for the presence of a recent upper respiratory infection, exposure to passive smoke, use of a pacifier, vector exposure in a child-care setting, low socioeconomic profile, and other factors that might contribute to the underlying condition. Rule out the presence of craniofacial distortions, such as clefts of the hard or soft palate, that may not be apparent upon observation but that may contribute to otitis media or other hearing disorders.

Check for signs of infection

The physician should make every attempt to isolate cases that have clear signs and symptoms of acute, progressive infection. These cases usually cannot be successfully treated using conservative care and may constitute a danger to the patient.

Table 1. Risk factors for otitis media

- Season. There is a higher incidence of otitis media reported during the winter months.[28]
- Dairy. There are data to support the correlation of childhood consumption of dairy products, specifically cow's milk, and increased likelihood of middle ear infections.[1,29,30]
- Infant feeding. Breast-fed infants are far less likely to experience an episode of otitis media (6%) than milk fed infants (26%).[29] The practice of bottle feeding infants has been shown to increase the likelihood of otitis media.[24] It has been shown that the use of pacifiers is responsible for 25% of the cases of otitis media in children younger than 3 years.[31]
- Craniofacial distortions. There is a higher occurrence of otitis media in children with fetal alcohol syndrome, Down syndrome, and other conditions causing craniofacial distortions. Otitis media occurs in as many as 93% of children with fetal alcohol syndrome and 60% of children with Down syndrome.[32,33]
- Allergies. Children with allergies or a family history of allergies are more likely to contract middle ear inflammatory disorders. The role of food allergies in serous otitis media has been suggested, but the exact incidence is unknown.[30,34,35]
- Day care. Children attending day care are twice as likely to experience middle ear infections as those who are cared for at home. Some early population-based studies indicate the rate for day-care children three- to fourfold higher.[36]
- Socioeconomic status. Children raised in poverty conditions are more likely to contract otitis media.[26]
- Diet. Children deficient in certain nutrients are at risk for otitis media. The nutrients most frequently implicated are vitamin A, zinc, and essential fatty acids.[37–40]
- Secondary smoke. Children exposed to an environment where tobacco use is common are three to four times more likely to develop otitis media than children from a nonsmoking environment.[13]

Check vital signs

Fever over 101°F in adults and 102°F in children and/or chills may indicate the presence of infection (bacterial or viral) and warrant further investigation and/or referral for consideration of antibiotics. Elevated temperatures in general have limited value for determining etiology, severity, prognosis, management choices, or outcome.

Inspect the head, neck, and ears for symmetry and signs of infection

Palpation is imperative, especially of the cervical lymph nodes and the auricular lymph nodes that overlay the mastoid process. Infection of the ear will usually drain through the retropharyngeal and deep cervical lymph nodes. Lymph nodes that are large, fixed or immobile, inflamed, or tender usually indicate some problem.

Tenderness is almost always indicative of inflammation. Nodes become warm or tender to the touch, matted, and much less discrete in the presence of infection.[41(pp502–503)] Digital pressure over the mastoid process will be painful if there is involvement of the mastoid air cells, which is common in mastoiditis.[20]

Evaluate the external ear

Pain elicited by tugging the pinna of the ear may indicate an external ear problem.[42(p534)] External ear complaints can be diagnostically subdivided into disorders of the auditory canal and disorders of the external ear. Disorders of the canal include cerumen impaction and the myriad manifestations such as swimmer's ear, cholesteatoma, polyps, otomycosis, and furunculosis. The second category, disorders of the external ear, includes hematomas, frostbite, benign tumors (senile keratosis, gouty tophi, rheumatoid nodules, and sebaceous cysts, etc), and malignant tumors (basal cell and squamous cell carcinoma and melanoma). Because of the accessibility of these externalized lesions, they are easier to diagnose than those of the middle ear.

Evaluate the middle ear

Bacterial, suppurative otitis media can be definitively diagnosed only when fluid in the middle ear is analyzed by laboratory procedures following a myringotomy. Owing to the invasive nature and cost of myringotomy, it is not routinely performed. Therefore, indirect methods are used in the

Table 2. Key symptoms and signs of acute suppurative otitis media

Best indicator: Otoscopy shows bulging, cloudy tympanic membrane with distinctly impaired mobility.[41]

Other symptoms and signs:
- Otorrhea with perforation of tympanic membrane.
- Hyperemic vascular strip or distorted/obliterated light reflex.
- Absent or poor mobility of tympanic membrane demonstrated with pneumatic otoscopy.
- History of recent upper respiratory tract infection.
- Severe otalgia (may throb in conjunction with arterial pulse).
- Fever above 101°F in adults and 102°F in children.
- Conductive hearing loss.
- Sleep disturbance and irritability. (These symptoms are common, and nausea, vomiting, and diarrhea may also be present.)

Table 3. Key symptoms and signs of serous otitis media

Best indicator: Otoscopy shows tympanic membrane to be normal or retracted or uncovers the existence of air bubbles in the fluid within the middle ear. The fluid behind the membrane may appear as a meniscus.[41]

Other symptoms and signs:
- Minor or absent hyperemia, bulging, and/or thickening of the tympanic membrane.
- Normal mobility or moderate hypomobility of tympanic membrane demonstrated with pneumatic otoscopy.
- History of recent upper respiratory tract infection.
- Mild or moderate otalgia (may be more constant and less throbbing).
- Fever, if present, below 101°F in adults or 102°F in children (more commonly it is absent altogether).
- Conductive hearing loss.
- Subjective "fullness" or stuffiness reported.
- Popping or crackling noise in patient's ears upon swallowing or yawning.
- Pressure discomfort within ears upon changing attitude (bending forward or to the side).

Note: Serous otitis media has numerous clinical designations: otitis media with effusion, secretory otitis media, glue ear, fluid ear, tubotympanitis, exudative catarrh, tympanic hydrops, barotrauma, and eustachian tube dysfunction.[11] It is not uncommon for serous otitis media to present as a sequela of an acute otitis media infection. The patient may be asymptomatic or present with milder signs and symptoms.

---

diagnosis of otitis media of undetermined origin. These indirect methods can involve the following procedures.

Pneumatic otoscopy is necessary for a proper diagnosis. This protocol requires the physician to inspect the tympanic membranes while varying the air pressure within the auditory canal. A good seal around the auditory meatus is required in order to achieve the clinical objectives. A bulbous-tipped speculum is helpful in achieving a proper seal. Once a proper seal is obtained, the clinician introduces air into the canal by blowing into a tube connected to the scope or by compressing an insufflation bulb attached to the otoscope. The examiner should observe the relative movement of the tympanic membrane as the change in air pressure occurs. If normal, the tympanic membrane will move briskly in and out with ease. A sluggish or absent response suggests the presence of fluid behind the membrane. When fluid is present, mobility is inhibited. A tympanic membrane affected by negative middle ear pressure moves out with negative pressure, then passively returns without the need of positive pressure. The mobility of the tympanic membrane in infants younger than 7 months is below the norm for children and adults, and pneumatic otoscopy may not be reliable.[4,8,9]

Studies have shown that otoscopy alone produces predictive values (for visible tympanic membrane characteristics) that range widely and is thus not recommended as the sole evaluative method. Pneumatic otoscopy has been widely credited as an advance over otoscopy alone and is recommended for diagnostic evaluation in suspected otitis media presentations. In one study, pneumatic otoscopy was shown to have a sensitivity of 85% to 90% and a specificity of 70% to 79%.[43] In another study, positive and negative predictive values of pneumatic otoscopy for middle ear effusion were found to be 91% and 84%, respectively.[44]

Autoinflation of the middle ear may be used to evaluate the patency of the eustachian tube. This maneuver is performed during an otoscopic examination to observe tympanic membrane movement. If the patient is able to easily "clear" his or her ears by performing a Valsalva maneuver with the nose and glottis closed, the eustachian tube may be assumed to be patent.

Evaluate neck biomechanically

Assess the cervical spine for normal range of motion and the existence of fixations/subluxations. The osteopathic and chiropractic literature on manipulation and otitis media is limited and not of good quality. It does suggest, however, that a correlation may exist between otitis media and fixations/subluxations in the occiput/C1/C2 region.[45,46]

Check for possible sources of referred pain

If there is no evidence of otitis media or other ear pathology, you must look for other sources of the ear pain. Particular attention should be given to the temporomandibular joint. Dysfunction of this joint has been implicated in cases of ear pain and dysfunction.[5,20] Secondary otalgia can also arise from cranial nerve V, VII, IX, and X involvement as well as disorders of the temporal bone, mastoid, larynx, teeth, and tongue.[5,20] Myofascial trigger points in the lateral and medial pterygoid, masseter, and sternocleidomastoid may refer pain to the ear.[47] Referred otalgia commonly occurs with tonsillitis, pharyngitis, and carcinoma of the hypopharynx and larynx.[5]

Perform ancillary studies

There are a number of diagnostic procedures involving the use of more sophisticated technology that provide valuable information for the physician. Two of the most common are tympanometry and audiometric testing. Based on limited scientific evidence and expert opinion, tympanometry is an option for use as a confirmatory test for otitis media with effusion.[44,48,49] Pneumatic otoscopy gives only a qualitative measure of tympanic membrane mobility, whereas tympanometry gives a quantitative measure of this variable. Performing pneumatic otoscopy provides information about the ear anatomy and mobility of the tympanic membrane that is essential for an accurate diagnosis. The Agency for Health

Care Policy and Research (AHCPR) guidelines panel recommends pneumatic otoscopy as the primary diagnostic protocol and tympanometry as a confirmatory test.[25,50–52]

Audiometric testing is commonly used to assess hearing loss, which can be an indicator of the presence of otitis media with effusion. AHCPR guidelines recommend hearing evaluation in a child who has had bilateral otitis media with effusion for a total of 3 months. For clinical presentations of less than 3 months duration, audiometric hearing evaluation is an option.[2]

Please note that there have been no epidemiologic studies to determine the true incidence or prevalence of the complications of otitis media using all patients with otitis media as the denominator. However, the percentage of complications is quite low.[8] Mastoiditis,[53] petrous apicitis,[20] otogenic skull base osteomyelitis,[21] facial paralysis,[54] sigmoid sinus thrombosis,[55] and central nervous system infection,[56] although uncommon, each seriously compromise a patient's health and require referral to an appropriate allopathic physician.

MANAGEMENT OF OTITIS MEDIA

Much of what has historically been diagnosed as otitis media and subsequently treated with antibiotics was, in fact, a condition of lesser severity and would have responded to a more conservative management approach. The data available today clearly suggest a more prudent approach.[17,19,57]

In light of increasing worldwide resistance of bacteria to antimicrobial drugs and the subsequent higher morbidity, mortality, and costs, it is not surprising the health care community is concerned about the use of these drugs in the management of otitis media. In a recent article published in the *British Medical Journal,* the authors concluded that

> existing research offers no compelling evidence that children with acute otitis media routinely given antimicrobials have a shorter duration of symptoms, fewer recurrences, or better long-term outcomes than those who do not receive them. It is also not clear that routine compared with selective use of antimicrobials prevents complications. Thus it is prudent to reconsider routine use of antimicrobials for otitis media and to consider other approaches.[58]

Simply put, watchful waiting is now the recommended approach to the overall management of earaches and conductive hearing disorders.[2]

The literature clearly suggests that many of these cases will spontaneously resolve without the need for more invasive procedures such as antibiotic therapy, tympanostomy, myringotomy, or surgery.[2,17–19,57] However, given the prevalence of this disorder and the high rate of recurrence,[17] the employment of conservative interventions may decrease the likelihood of further infectious episodes, relieve pain, and facilitate the healing process.

Table 4 identifies the major therapeutic objectives in caring for patients with otitis media. Cases of otitis media that present with signs and symptoms of acute progressive infection should be referred for appropriate medical attention. After the acute, active phase of the infection has been controlled, conservative care may minimize the likelihood of recurrence or chronicity (see section entitled "Management and Prevention of Recurrent Acute Otitis Media and Serous Otitis Media").

Serous otitis media—although similar to an active, progressive infection—has a presentation that allows the physician to both "watchfully wait" and intervene conservatively. For patients diagnosed with nonsuppurative otitis media, the physician can employ conservative management protocols immediately.

If the patient has serous otitis media for more than 3 months (chronic otitis media with effusion) and it is not responding to conservative therapy, consider a referral or consult.[59] Unilateral serous otitis media in an adult should raise suspicion of a noninfectious process (eg, tumor).[60]

METHOD FOR REVIEWING CONSERVATIVE TREATMENT STRATEGIES

Given the limitations in evidence regarding a number of conservative treatment options, Western States Chiropractic College (WSCC) convened a consensus panel to review available literature and determine which options may have the most value and should be applied in the college clinics. The panel was composed of full-time WSCC clinicians who staffed the college's three clinics and a representative from the research department. The original draft was the result of an exhaustive review of available chiropractic and medical literature as well as established guidelines such as those promulgated by the AHCPR. Using a modified nominal group process, the panel met weekly for approximately 20 weeks to evaluate the draft and revise it based on the members' combined clinical experience. Selected sections were also reviewed by on-campus subject-matter experts.

CONSERVATIVE TREATMENT OPTIONS

The decision to conservatively manage a patient with ear pain depends greatly upon the progression and severity of

---

Table 4. Specific therapeutic objectives

- Address the patient's symptoms.
- Improve drainage from the middle ear.
- Identify risk factors and take steps to eliminate their impact.

the patient complaints. A number of conservative interventions that fall within the scope of chiropractors' expertise have been used to treat patients with otitis media. Although well-designed outcomes studies are still lacking, there is good reason for using manual procedures in many cases of infection instead of antibiotics. If there are obvious signs of acute, progressive infection or the tympanic membrane has ruptured, the patient should be under the care of a primary care physician. If, however, the signs and symptoms warrant conservative intervention, the chiropractor may employ various approaches, depending on his or her training and experience. Table 5 lists several common interventions chiropractors can consider. The rationales for their use follow.

It is important to monitor patients on a daily basis during the acute phase of otitis media and while conservative interventions are being used. All of the conservative interventions listed in Table 5 can be administered daily or every other day during the acute phase, which usually lasts 3 to 5 days. Soft tissue massage, autoinflation, and home care therapies (warm oil, local heat, analgesics) can be administered as needed.

If the signs and symptoms do not resolve, diminish, or stabilize in 3 to 5 days, or if the symptoms progress, the patient should be referred for further evaluation. Following further evaluation or medical intervention, the patient should consider conservative management protocols to minimize the likelihood of recurrent infections. When to employ preventive, conservative management interventions is a clinical decision best made by the attending physician.

During an otitis media episode, there are essentially two approaches a patient may take. Either begin preventive, conservative management immediately following resolution of the acute phase or begin conservative interventions after the patient experiences a recurrent episode. Treatment options can include manual therapy (manipulation/adjustment, soft tissue work, endonasal procedures, tympanic ventilation), physiotherapeutics (warm oil or local heat), symptom control with over-the-counter analgesics or anti-inflamatory medications, and other forms of self-care (reduction of risk factors, warm oil, lymphatic drainage, autoinflation).

MANUAL THERAPY

Cervical manipulation

Found in the osteopathic and chiropractic literature were only two studies, of limited design, that addressed the impact that manipulation/adjustment of the upper cervical spine and/or occiput may have in the management of otitis media.[45,61] The more recent was a chiropractic study that used a nonrandomized, retrospective cohort of 46 children aged 5 or under.[61] Ninety-three percent of the cases resolved successfully, with 75% taking less than 10 days and 43% requiring only one or two treatments. The study's main limitation was the lack of comparison and natural progression groups; however, the results were promising regarding the symptom relief associated with the administration of cervical adjusting. Better outcomes were correlated with younger age, no history of antibiotic use, and initial (vs recurrent) episodes. The consensus of the Western States Chiropractic College Clinical Standards, Protocols, and Education Committee was that cervical adjusting by an experienced practitioner was a reasonable form of intervention.

Auricular adjusting

Use of auricular adjusting is also supported by the Western States Chiropractic College Clinical Standards, Protocols, and Education Committee. Although there are no data available to support this intervention, it is commonly used by practitioners in conjunction with the endonasal technique. The adjustment is performed differently by different physicians, and consideration of its use is part of the clinician's decision-making process. One way to perform this maneuver is to grasp the patient's ear and traction it in a full complement of directions. Following this procedure, the physician may perform an optional forceful tug to the ear. One way this is achieved is by placing the physician's index finger behind the ear and the corresponding thumb along the antitragus and antihelix. The direction of the forceful tug is generally away from the head and toward the anterior. The rationale is that the possible traction of the external auditory meatus and tympanic fascia as well as the potential stretching of the intrinsic neck musculature that surrounds the eustachian tube

Table 5. Conservative treatment options for ear pain and otitis media

- Consider adjustment of the cervical spine for fixations or subluxations. Particular attention to the upper cervical area (C1-C3) may be warranted.
- Endonasal technique and/or auricular adjustment may impact muscle tone surrounding the middle ear pressure affecting drainage.
- Self-care instruction to autoinflate the affected ear(s) may be helpful for older children.
- Consider soft tissue massage and instructing the patient on self-massage for the soft tissue structures of the neck to promote lymphatic drainage.
- For those patients experiencing significant or intractable pain, warm oil or hot air may provide relief.
- For patients with severe pain, consider the use of OTC analgesics and/or anti-inflammatories.
- Recommend and properly instruct the patient on appropriate self-care interventions.

may facilitate drainage of the middle ear. Positioning for cervical adjusting may also stretch this musculature.

Soft tissue manipulation

Soft tissue manipulation is a third intervention accepted by the Western States Chiropractic College Clinical Standards, Protocols, and Education Committee. The two basic approaches are differentiated primarily by the degree of invasiveness. Soft tissue manipulation can be conducted either by the physician or by the patient following self-help instruction.

One massage technique involves the insertion of two fingers into the sulcus created by the anterior aspect of the mastoid process and the posterior angle of the jaw. From a point in the sulcus, place a finger anterior and a finger posterior to the ear lobe of the involved ear. Apply moderate to deep pressure as the two fingers are swept inferiorward along the anterior margin of the sternocleidomastoid muscle. The process can be performed periodically but frequently for up to 2 minutes per intervention throughout the remainder of the day following employment of the endonasal technique. This soft tissue manipulation is intended to *milk* the eustachian tube and promote evacuation of fluid accumulation from the middle ear chamber.

A gentler massage of the anterior and posterior soft structures of the neck is intended to promote lymphatic flow away from the involved lymphoid tissues. A superficial, slow, and mild stroking massage can be administered by the physician or can be demonstrated to the patient for home care. The number of strokes varies, as does the time between strokes, but one stroke every 10 seconds is probably the mean. The massage is usually discontinued when local skin redness appears or the patient experiences symptomatic relief.

Endonasal technique

The endonasal technique[62–65] involves intraoral massage of selected nasopharyngeal musculature. Typically, introduction of a gloved finger, palmar surface upward, is made into the mouth, past the uvula into the nasopharynx and laterally outward and upward to the fossa of Rosenmüller. Minimizing direct contact with the uvula is important to diminish chance of a gag reflex. A sweep of the fossa is made, and a tractional tug of the inferior tissues is applied as the finger is withdrawn. Antiseptics such as dilute solutions of phenolated iodine, Chloraseptic, or chlorophyll astringent can be applied to the gloved finger to minimize bacterial inoculation of the fossa. Having the patient gargle with a mild antiseptic mouthwash or warm saltwater after the procedure may decrease the risk of spreading infection as well. The endonasal technique can be performed daily or every other day as a therapeutic trial for the treatment of otitis media. If reduction of symptoms is not achieved after three treatments, it is unlikely that further treatments will result in a positive response. The endonasal technique should not be done when there is evidence of an acute throat infection as exudates may be transmitted from the nasopharynx to the middle ear.

Tympanic ventilation

Tympanic ventilation, a conservative intervention used in the management of serous otitis media, involves the forceful administration of air through the eustachian tube into the middle ear space.[10,11,66–68] Resolution of negative intratympanic pressure through tympanic ventilation has been shown to be up to 91% effective in cases of serous otitis media.[67] Normalization of middle ear pressure can be achieved by autoinflation, a modified Valsalva maneuver, or by politzerization (use of an inflation bulb).

Autoinflation is done by having the patient occlude the nostrils by pinching the nose. The patient closes the glottis and blows gently as if trying to blow up a balloon. The patient continuously blows until a "popping" in the ear(s) or a noticeable change in the middle ear pressure is felt.[10,68]

Politzerization requires an external instrument that introduces positive air pressure through the nose during deglutition. The most common instrument is a small, 1-ounce rubber bulb. The bulb tip is placed into one nostril while the other is manually occluded. Air is squeezed from the bulb in synchrony with the act of swallowing.[67] This procedure is usually done following the endonasal technique. Autoinflation can be performed at regular intervals throughout the day. Tympanic ventilation will cause the patient to experience a feeling of fullness or pressure in the middle ear. Existing data suggest that, following tympanic ventilation, the middle ear pressure will normalize in approximately one-half hour.[67] Once the pressure in the middle ear has normalized, ventilation can be performed again. This time frame might provide some guidance for establishing appropriate ventilation intervals. Politzerization can be employed until the ear appears to have permanently cleared.

PHYSIOTHERAPEUTIC MODALITIES

Warm oil application

If there is no perforation in the tympanic membrane, heated oil drops (mineral oil, castor oil, mullein oil, garlic oil, etc) may be placed in the affected ear for pain relief. It should be repeated every hour until relief is achieved.[69–71] Before administering the heated oil to an infant or small child, test the temperature of the oil by placing a drop on the sensitive skin of the anterior wrist.

Local heat

The application of local heat has been used frequently for the relief of localized pain associated with earaches.[46,70] It is a simple technique that affords an immediate decrease in pain and is especially beneficial in the treatment of infants and small children awakened in the middle of the night with an earache, for they are usually uncooperative, distressed, and difficult to manage. Application of a heating pad or hot air from a hair dryer directly on the affected ear will usually calm the patient and return him or her to sleep. Be sure to monitor the level of heat to ensure that the temperature does not rise too high. Application of heat is a simple, noninvasive, and quick intervention that can be used effectively for temporary relief.

Even though the symptoms may disappear entirely, there is a possibility that underlying problems remain. In such cases, further evaluation of the patient by a clinician should be based on severity of the initial episode, objective findings at the time of presentation, and/or likelihood of recurrent episodes due to risk factors.[46,69,70]

OVER-THE-COUNTER MEDICATIONS

Analgesics and anti-inflammatories

The use of over-the-counter medications (OTCs) for the management of pain and/or inflammation is an option for the clinician. More conservative, less invasive options should be tried before an OTC intervention is considered. The decision to use OTCs should be based on the severity of the patient's complaint and/or objective findings. There are numerous studies that support wide use of analgesics for pain control as well as suppression of inflammation for a variety of human disorders, and analgesics may be applicable to otitis media. However, there are only a few studies that specifically address OTC use for otitis media. Those studies identified ibuprofen, topical anesthetics, and sodium naproxen as effective in the management of otitis media.[72-75]

Physicians considering a recommendation of a pharmaceutical intervention should apprise themselves of the clinical indications, contraindications, and adverse side effects or reactions. It is now understood by most physicians that the use of aspirin in a febrile infant or child is contraindicated. Otitis media presents its own unique set of symptoms that require caution by the treating physician before pharmaceutical agents are employed.

Nasal decongestants and antihistamines

Antihistamine and decongestant agents are not recommended for treatment of otitis media with effusion, according to a recent US government study. This conclusion, by the AHCPR, was based on an expert panel review of evidence and was felt to be generalizable to children of all ages.[2] Four randomized controlled studies of antihistamine or decongestant therapy failed to show a statistically significant effect of these medications in resolving otitis media with effusion. Additionally, these agents may cause adverse side effects such as insomnia, drowsiness, behavioral changes, and seizures.[22,76-78]

General self-care advice

Home care advice for the management of the acute phase of ear pain should address the identified risk factors identified previously (see Table 1). The provider should specifically discuss elimination of dairy products from the diet, discontinuation of the use of pacifiers, prevention of exposure to secondary smoke, and increase of fluid intake.

Patients and/or parents can place warm oil in the affected ear to help soothe earache pain or apply heat locally, as described in the section "Physiotherapeutic Modalities." Lymphatic drainage (see "Soft Tissue Manipulation") and autoinflation (see "Tympanic Ventilation") may also be self-administered or applied by a parent according to the provider's instructions.

Considerations for referral or consult

A short trial of conservative therapy should be able to determine if the patient will respond. Failure to respond in 3 to 5 days—that is, if conservative measures fail to stem the progression of symptoms such as progressive/persistent listlessness, pain, fever, or congestion—warrants consideration of medical referral. Fever above 101°F in adults and 102°F in children suggests a more serious infection, as do signs of mastoiditis (eg, extreme mastoid tenderness) or other progressive infectious disorders.

If otoscopic examination reveals rupture or imminent tympanic membrane rupture (red, bulging, "angry" in appearance), referral should be sought. Chronic otitis media with effusion (serous otitis media lasting longer than 3 months) that is not responding should also be referred.

MANAGEMENT AND PREVENTION OF RECURRENT ACUTE OTITIS MEDIA AND SEROUS OTITIS MEDIA

Conservative methods to prevent recurrent otitis media include many of the same procedures used in the management of the initial acute episode of otitis media. However, there are several additional procedures that can help prevent future episodes, facilitate the healing process, decrease the virulence of the pathogen, or increase the resistance of the patient host (see Table 6). Endonasal techniques, spinal manipulation, and nasal specifics are also applicable and may be applied as described previously. Dietary and nutritional modification as well as a number of self-care options may also be useful.

Dietary and nutritional considerations

Testing for specific food sensitivity may be of value for those patients experiencing chronic or recurrent otitis media. If particular foods are identified as irritants, subsequent di-

Table 6. Conservative management protocols for managing and preventing recurrent acute otitis media and serous otitis media

- Manual therapies
  - Nasal specifics
  - Endonasal technique
  - Spinal manipulation
- Dietary and nutritional considerations
  - Food allergy testing
  - Vitamin A, zinc, essential fatty acid deficiencies
  - Delay of solid food for infants
  - Encouragement of breast-feeding
  - Restrictions on the use of pacifiers
- General self-treatment
  - Self-massage
  - Tympanic ventilation
  - Control of secondhand smoke
  - General nutrition and lifestyle
  - Evaluation of impact of day-care exposure

---

etary changes should be encouraged, including elimination of the foods at fault. Cow's milk, wheat, egg white, peanuts, soy, corn, oranges, tomatoes, chicken, and apples are the most frequently identified foods causing allergic responses in children.[28] Additional factors, including vitamin and mineral deficiencies and supplementation, are listed in Table 7.[36-39]

Self-care summary

Self-care instructions are also important in chronic and recurrent cases, and the strategy is the same as that described for acute management (see also Table 8).

CONCLUSION

Otitis media is a condition that has routinely been medically treated with antibiotics. New evidence suggests that other conservative measures may be more useful and may have better long-term outcomes. However, detailed evidence demonstrating that conservative interventions are the most appropriate remains to be gathered.

Chiropractors have long approached patient care with a variety of conservative manual, dietary, and lifestyle interventions and have reported utility in applying them with patients suffering from otitis media. Although use of such interventions has been the source of controversy in the past, new evidence has spawned greater interest in them. In the absence of definitive studies on many conservative interventions, the Western States Chiropractic College Clinical Standards, Protocols, and Education Committee used a formal process to gather and appraise available literature and identify conservative options likely to be of greatest value. Manipulation to relax musculature, other manual methods to promote middle ear drainage, reduction of risk factors, self-care instructions, and dietary or lifestyle changes may help reduce morbidity and promote resolution of this common problem, and these are all tools that chiropractors are qualified to employ.

Table 7. Potential dietary and nutritional considerations in treating chronic otitis media

- Food allergies may play a role in chronic cases or in cases of nonresponse to treatment.
- Vitamin A, zinc, and essential fatty acid deficiencies have been associated with otitis media.
- RDA dosage supplementation is recommended for all children who have a history of otitis media.
- Delay until at least 6 months of age the introduction of solid foods to nursing infants.
- Encourage breast-feeding. Breast-feeding (as opposed to formula feeding) should continue for at least the first 6 months of life.
- Restrict the use of pacifiers to the first 10 months of life, when otitis media in children is more uncommon.

Table 8. Self-care instructions for otitis media

- Encourage elimination or reduction of exposure to risk factors including use of dairy products, pacifiers, and exposure to second-hand smoke. Educating patients about socioeconomic factors, such as nutrition and lifestyle habits may be useful. Discussion of resources available through various social and welfare agencies may help provide assistance.
- Increase fluid intake.
- Warm oil placed in the affected ear and/or application of local heat may soothe discomfort.
- Encourage patient to perform self-massage and/or instruct parent in gentle soft tissue manipulation of the cervical musculature to promote drainage.
- During acute recurrent episodes, encourage daily, routine tympanic ventilation of the middle ear to promote drainage of accumulated fluid.

REFERENCES

1. Shapiro AM, Bluestone CD. Otitis media reassessed. *Postgrad Med.* 1995;97:73–82.
2. Demlo LK, ed. *Otitis Media with Effusion in Young Children.* Rockville, MD: US Department of Health and Human Services, Agency for Health Care Policy and Research; 1994.
3. Cantekin EI, Casselbrant ML, Doyle WJ, Brostoff LM. Eustachian tube function: prospective study of eustachian tube function and otitis media. Recent Advances in Otitis Media: Proceedings of the Fourth International Symposium. Philadelphia, PA: BC Decker; 1987.
4. Casselbrant ML, Cantekin EI, Dirkmaat DC, Doyle WJ, Bluestone CD. Reversible functional obstruction of the eustachian tube. Recent Advances in Otitis Media: Proceedings of the Fourth International Symposium. Philadelphia, PA: BC Decker; 1987.
5. Koufman JA. *Core Otolaryngology.* Philadelphia, PA: JB Lippincott; 1990.
6. Casselbrant ML, Brostoff LM, Cantekin EI. Otitis media with effusion in preschool children. *Laryngoscope.* 1985;95:428–436.
7. Berkow R, ed. *The Merck Manual.* 16th ed. Rahway, NJ: Merck Sharp & Dohme Research Laboratories; 1992.
8. Eden AN, Fireman P, Stool S. Otitis media with effusion: sorting out the options. *Patient Care.* 1995;15:52–56.
9. Taylor RB, ed. *Family Medicine: Principles and Practice.* New York, NY: Springer-Verlag; 1993.
10. Shea JJ. Autoinflation treatment of serous otitis media in children. *J. Laryngol Otol.* 1971;85:1254–1258.
11. Bluestone CD. Current concepts in otolaryngology. *N Engl J Med.* 1982;306(23):1399–1404.
12. Eden AN, Fireman P, Stool S. The rise of acute otitis media. *Patient Care.* 1995;15:22–51.
13. Kraemer MJ, Richardson MA, Weiss NS. Risk factors for persistent middle ear effusions: otitis media catarrh, cigarette smoke exposure and atopy. *JAMA.* 1983;249:1022–1025.
14. Ostfeld E, Segal J, Kaufstein M, Gelernter I. Management of acute otitis media without primary administration of systemic antimicrobial agents. Recent Advances in Otitis Media: Proceedings of the Fourth International Symposium. Philadelphia, PA: BC Decker; 1987.
15. Rosenfeld RM, Post JC. Meta-analysis of antibiotics for the treatment of otitis media with effusion. *Otolaryngol Head Neck Surg.* 1992;106:378–386.
16. Schloss MD, Dempsey EE, Rishof E, Sorger S, Grace MGA. Double blind study comparing erythromycin-sulfisoxazole (Pediazole) t.i.d. to placebo in chronic otitis media with effusion. Recent Advances in Otitis Media: Proceedings of the Fourth International Symposium. Philadelphia, PA: BC Decker; 1987.
17. van Buchem FL, Dunk JH, van't Hof MA. Therapy of acute otitis media: myringotomy, antibiotics, or neither? *Lancet.* 1981;24:883–887.
18. Cantekin EI, McGuire TW, Griffith TL. Antimicrobial therapy for otitis media with effusion (secretory otitis media). *JAMA.* 1991;266:3309–3317.
19. Frenkel M. Acute otitis media: does therapy alter its course? *Postgrad Med.* 1987;82(5):85–86.
20. Tierney LM, McPhee SJ, Papadakis MA, Schroeder SA, eds. *Current Medical Diagnosis and Treatment.* Norwalk, CT: Appleton & Lange; 1993.
21. Beneke JE. Management of osteomyelitis of the skull base. *Laryngoscope.* 1989;99:1220.
22. Cantekin EI, Mandel EM, Bluestone CD. Lack of efficacy of a decongestant-antihistamine combination for otitis media with effusion (secretory otitis media) in children: results of a double-blind, randomized trial. *N Engl J Med.* 1983;308: 297–301.
23. Kenna MA. Incidence and prevalence of complications of otitis media. *Ann Otol Rhinol Laryngol Suppl.* 1990;149:38.
24. Teele DW, Klein JO, Rosener BA. Epidemiology of otitis media in children. *Ann Otol Rhinol Laryngol Suppl.* 1980;89:5–6.
25. Roland PS, Finitzo T, Friel-Patti S, Brown KC, Stephens KT, Brown O, Coleman JM. Otitis media: incidence, duration, and hearing status. *Arch Otolaryngol Head Neck Surg.* 1989;115:1049–1053.
26. Biles RW, Buffer PA, O'Donell AA. Epidemiology of otitis media: a community study. *Am J Public Health.* 1980;70:593.
27. Saarinen U. Breastfeeding prevents otitis media. *Nutr Rev.* 1983; 41(8):241.
28. Nsouli TM, Nisouli SM, Linde RM, et al. Role of food allergy in serous otitis media. *Ann Allergy Asthma Immunol.* 1994;73:215–219.
29. Niemela M, Uhari M, Mottonen M. A pacifier increases the risk of recurrent acute otitis media in children in daycare centers. *Pediatrics.* 1995;96:884–888.
30. Church MW, Gerkin KP. Hearing disorders in children with fetal alcohol syndrome: findings from case reports. *Pediatrics.* 1988;82:147–154.
31. Schwartz DM, Schwartz RH. Acoustic impedence and otoscopic findings in young children with Down's syndrome. *Arch Otolaryngol.* 1978;104:652.
32. Bahna SL, Myer CM. Food allergy for the pediatrician. *Int Pediatr.* 1988;3:245–249.
33. Hurst DS. Allergy management of refractory serous otitis media. *Otolaryngol Head Neck Surg.* 1990;102:664–669.
34. Backman A, Bjorksten F, Ilmonen S, Juntunen K, Suoniemi I. Do infections in infancy affect sensitization to airborne allergens and development of atopic disease? A retrospective study of seven year old children. *Allergy.* 1984;39:309–315.
35. Roberts JE, Burchinal MR, Collier AM, et al. Otitis media in early childhood and cognitive, academic, and classroom performance of the school-aged child. *Pediatrics.* 1989;83(4):477–485.
36. Chole RA. Squamous metaplasia of the middle ear mucosa during vitamin A deprivation. *Otolaryngol Head Neck Surg.* 1979;87:837–844.
37. Bondestam M, Foucard T, Gebre-Medhin M. Subclinical trace element deficiency in children with undue susceptibility to infections. *Act Paediatr Scand* (case series). 1985;74:515–520.
38. Hussey GD, Klein M. A randomized controlled trial of vitamin A in children with severe measles. *N Engl J Med.* 1990;323:160–164.
39. Jung TTK. Prostaglandins, leukotrienes, and other arachidonic acid metabolites in the pathogenesis of otitis media. *Laryngoscope.* 1988;98:980–993.
40. Karma PH, Penttila MA, Sipila MM, Timonen MS. Diagnostic value of otoscopic signs in acute otitis media. Recent Advances in Otitis Media: Proceedings of the Fourth International Symposium. Philadelphia, PA: BC Decker; 1987.

41. Seidel HM, Ball JW, Dains JE, Benedict GW. *Mosby's Guide to Physical Examination.* St Louis, MO: Mosby; 1987.
42. Rakel RE. *Textbook of Family Practice.* Philadelphia, PA: WB Saunders; 1990.
43. Kaleida PH, Stool SE. Assessment of otoscopists' accuracy regarding middle ear effusion. *Am J Dis Child.* 1992;146:433–435.
44. Toner JG, Mains B. Pneumatic otoscopy and tympanometry in the detection of middle ear effusion. *Clin Otolaryngol.* 1990; 15(2):121–123.
45. Pintal WJ, Kurtz ME. An integrated osteopathic treatment approach in acute otitis media. *J Am Osteopath Assoc.* 1989;89:1139–1141.
46. Thrash AM, Thrash CL. *Home Remedies: Hydrotherapy, Massage, Charcoal, and Other Simple Treatments.* Seale, AL: Thrash Publications; 1981.
47. Travell JG, Simons DG. *Myofascial Pain and Dysfunction.* Baltimore, MD: Williams & Wilkins; 1983;1:166.
48. Babonis TR, Weir MR, Kelly PC. Impedance tympanometry and acoustic reflectometry at myringotomy. *Pediatrics.* 1991;87(4):475–480.
49. Dempster JH, MacKenzie K. Tympanometry in the detection of hearing impairments associated with otitis media with effusion. *Clin Otolaryngol.* 1991;16(2):157–159.
50. Tos M, Poulen G, Borch J. Tympanometry in 2-year-old children. *ORL J Otorhinolaryngol Relat Spec.* 1978;40(2):77–85.
51. Fiellau-Nikolajsen M. Serial tympanometry and middle ear status in 3-year-old children. *ORL J Otorhinolaryngol Relat Spec.* 1980;42(4):220–232.
52. Fiellau-Nikolajsen M. Tympanometry in 3-year-old children: prevalence and spontaneous course of middle ear effusion. *Ann Otol Rhinol Laryngol Suppl.* 1980;89:223–227.
53. Farrior J. Complications of otitis media in children. *South Med J.* 1990;83:645.
54. Moore GF. Facial nerve paralysis. *Prim Care.* 1990;17:437.
55. Kelly KE, Jackler RK, Dillon WP. Diagnosis of septic sigmoid sinus thrombosis with magnetic resonance imaging. *Otolaryngol Head Neck Surg.* 1991;105:617.
56. Freidman EM, McGill TJI, Healy GB. Central nervous system complications associated with acute otitis media in children. *Laryngoscope.* 1990;100:149.
57. Browning GG, Bain J. Childhood otalgia: acute otitis media. *BMJ.* 1990; 300:1005–1007.
58. Nelson WE, Behrman RE, Vaughan VC III, eds. *Nelson Textbook of Pediatrics.* 15th ed. Philadelphia, PA: WB Saunders; 1996.
59. Froom, J, Culpepper L, Jacobs M. Antimicrobials for acute otitis media? A review from the International Primary Care Network. *BMJ.* 1997;315:98–102.
60. Isselbacher KJ, Martin JB, Braunwald E, et al., eds. *Harrison's Principles of Internal Medicine.* 13th ed. New York: McGraw-Hill; 1994.
61. Froehle RM. Ear infection: a retrospective study examining improvement from chiropractic care and analyzing for influencing factors. *J Manipulative Physiol Ther.* 1996;19(3):169–177.
62. Gillett CF. *A Manual for Eye, Ear, Nose, and Throat.* San Francisco: Kohnke Printing Co; 1928.
63. Finnell FL. *Constructive Chiropractic and Endonasal-Aural and Allied Office Techniques for Eye-Ear-Nose and Throat.* Portland, OR: Ryder Printing; 1951.
64. Lake TL. *Endo-Nasal, Aural and Allied Techniques: Ear, Eye, Nose and Throat.* 5th ed. Philadelphia, PA: WB Saunders; 1942.
65. Finnell FL. *Manual of Eye, Ear, Nose and Throat.* Portland, OR: Oak Grove Press; 1951.
66. Williams HR. A method for maintaining middle ear ventilation in children. *J Laryngol Otol.* 1968; 82:921–926.
67. Schwartz DM, Schwartz RH, Redfield NP. Treatment of negative middle ear pressure and serous otitis media with Politzer's technique. *Arch Otolaryngol.* 1978;104:487–490.
68. Chan KH, Cantekin EL, Karnavas WJ, Bluestone CD. Autoinflation of eustachian tube in young children. *Laryngoscope.* 1987; 97:668–674.
69. Cameron M. *Treasury of Home Remedies.* Englewood Cliffs, NJ: Prentice Hall; 1987.
70. Tkac D, ed. *The Doctor's Book of Home Remedies.* Emmaus, PA: Rodale Press; 1990.
71. Hansen RA. *Get Well at Home.* Wildwood, NJ: Shiloh Medical Publications; 1980.
72. Francois M. Efficacy and tolerance of a local application of phenazone and chlorhydrate lidocaine (Otipax) in infants and children with congestive otitis [in French]. *Annales de Pediatrie.* 1993;40(7):481–484.
73. Campos L, Diaz Gomez M, Ondiviela R, Masorra F. Naproxen sodium in the treatment of otitis [in Spanish]. *Atencion Primaria.* 1992;9(6):316–317.
74. Diven WF, Evans RW, Swarts JD, Burckart GJ, Doyle WJ. Effect of ibuprofen treatment during experimental acute otitis media. *Auris Nasus Larynx.* 1995;22(2):73–79.
75. Diven WF, Evans RW, Alper C, Burckart GJ, Jaffe R, Doyle WJ. Treatment of experimental acute otitis media with ibuprofen and ampicillin. *Int J Pediatr Otorhinolaryngol.* 1995;33(2):127–139.
76. Haugeto OK, Schroeder KE, Mair IW. Secretory otitis media, oral decongestant and antihistamine. *J Otolaryngol.* 1981;10(5):350–362.
77. Dusdieker LB, Smith G, Booth BM, Woodhead JC, Milavetz G. The long-term outcome of nonsuppurative otitis media with effusion. *Clin Pediatr.* 1985;24(4):181–186.
78. Mandel EM, Rockette HE, Bluestone CD, Paradise JL, Nozza RJ. Efficacy of amoxicillin with and without decongestant-antihistamine for otitis media with effusion in children: results of a double-blind, randomized trial. *N Engl J Med.* 1987;316:432–437.

5

Chiropractic Management of the Special Needs Child

Tracy Barnes

Children with special needs can present unique challenges to any physician involved in their care. This chapter outlines conditions most likely to be seen in chiropractic practice, along with approaches for management. It reviews assessment strategies and discusses specific assessment techniques and modifications that may assist in the work-up of these children. Cerebral palsy, autism, and Down syndrome are the special needs conditions that most frequently present at the Kentuckiana Children's Center in Louisville, Kentucky, and they are thus likely to be periodically confronted in general chiropractic practice.

The term *special needs* is a contemporary and sensitive substitute for historical terms such as *handicapped, retarded,* and *disabled.* The term typically encompasses children who have profound difficulties in both physical and mental arenas. Special needs conditions can be divided into disorders of neurologic and muscular systems; bone and joint; kidney and urinary tracts; behavioral and psychosocial origin; ear, nose and throat; and so on. This article focuses primarily on the management of children with cerebral palsy, autism, and Down syndrome.

CLINICAL HEALTH HISTORY CONSIDERATIONS

The axiom that "90% of diagnosis comes from the history" holds true for the pediatric as well as the adult population. Children with special needs often have very extensive histories replete with multiple tests, imaging studies, and a variety of assessments from previous evaluations. Table 1 outlines key historical concerns for different age groups that need to be addressed. History taking with these children is oriented less toward discovering new information than toward delineating the most pertinent data from a wealth of material. A useful approach is to take the most complete history possible prior to reading any evaluations the parents may bring in from outside agencies. This allows for an opinion to be formulated independent of influence from previous diagnoses and prognoses.

Although some information is gleaned directly from the child, a chiropractor's complete health history of the special needs child should begin with a detailed account of any chief complaints gleaned from a parent. "When did you first notice there was a problem with your child?" is a productive way to begin discussion. Some parents of special needs children are more reliable historians than others. Many have recounted their child's problems so often that they tell their story somewhat mechanically. Others have become such experts in their child's condition that they may overwhelm the doctor with extraordinary clinical details. Remaining patient and persistent is the key to handling these situations.

An important step in the history-taking process is to ascertain the parent's goal in managing the child's condition. Certainly parents wish to foster a vision of complete health, happiness, and well-being for their children. However, this may not be an attainable outcome for some children with special needs. The parent of a child with spastic quadriplegic cerebral palsy, for example, may want, as a first goal, the child to walk, gain bladder control, or be able to feed him- or herself. Or the primary desire may be that the child becomes free of a constant cold and runny nose. Whether the goal is to improve attention span, decrease seizure frequency, or eliminate ear infections, the clinician should have an understanding of the family's desires before offering opinions or initiating care. In cases where the child is able to communicate effectively, it is important to involve him or her in the history-taking and goal-setting process.

Reprinted from *Top Clin Chiro* 1997; 4(4): 9–18
© 1997 Aspen Publishers, Inc.

In addition to recording details concerning the child's chief complaint, the health history should illuminate all developmental periods, including the mother's prenatal history. Mailing a written patient history form to the family before their appointment can save time for both parents and the doctor. It will also minimize the problem of children becoming uncomfortable and perhaps disruptive while waiting in the doctor's office. Providing a children's corner in the reception area, with quiet toys and books, is always helpful. The interview should allow adequate time to address parents' concerns and to answer any questions.

EXAMINATION CONSIDERATIONS

Performing a detailed examination on a child with special needs requires a great deal of flexibility on the part of both doctor and staff. The exam is a time to expect the unexpected. For example, an examination of an ambulatory child is a very different matter than an examination of a nonverbal child who is bound to a wheelchair and prone to seizure. This latter child may be unable to assume a prone or supine position comfortably and may need to be examined while seated. Another child may be unable to verbally communicate where he or she feels discomfort. Nonverbal communication such as hand gestures or constant touch of a particular body part (rubbing the head, tugging the ears, holding the abdomen) may help in uncovering dysfunction or discomfort. A child in diapers may be unable to give a urine sample. Cursory information may need to be obtained by sampling a wet diaper.

A fearful child may be comforted by a compassionate and friendly staff person who reads a book to or plays a simple game with the child before the exam begins. Extra time should always be allotted for such unforeseen delays. In addition, staff members who will work with the child should be given as much information as possible about the child's condition prior to the appointment. Knowledge about what to expect may alleviate any apprehension about working with many of these children. It is important to stress to staff members that the inherent dignity of each child, regardless of appearance or behavior, should be acknowledged through conveying the respect and compassion any child deserves. As much communication as possible should be directed to the child even if the child appears unable to understand. Never underestimate what a child may be able to perceive. Outward appearance may reveal little of inward ability.

Children with special needs who have been through myriad tests and exams, some perhaps painful, may be hesitant to undergo yet another evaluation. For this reason the doctor must work to establish good rapport with the child before beginning the exam. The doctor should greet the family in the waiting room and make sure to introduce him- or herself directly to the child.

Many children are frightened by the appearance of anyone in a white uniform. Those offices that require staff to wear uniforms may find it helpful to opt for a more colorful or playful approach, such as a dinosaur print jacket or simply no uniform at all on the day of the exam. Making direct eye contact with the child and explaining exam procedures in a nonthreatening manner ahead of time can also alleviate fears. Some form of friendly contact with a child should occur prior to any hands-on procedures. An exam procedure known to be painful should be revealed to the child before it is done. An honest approach will foster trust. Confronting a child's fears about injections is recommended. Use language that directly addresses the child's potential concerns, such as, "Sally, before we get started, I want you to know that we don't like shots either. We won't be using any needles or taking any blood today."

Allowing the child to play with exam tools such as the otoscope, reflex hammer, and stethoscope may engage the child in the process and help to alleviate fear. It may also be helpful to have the child look in the doctor's ears or listen to his or her own heart beat. Having stuffed toys available and adopting a playful attitude can make the process a very positive experience for both child and doctor. For example, instead of just listening to the abdomen, the doctor might explain to the young child that he or she is listening to hear what the child had for breakfast. Guessing outlandish combinations, such as green eggs and ham or liver and onions, can delight the child. Although elementary, these simple ways of making the exam fun can go a long way in establishing patient compliance for the future. Table 2 provides an inventory of some items that can add to the "child-friendliness" of the clinical environment.

The decision to have a child's parent present while performing the exam should be made on an individual basis. The child's preference should take priority when possible. It is always best to have another person, such as a doctor's assistant, in the room throughout the examination. In some cases, the child may present a different picture when alone than the picture painted by the parents. Some parents, perhaps in an effort to protect, may underestimate the ability of their child. One parent, for example, had to offer a monetary inducement to her 14-year-old daughter in order for her consent to be examined. The chiropractor was told that this child absolutely hated doctors and would not comply with any requests made of her. The child's chief complaint was violent and out-of-control behavior. Police had often been called to the home for multiple instances of fire setting, attempts to strangle the mother, and animal abuse. The doctor however was able to connect with the child through a mutual interest in martial arts. By the end of the successful exam, this "noncompliant" child was entertaining staff members with karate demonstrations and the "bribe" was returned to the mother. Of course, not all parents underestimate their children, but such misperception should be taken into consideration as a possibility.

Table 1. Essential items for the health history of a special needs child

Prenatal history
- Number of previous pregnancies, miscarriages, or stillbirths
- History of maternal involvement in motor vehicle accidents
- Duration of mother's prenatal care
- Mother's participation in delivery preparation classes
- Length of gestation period
- Status of mother's physical and emotional health during pregnancy
- Maternal exposure to X-rays, smoke, alcohol, caffeine, and medications (both prescribed and over-the-counter)
- Frequency and outcome of prenatal interventions (eg, ultrasound, amniocentesis, and chorionic villi sampling)
- Mother's nutritional status
- Family attitude toward pregnancy

Natal history
- Duration, progression, and location of labor and delivery
- Delivery interventions (eg, labor induction, artificial rupture of membranes, use of forceps, and vacuum extraction methods)
- Presence of physician, nurse, or lay midwife at delivery
- Infant's presentation at delivery (head first, breech, transverse)
- Birth weight and length
- Condition of the child after birth, including APGAR scores

Neonatal history
Was there evidence of any of the following?
- Fever
- Convulsions
- Cyanosis
- Jaundice
- Infections
- Rash
- Breathing problems
- Sucking difficulty
- Congenital anomalies

Infancy history
- Method and duration of infant feeding (breast or bottle)
- Digestive disturbances (eg, colic, projectile vomiting, excess crying)
- Time of introduction to solid foods
- Suspected allergic reactions
- Infant and maternal nutritional supplementation
- Infant's appetite and attitude toward food
- Age at developmental milestones
  —Response to sound
  —Ability to follow objects with eyes
  —Head control
  —Ability to sit unaided
  —Ability to crawl
  —Ability to walk
- Presence of abnormal crawl pattern
- Sleep patterns
- Habits (eg, nail biting, rocking, thumb sucking, head banging, masturbation, pica)

Childhood/adolescent history
- Sexual development (presence of secondary sex characteristics)
- Age of menarche
- Current discipline status and family intervention methods
- Social adjustment (eg, separation anxiety, independent, shy, friendly)
- Involvement in sports, hobbies
- Current eating habits (eg, number of daily meals and snacks, picky, constant eater, junk food consumer)
- Preference for sweet or salty foods
- Amount of Nutrasweet in diet
- Preference or distaste for certain food textures
- Favorite food preference

Review of systems
- Special senses: smell, sight, hearing, speech, touch
- Dentition: cavities, material used in filling cavities, discolored teeth, braces, special dental care
- Cardiovascular: dyspnea, cyanosis, edema, precordial pain, syncope, murmur
- Respiratory: cough, congestion, upper respiratory infections, allergies, ear infections, tubes in the ears
- Genitourinary: enuresis, encopresis, yeast infections
- Nervous system: convulsions, nervous, stare, seizures, number of hours sleep per night, restless, sleepwalking, nightmares, wakes often
- Musculoskeletal: muscle paresis, paralysis, spasticity, growth spurts, joint pain
- Gastrointestinal: constipation, diarrhea, irritable bowel syndrome, ulcer, reflux, number of bowel movements each day, stool consistency

Medical history
- History of childhood disease
- Specific immunizations received, any reaction
- Past illnesses or conditions
- Hospitalizations
- Medications
- Supplements
- Injuries (eg, falls, stitches to head, fractures, knocked unconscious)
- School (eg, not attending, regular class, special class, home schooling, grade, progress)
- Does anyone else besides parent take care of the child on a regular basis?
- Is the child exposed to secondhand smoke on a regular basis?

Family health history
- Birth order of child
- Family status at child's birth
- Current status
- Do all family members reside at same address?
  —Natural mother's age and health (eg, doctor-provided care, surgeries, chronic illness, mental health care, emotional instability)
  —Natural father's age and health (eg, doctor-provided care, surgeries, chronic illness, mental health care, emotional instability)
  —Sibling's age and health
  —Significant family history of disease

CEREBRAL PALSY

There are more individuals with cerebral palsy in the United States than those with any other developmental disability, including Down syndrome, epilepsy, and autism.[1] Approximately 2 out of every 1,000 children in this country have some type of cerebral palsy.[1] The term is only loosely descriptive and covers a variety of nonprogressive motor disorders affecting a child's ability to move and to maintain posture and balance. William John Little, an English orthopaedic surgeon, was the first person to formally study children with cerebral palsy. In 1861 he published a paper describing the neurological problems of children with spastic diplegia.[1] The disorder is still occasionally called Little's disease. Also, Sigmund Freud published some of the earliest papers on cerebral palsy.[1]

The etiology of cerebral palsy is often difficult to establish, but in utero disorders, birth trauma, maternal seizures, neonatal asphyxia, infections during pregnancy, and neonatal jaundice play important roles.[2] Prenatal exposure to methylmercury has also been linked to increased incidence of cerebral palsy.[3] Children born with Rh incompatibility, stroke/intracranial hemorrhage, abnormal birth presentations (breech, face, or transverse lie), and low birth weight (less than 5 pounds, 7 ounces) and those born premature (less than 37 weeks) are more likely to suffer from cerebral palsy.[4] Cerebral palsy is generally thought to be a lifelong disability.

Four broad categories are used to classify cerebral palsy according to the type of movement disturbance present: spastic, athetoid, ataxic, and mixed forms (see Table 3). Other problems that are commonly associated with cerebral palsy are found in Table 4.

Treatment

Although the presentation of cerebral palsy may vary, several common treatment approaches from a chiropractic perspective exist. In the author's clinical experience, atlanto-occipital subluxations are commonly found, a fact concurred by McMullen.[5] McMullen observed that children who have difficulty with sleeping, personality disturbances, and hypertonic musculature often have dramatic changes after the adjustment of the atlanto-occipital area.

No formal studies appear to exist on the role chiropractic may have in alleviating any problems or symptoms cerebral palsy patients may have. However, one case report described clinical improvements experienced by a 5-year-old male with quadriplegic cerebral palsy following an upper cervical spine adjustment.[6] Changes were observed in electromyographic patterns taken of lower cervical paravertebral muscles and wrist extensors. Postadjustment findings indicated a decrease in the patient's cervical tonic/clonic contractures and elimination of wrist extensor spasms. The authors also reported the presence of a placing reaction or automatism in the child's lower extremities that was not possible prior to the upper cervical adjustment.

Cranial dysfunction, primarily at the sphenobasilar junction, have been reported in those children who have history of birth trauma or head injury.[7] Phillips comments that children with cerebral palsy frequently appear to have cranial malformations around the brainstem. Motor tracts of the medulla may be compromised by malposition of occipital condyles, which changes the shape of the foramen magnum.[7] Accompanying this sphenobasilar lesion may be a dysfunction of the temporomandibular joint (TMJ). Children who drool excessively may benefit from manual release of TMJ-related muscles, such as the masseter and temporalis.

Clinical observation suggests that other common areas of muscle contracture for children with spastic cerebral palsy include the paraspinals, lateral thigh muscles, lower extremity adductors, Achilles tendons, and wrist extensors. The use

Table 2. Helpful items for a child-friendly exam

Stickers
Bubbles
Infant scale
Child-sized gowns
Colorful exam gloves
Hand/finger puppets
Infant teething biscuits
Pediatric adjusting table
Covers for electric plugs
Brightly colored lab coat
Model of pediatric spine
Coloring books and crayons
Colorful tongue depressors
Pediatric blood pressure cuff
Cervical pillow for infants to rest in
Wall chart for height measurement
Extra infant diapers/diaper wipes
Toys and books that make sounds
Disinfectant spray for cleaning tables
Anthropometric charts for boys and girls
Brightly colored toys to use as distraction
Pediatric eye chart (uses pictures instead of letters)
Instant hand-washing soap or germicidal hand wash
Camera/video in office (great for recording changes!)
Toys to assess small-motor control or sequential thought
Change of clothing for the doctor (expect the unexpected)
Air mattress for performing exam on special needs children
Ear bear with anatomically correct ears for real-life inspection
Child's flashlight, child-size otoscope, or pediatric speculum tips
Cinnamon instead of coffee when testing for olfaction
Age-appropriate pain assessment charts (charts using facial expressions are available for children)

Table 3. Cerebral palsy classifications

Spastic
Most common type, affecting 70% to 80% of cases
- Presents with stiffness, weakness, increased deep tendon reflexes, "scissors gait," and toe-walking
- Upper motor neuron involvement
- Further categorized according to limbs affected

Athetoid or dyskinetic
- Affects 10% to 20% of cases
- Characterized by uncontrolled, slow writing movements
- Emotional stress often increases symptoms
- Basal ganglia involvement

Ataxic
- Rare
- Balance and coordination are affected
- Cerebellum involvement

Mixed
- Combines spastic and athetoid movements

---

of myofascial release in these areas of contractures may assist in decreasing the severity of spinal distortion and aid in stabilizing gait patterns in some children with cerebral palsy. Lateral thigh muscle stimulation is especially important for those children prone to a scissoring gait, frequently seen in those with spastic diplegia. Parents and patients can be taught to perform stretching exercises and trigger point stimulation in those areas in need of home therapy.

Case study 1

A 9-year-old girl presented to the Kentuckiana Children's Center with previously diagnosed spastic paraplegic cerebral palsy. She had worn lower extremity twister cable braces for 4 years. She was referred to the center by a local chiropractor. The mother's primary concern was the diagnosis of "S-shaped curve" scoliosis and a functional short right leg.

The child's health history revealed a 13-week premature traumatic birth with a Caesarean section delivery due to a transverse lie position. Immediately after delivery the child was placed on supplemental oxygen. She weighed 2 lb. 14 oz., and was 11 inches long at birth. She had multiple neonatal problems, including sucking and breathing difficulties, patent ductus arteriosus, and pathologic jaundice. She received two blood transfusions and was given cardiac medication for 6 months. After 3 weeks in neonatal intensive care, she was finally allowed to be held by her mother. She was fed expressed breast milk for 2 months and then switched to infant formula. Early feedings were accomplished by feeding tube. Her stay in the hospital lasted 2 and a half months. She was then monitored at home for sleep apnea and bradycardia.

All developmental milestones were significantly delayed. When the child was 7 months old, she was unable to sit, squat, or crawl. An orthopaedist was consulted, and the child was periodically observed every 3 to 6 months. The orthopaedist noted developmental delay, habitual toe walk, bilateral heel cord tension, and internal femoral torsion. The mother was advised to discourage the child from sitting in the "TV" (reverse talar) position and was given heel cord stretches for the child to perform daily. She was also told to have the child wear high top, stiff-soled shoes. At 4 years of age the child was said to have 90° of internal rotation at both hips and no external rotation. Her orthopaedic doctor ordered bilateral lower extremity braces with twister cables to be worn 24 hours a day. She was restricted from routine activities such as bicycle riding and roller skating. She wore the braces until age 7 years, when they were removed for approximately 9 months. Her toes, however, began to noticeably turn in with walking. Surgical osteotomies were recommended if additional bracing was unsuccessful.

Her history also revealed allergic reactions to milk, green leafy foods, cats, and house dust. She had previous problems with calcium urate crystal development, and she had myringotomy tympanotomy surgery twice. She complained of headaches combined with blurred vision when fatigued.

Physical examination findings

Upon physical examination, a slow, staggered gait was noted, possibly related to the braces she wore; slight right thoracic scoliosis; winging of left scapula; and a functional right short leg. A need for optometric and audiometric evaluation was also noted. Radiographic findings included cervical and lumbar hyperlordosis, rotation of atlas and axis, and bilateral hypertrophy of the C-7 transverse processes. There was a 4° right thoracic scoliosis with apex at T-7. A grade 2 spondylolisthesis of L-5 was present. She also had an interruption of Shenton's line and increased femoral angles bilaterally. The patient showed no sign of mental impairment and had no history of seizure activity.

Management

Chiropractic adjustments (consisting of full-spine manual diversified adjusting and pelvic blocking) were initiated at a frequency of twice per week and reduced over time. Manual

---

Table 4. Other problems associated with cerebral palsy (all types)

Seizures
Mental retardation
Learning difficulties
Failure-to-thrive syndrome
Attention deficit hyperactivity disorder (ADHD)
Sensory, visual, auditory, and speech impairments

toggle recoil-style adjustments using a pediatric drop head piece were also used on upper cervical spine subluxation areas. The patient was given home stretching exercises for bilateral Achilles tendon and calf muscle areas. She was also fitted for orthotic supports. After 7 months, follow-up radiographic films were taken, and these indicated a reduction of the femoral angles and Shenton's line. According to the mother's report, the child's orthopaedist reviewed the chiropractic radiographs and indicated that the "spontaneous remission" allowed for removal of the braces and discharge from further orthopaedic management. The patient continues to be seen on a PRN basis for chiropractic care.

AUTISM

Autism was once thought to be a psychological problem that was the result of "faulty mothering." The disorder however, is currently accepted as a biological problem with roots in a variety of areas, such as the immune, alimentary, and central nervous systems. Metabolic defects, genetics, and biochemical peculiarities are also suspected as possible causes. Individuals with autism have a wide spectrum of developmental, perceptual, behavioral, and attentional problems. Language and social disorders are common to all affected.[8] Diagnostic criteria for autism includes qualitative impairment in reciprocal social interaction, verbal and nonverbal communication, and imaginative activity. Autistic individuals commonly display a markedly restricted repertoire of activities and interests. Some show stereotyped body movements such as hand flicking, rocking, or spinning. Some children with autism may display unique skills in music or mathematics or in using spatial concepts (eg, in working jigsaw puzzles). Table 5 lists the classical signs of autistic behavior. The disorder is commonly diagnosed before age 3. It occurs in approximately 5 out of every 100,000 births and is four times more common in males than in females.[9] The cause for autism has not been determined.

Treatment

Conventional treatment generally involves a combination of highly structured education, supportive family counseling, and behavior modification training (see Tables 6 and 7). Medications are also commonly prescribed. At present there is no known cure for autism. However, studies in six different countries have shown benefits from the high-dosage supplementation of vitamin B_6 and magnesium.[10] Other interventions that have been successful for some children include the elimination of gluten, casein, and yeast from the diet. Supplementation with dimethyl glycine and megavitamins and the use of antifungal medication such as nystatin or fluconazole (Diflucan) have also shown promise.[8] Auditory and sensory integration therapies have been employed successfully in some cases.[11]

The use of chiropractic care in the treatment of individuals with autism is highlighted in four published works,[12–15] none of which are found in peer-reviewed literature sources.

Table 5. Common signs of autistic behavior

A child who exhibits seven or more of the following signs and symptoms is likely to be given the diagnosis of autism. In a child who is autistic, these abnormal behavior patterns will be constant and age inappropriate.
- Difficulty in mixing with other children
- Acts as if deaf, visually impaired, or blind
- Resists learning
- Displays fear of real dangers or no fear
- Resists change in routine
- Lacks gestures
- Engages in inappropriate laughing and giggling
- Avoids physical touch
- Demonstrates marked physical overactivity
- Avoids eye contact
- Has inappropriate attachments to objects
- Spins objects
- Sustains odd play
- Has standoffish manner

Table 6. Treatment guidelines for children with autism

Chiropractors who provide care for individuals with autism may benefit from the following guidelines.
- *Establish consistent treatment routines.* Since many of these children are disturbed by change, it is best to maintain a general sameness in the way each child is greeted, treated, and sent home from visit to visit.
- *Avoid any loud disturbances during treatment.* Hypersensitivity to sound is a common problem and may even interfere with simple otoscopic procedures or X-ray examinations. Some children with autism have been known to be disturbed by the buzz from fluorescent lighting. A relaxed, quiet environment will promote effective care.
- *Distraction is key.* Having an assistant distract the child with finger puppets, flashlights, story books, and so on, may allow the doctor to work more efficiently.
- *Be alert for nonverbal cues of discomfort from the child.* These may be areas in need of attention.
- *Question parents about changes in behavior patterns.* Significant changes for a child with autism may include the cessation of curious behaviors such as doing headstands, spinning objects, and tugging at underclothing. Positive change may also be indicated by an increase in repertoire of foods the child will eat or an improved use of vocabulary.

Table 7. Autism informational resources

Autism Research Institute, 4182 Adams Avenue, San Diego, CA 92116. Tel: (619) 281-7165. Conference information and educational materials available for parents and professionals on many topics relevant to the autistic spectrum of disorders. Founded by Bernard Rimland.

Autism Society of America, 1234 Massachusetts Avenue NW, Suite 1017, Washington, DC 20005. Tel: (202) 783-0125; fax: (202) 783-7435.

CAN (Cure Autism Now), 5225 Wilshire Boulevard, Suite 503, Los Angeles, CA 90036. Tel: (213) 549-0500; fax: (213) 549-0547; e-mail: CAN@primenet.com. CAN is an organization founded by parents dedicated to finding effective biological treatments and a cure for autism.

The Georgiana Organization, Inc, PO Box 2607, Westport, CT 06880. Tel: (203) 454-1221. This organization encourages the practice of auditory integration therapy.

Indiana Resource Center for Autism, 2853 East Tenth Street, Bloomington, IN 47408-2601. This nonprofit organization is affiliated with Indiana University. It publishes a quarterly newsletter and sponsors educational conferences on autism.

Institutes for the Achievement of Human Potential, 8801 Stenton Avenue, Philadelphia, PA 19118. Tel: (215) 233-2050; fax: (215) 233-1530. The Better Baby Store can be reached at same phone number.

Judevine Center for Autism, 9455 Rott Road, St Louis, MO, 63127. Tel: (314) 849-4440. This organization offers an intensive three-week outpatient program on behavior modification techniques for parents and children.

Latitudes, 1120 Royal Palm Beach Boulevard #283, Royal Palm Beach, FL 33411. Tel: (407) 798-0472. *Latitudes,* a bimonthly newsletter of the Alternative Therapy Network, is devoted to alternative therapies for attention deficit hyperactivity disorder, Tourette's syndrome, and autism.

MAAP Services, Inc, PO Box 524, Crown Point, IN 46307. Tel: (219) 662-1311. MAAP is oriented toward *more advanced autistic people.*

Option Institute, 2080 South Under Mountain Road, Sheffield, MA 02157. Tel: (413) 229-2100. This organization was founded by the Kaufman family after having success with their son Raun. Barry Kaufman authored *Son-Rise* and other books on their experience.

Three of the four papers are single case studies, and one is a case review of six children with autism who were given chiropractic care. The subjects were recruited from a Kansas City area facility and were given a systematic series of chiropractic adjustments for a period of 3–6 months. Areas of subluxation varied in each child but involved either the first or second cervical vertebrae and multiple midthoracic regions. Subjects were seen twice a week and were adjusted as needed using diversified manual technique. Information about educational and behavioral progress was gathered from the subjects' classroom teachers. Improvements were observed in such diverse areas as picking up toys, use of sign language, reduction in self-abuse, and appropriate use of language.[12] Although this study noted positive change in the subjects, the small sample size and lack of control group brings the validity of its conclusions into question. Certainly more in-depth studies are required in this area.

Case study 2

A 16-year-old boy with high-functioning autism presented to a chiropractor's office with a chief complaint of daily encopresis. The mother stated that the chiropractic approach was a "last resort," as they had been to countless medical professionals to no avail. The problem had progressed to the point where the child was soon to be removed from the third after-school program he had attended. He was unable to enjoy overnight activities or extended visits outside the home due to the unpleasantness of his problem. On initial consultation, the boy was found rocking in the doctor's waiting room, clutching a small stuffed dog. Although he was unable to carry on a normal conversation and spoke in an extremely loud voice, he could recite the entire season's scores for his favorite college basketball team.

Clinical health history

Clinical health history information obtained from the mother detailed the child's 6-month 3-week gestational-age forceps delivery. He weighed 3 lbs. 5 oz at birth and was 12 inches long. He had neonatal breathing problems, physiologic jaundice, and mild hydrocephalus. Heart surgery, for reasons unknown to the mother, was performed when the boy was 2 days old. Before age 3 years he experienced approximately 15 ear infections, which were all treated with antibiotic therapy. He sustained a minor head injury at age 3 years when he tripped and fell into a wall. He developed a raised bruise over the left temporal bone and had a small cut under the chin. Cranial radiographs were negative for fracture following the injury. A double inguinal hernia operation was done at age 4 months and surgery to correct for poor eye muscle control was performed at age 10 years. The child had a negative history for broken bones and fractures and had never been involved in a motor vehicle accident. All his vaccinations were up to date. He suffered single bouts of chicken pox and measles. He said his first word at 16 months. He did not crawl but rose instead at 13 months and began to walk. The child gained bladder control at age 5 years and bowel control at age 8 years. His problem with involuntary bowel movements began insidiously, approximately 2 years prior to the initiation of chiropractic care.

The child had known allergies to dust and mold and had been receiving weekly allergy shots for approximately 2 years. His mother commented that he had a constantly stopped up head. He had previously been on Ritalin, lithium and Dexedrine medication for hyperactive behavior and was taking 1 mg of risperdal three times per day to calm him down, according to the mother.

Physical exam

Exam findings showed a 5-foot 9-inch male weighing 184 pounds, with a pulse rate of 72 beats per minute and supine blood pressures of 130/60 on the right and 132/66 on the left. The young man had been injured in a basketball game the day before the exam and presented with a bruise around his right nostril. His heart sounds were within normal limits. Decreased bowel sounds were noted in all four quadrants. Multiple scars were noted on the anterior chest as evidence of previous thorax surgery.

Postural analysis found a left low occiput, right low shoulder, and left low pelvic crest. Analysis of active range of motion in the cervical spine found all ranges to be within normal limits except for a slight decrease in right rotation as measured by visual inspection. Thoracolumbar active range of motion noted 90° of flexion, approximately 20° of right lateral flexion, and approximately 10° of left rotation. Thoracolumbar extension and right rotation were within normal limits. Motion and static palpation showed right lateral rotary subluxations at the second and third cervical vertebral complexes, anteriority of the midthoracic region between the fifth and seventh thoracic vertebrae, and a left rotation fixation of the fourth and fifth lumbar segments. Right posterior superior iliac spine was posterior, and the sacral apex was shifted left. Cranial palpation found a flattening of the left occipital region and fixation at the sphenobasilar junction.

Management

Chiropractic care began at a frequency of twice a week for 1 week, decreasing to once a week for 2 months. His care schedule was then changed to once every 2 weeks for 1 month and then once every 3 weeks for 2 months. His care involved adjustment of the subluxations found on the physical exam. Diversified manual adjusting, pelvic blocking, and Upledger cranial methods were used. Trigger point massage work was done in bilateral lumbar paraspinal, piriformis, and tensor fascia lata muscles. He was also given nutritional supplementation of acidophilus and a B vitamin complex. He was admonished to decrease his consumption of caffeinated beverages and fried foods.

After four visits the young man's encopresis incidents had decreased to one per week. During the 5th week of care his mother reported that it appeared as if his "thought processes" were clearer. On the 8th visit the mother reported that bowel accidents had decreased to once every 2 weeks, and by the 9th visit the accidents had decreased to once every 3 weeks. On the 13th chiropractic visit, the boy returned to the office wearing a staff shirt from the after-school facility program from which he had previously been removed. His bowel accidents had not occurred in 2 months. His care was halted at this point, as the family moved and became involved in multiple outside activities. He was not seen for 7 months. He then returned for chiropractic care, and it was noted on reevaluation that a bowel accident had not occurred in those 7 months. The young man was still employed and was scheduled to attend 5 weeks of a summer camp program.

DOWN SYNDROME

In 1866, John Langdon Down, an English physician, made note of a unique group of children who shared the common features of small nose; broad face; and straight, thin hair. In the early 1930s, children with Down syndrome were discovered to have a genetic abnormality, later found to be an addition at chromosome 21.[16] Table 8 describes characteristics found in these children. The incidence of Down syndrome in the United States is approximately one in every 800–1100 live births. The exact cause of the disorder is currently unknown, but an increase in maternal age may be a factor. Most children affected by Down syndrome have a variety of delays in physical, intellectual, and language development.[17]

Nearly 60% of all children with Down syndrome suffer from otitis media and chronic congestion. This large percentage may be due to a congenital narrowing of nose and ear passages.[18] In addition, defects in immune function may compound the problem. Supplementation with zinc, vitamin C, selenium, folic acid, and amino acids has been shown to be helpful in multiple studies of children with Down syndrome.[19–23] A 1991 study noted that high-dose, broad-spectrum vitamin supplements have improved the IQ of Down syndrome children by an average of 10 points.[24] Dixie Lawrence, the executive director of Trisomy 21 Research, is the mother of a child with Down syndrome and has been a driving force in researching nutritional treatment approaches for these children. Lawrence describes reports of improved

---

Table 8. Common characteristics of children with Down syndrome

There are over 50 possible characteristics of children with Down syndrome. The most common are these:
- Hypotonia
- Low set ears
- Heart defects
- Microcephaly
- Mental retardation
- Shallow oral palate
- Small hands and feet
- Short physical stature
- Brushfield spots on the iris
- Simian crease in palms of hands
- Short fifth digit, often with only one joint
- Almond-shaped eyes with persistent epicanthus

intelligence, improved motor skills, and altered physical characteristics such as facial features following initiation of a nutritional protocol.[18]

Atlantoaxial instability is another common feature found in children with Down syndrome. This instability is due to laxity of the transverse atlantal ligament or an anomalous axis formation. Chiropractors using upper cervical manipulation will want to carefully evaluate this region before any care is provided. In 1990, La Francis published a useful review on this subject in the *Journal of Manipulative and Physiologic Therapeutics*.[25]

CONCLUSION

Genetic disorders remain incurable. However, some management strategies may be of benefit in controlling symptoms, slowing progression (or the disability associated with progression), and perhaps improving attributes related to the quality of life. The effects of chiropractic care on genetic disorders remain poorly studied, but some case reports and numerous clinical anecdotes exist that suggest conservative management may be of value. Although such reports are typically positive, more dedicated study is necessary in order to draw generalizable conclusions.

Chiropractors who work with children with special needs should be aware of many unique attendant circumstances. Progress monitoring, modification of examination and care procedures, and the psychosocial needs of the children and their families may require special attention. The experience of caring for these individuals can be extremely rewarding, particularly given the limitations of treatment options and the difficulties that must be overcome.

REFERENCES

1. Geralis E. *Children with Cerebral Palsy: A Parents' Guide.* Kensington, Md: Woodbine House; 1991.
2. Berkow R, et al. *The Merck Manual of Diagnosis and Therapy.* Rahway, NJ: Merck Sharp & Dohme Research Laboratories; 1987.
3. Ziff S, Ziff M. *Infertility and Birth Defects.* Orlando, FL: Bio-Probe; 1987:65, 154.
4. National Institute of Neurological Disorders and Stroke (NINDS). Pamphlet. *Cerebral Palsy—Hope through Research.* Bethesda, Md: National Institutes of Health; 1993. NIH publication 93-159.
5. McMullen M. Chiropractic and the handicapped child: cerebral palsy. *ICA Rev.* September–October 1990:39–45.
6. Hospers L, Daso J, Steinie L. Electromyographic patterns of mentally retarded cerebral palsy patients after life upper cervical adjustment. *Today's Chiro.* September–October 1986:13–14.
7. Phillips C. Birth trauma—antibiotic abuse—vaccine reaction: a single case report. *ICA Rev.* September–October 1996:64–65.
8. Baker S, Pangborn J. DAN conference protocol. San Diego, Calif: Autism Research Institute; 1996.
9. National Institute of Neurological and Communicative Disorders and Stroke, Office of Scientific and Health Reports. *Autism Fact Sheet.* Bethesda, Md: National Institutes of Health; 1991.
10. Rimland B. *Autism Diagnosis.* San Diego, Calif: Autism Research Institute; 1991.
11. Stehli A, ed. *Dancing in the Rain.* Westport, Conn: The Georgiana Organization; 1995.
12. Sandefur R, Adams E. The effect of chiropractic adjustments on the behavior of autistic children: a case review. *J Chiro.* 1987;24(12):21–25.
13. Rubinstein H. Case study: autism. *Chiro Pediatr.* 1994;1(1):22–23.
14. Barnes T. Helping a child with autism. *Chiro Pediatr Newsletter.* Fall;1996:5–6.
15. Barnes T. The story of John . . . a little boy with autism. *ICA Rev.* November–December 1996:43–46.
16. Stray-Gunderson K, ed. *Babies with Down Syndrome: A New Parents Guide.* Kensington, Md: Woodbine House; 1995.
17. Up with Downs Organization brochure. Shreveport, La: Up with Downs Organization; nd.
18. Schmidt M. *Healing Childhood Ear Infections.* Berkeley, Calif: North Atlantic Books; 1996.
19. Growth delay in Down syndrome and zinc sulphate supplementation. *Am J Med Genet.* 1990;63(suppl 7):63–65.
20. Vitamin C and Down syndrome. *Minerva Pediatr.* 1989;41(4):189–192.
21. Selenium and Down syndrome. *Arch Dis Childhood.* 1990; 65(12):1353–1355.
22. Quillin P. *Healing Nutrients.* New York: Random House; 1989.
23. Lawrence D. Trisomy 21 Research, Inc, Gonzales, LA; 1994.
24. Megavitamins and mental retardation. *Am Acad Pediatr.* August 1991: News and Comments.
25. La Francis ME. A chiropractic perspective on atlantoaxial instability in Down's syndrome. *J Manipulative Physiol Ther.* March–April 1990: 159–160.

6

Infantile Colic: Identification and Management

Dorrie M. Talmage and Diane Resnick

Infantile colic is a challenging problem that plagues many families. As an entity, colic is both hard to define and manage. The word *colic* is derived from the Greek *kolikos*, an adjectival form of *kolon*, meaning the large intestine.[1] *The Boke of Chyldren*, published over 400 years ago, described colic as noise and "peine in the gut."[2,3] Many pediatricians and parents consider colic to be a painful disturbance of the gastrointestinal tract.[4] The basic definition is repetitive inconsolable bouts of crying in neonates, bouts that in some instances can last up to a year. Colic can make the parents feel like failures; it creates anxiety, fatigue, and fear that the crying may be a symptom of an underlying pathological condition. The disorder must receive an accurate diagnosis and appropriate management if the family is to cope with the crisis.

DEFINITION

Infantile colic is not a very well understood condition, nor is there a standard definition. Larsen[5] defines it as recurring violent and inconsolable fits of crying and screaming in an otherwise healthy child. Wessel and coworkers[6] base their definition of colic on the timing of the crying bouts; the infant must have paroxysms of crying more than 3 hours per day more than 3 days in 1 week for a minimum of 3 weeks. The attacks tend to occur within the first few weeks of life and last for 3 to 4 months, but some persist longer. The periods of crying are more likely to occur in the afternoon or evening but can occur any time of the day or night.[7] There are conflicting studies regarding colic and the timing involved. Brazelton[8] and others have documented that the median amount of crying in normal full-term infants at 6 weeks of age is about 2.75 hours per day, which is only .25 hours short of Wessel's definition. A study by St. James-Roberts[9] found 29% of Northamptonshire infants cried for more than 3 hours a day during the first 3 months of life. These studies support the hypothesis that colic represents the extreme of the normal spectrum of variability in crying.[7]

Etiology

At this point, colic has no clear etiology. Many doctors believe it can result from any one of many factors, including biomedical, social, and psychological factors.[5]

Biomedical causes

There are a number of possible biomedical causes, especially gastrointestinal causes. Suspected gastrointestinal causes include hypersensitivity response to certain foods, excessive intestinal gas, intestinal hypermotility, and hormonal factors (eg, an increase in basal motilin levels, which is known to stimulate gastric emptying and intestinal peristalsis).[4,7,10]

Other less accepted biomedical causes include exposure of the infant to fluoxetine hydrochloride (an adult antidepressant) via the breast milk[11]; carbohydrate intolerance (such as lactose intolerance) due to abnormal enzyme levels[7,10,12]; physical illnesses and structural anomalies (eg, incarcerated hernias, otitis media, hematomas); and gastrointestinal reflux.[10]

Another interesting biomedical hypothesis relates to intracellular calcium concentrations in the pineal gland. Colic appears to be more common farther away from the equator. The light quality near the equator may reduce pineal intracellular calcium concentrations during the day, leading to enhanced melatonin production at night, which would produce

Adapted from *Top Clin Chiro* 1997; 4(4): 25–29
© 1997 Aspen Publishers, Inc.

a calmer or sleepier infant in the evening hours. The longer period of daylight away from the equator during part of the year is detected by photo receptors in the eye, suppressing melatonin production and possibly creating a potentially more fussy infant.[13]

One additional hypothesis should be investigated. Recent research supports the idea that a newborn's nervous system is immature, and therefore selective screening of sensory stimulation is not possible, creating neurolabile colic. An infant can become overwhelmed by any type of excessive negative or positive sensory stimulation and begin crying episodes. Examples of negative stimuli include hunger, gas pains, temperature differences, and fatigue. Examples of positive stimulation are exposure to musical toys, television, voices, lights, faces, and excessive handling.[14–17]

Psychological and social causes

The evidence implicating nongastrointestinal factors can be grouped around three hypotheses: (1) that colic is one extreme of the normal range of crying, (2) that colic is a reflection of atypical parenting (usually maternal), and (3) that colic results from inappropriate maternal-infant interaction.[4]

Colic may be the far extreme of normal crying. Barr,[18] Brazelton,[8] and St. James-Roberts[19] did studies that provide evidence of a characteristic pattern of crying. The pattern is a progressive increase in crying that peaks in the second month of life and then gradually decreases and a diurnal rhythm typified by clustering during the evening hours. These studies suggest that so-called colicky infants may exhibit a variant of this normal pattern.

Spock,[20] in 1944, suggested that the transmission of emotional tension from mother to infant was a possible cause of colic. Stewart and colleagues[21] in a prospective study, reported that mothers of excessive criers had psychological conflicts regarding the maternal role, hostility toward their children, and an insensitive or inconsistent style in interactions with them. The crying was interpreted as the infants' response to tension secondary to unmet needs or inappropriate stimulation. However, their study's methodology has come into question. Wessel and colleagues[6] also reported a strong association between family tension and paroxysmal fussiness in infants. In both studies, retrospective analysis leaves open the alternative that family tension and maternal insecurity are the products rather than the causes of colicky crying.[10]

The third hypothesis is that crying is an attempt by the infant to communicate its needs and that crying continues because parents misinterpret or fail to respond correctly to the signal. This hypothesis entails that counseling to improve the effectiveness of parental responses can reduce bouts of crying.[10] Studies by Taubman[22] have shown that, with appropriate parental counseling and intervention, crying can be markedly reduced in colicky infants.

Incidence

The incidence of colic is difficult to determine owing to the lack of clarity of definition. Prospective studies have reported frequencies of 8% to 40%[2,8,23,24] and thus colic could affect over 700,000 infants in the United States each year.[2] Lehtonen and Kornenranta[25] found the incidence to be 13%, with no seasonal variation. Studies have shown that colic is more prevalent in breastfed than formula fed babies.[4,6,23,26,27]

Epidemiology

The mean onset of colic is 1.8 weeks of age,[27] and infants whose colic begins in the first 2 weeks of life seem to have a longer duration of symptoms than those whose symptoms start later.[2] The average duration of symptoms is 13.6 weeks.[27]

Clinical manifestations

The main clinical feature of infantile colic is inconsolable crying. Other signs include the drawing up of the legs, abdominal distention, and excessive gas.[12] Treem[7] found that, in addition to the problems uncovered by Kerner, 56% of the infants had feeding problems, including spitting up, vomiting, and crying with feeding; 50% were said to sleep poorly and were flushed; 86% were hypertonic; and 28% were actually inconsolable.

As these signs and symptoms can mimic a number of different entities, the clinician in charge of the infant must perform a thorough history on the symptoms via the parents and an accurate examination to rule out all other possible diagnoses. Once the history and examination have ruled out all of these diagnoses, a management plan can be initiated.

MANAGEMENT

A variety of drugs have been prescribed to address infantile colic. Most are sedatives, antispasmodics, or antiflatulents. Along with phenobarbital, the most frequently prescribed sedatives are hydroxyzine hydrochloride (Atarax) and chloral hydrate.[2] Hyoscyamine sulfate (Levsin) and Donnatal (a combination of hyoscyamine sulfate, atropine sulfate, scopolamine hydrobromide, and phenobarbital) contain 20% and 23% alcohol, respectively.[12] As noted by Weizman and colleagues,[28] infant alcohol consumption may result in hypoglycemia. Gastrointestinal tract irritation, drowsiness, general depression of the central nervous system, and lack of analgesic effect are other objections raised to the use of sedatives for the treatment of infantile colic.[3,29]

The antispasmodic dicyclomine hydrochloride (Bentyl) was effective in 63% of the infantile colic cases, versus 25% for the placebo group.[3] In another study, Oggero and co-workers[30] found dicyclomine hydrochloride less effective in relieving infantile colic than a diet in which cow's milk was replaced with hydrolyzed milk. In 1984, the use of dicyclomine hydrochloride was linked to incidences of respiratory collapse, apnea, seizures, coma, and death.[2] This drug is contraindicated for use in the treatment of infantile colic because of its serious potential side effects.

Among the antiflatulents prescribed for infants with colic, simethicone (Mylicon) produced varying results in the treatment of infantile colic.[31] Metcalf and associates[32] found simethicone no more effective than the placebo.

Herbal teas and gripe water have been used for years to calm colicky infants. Some of the more common components include chamomile, fennel, and balm-mint, all of which have proven antispasmodic activity.[33] Additional constituents may include papain, tincture of cardamom or ginger, dill water, dill or caraway oil, or sodium bicarbonate. The reported success of herbal tea preparations in the treatment of infantile colic has been mostly anecdotal. Health care providers and parents should be cautioned against the use of nonlicensed, nonformal herbs and herbal teas, such as Mother's Milk and Red Zinger, which contain digitalis or theophylline derivatives.[17]

Nutritional intervention is perhaps the method parents turn to first in an effort to console their infant. Sampson and Scanlon[34] suggested that 10% to 15% of infantile colic may be due to food allergy or intolerance. Therefore, a low allergen diet may lead to a decrease in symptoms. Unfortunately, contradictory approaches often lead to frequent formula changes and frustration. The majority of authors recommend one to two dietary changes at most.[3]

Several researchers have explored the postulated association between sensitivity or intolerance to cow's milk and infantile colic.[12,35,36] While the percentage of infants demonstrating allergic reaction to cow's milk varies greatly,[12] Iacono and colleagues[36] found remission of symptoms in 71.4% of cases when cow's milk protein was eliminated from the formula.

While soy may be an appropriate substitute for adults with cow's milk intolerance or sensitivity, the available data do not support the preferred use of soy.[12] Though Businco and associates[37] found decreased IgE for soy, one in four children sensitive to cow's milk may also be sensitive to soy.[12] The American Academy of Pediatrics Committee on Nutrition recommends that soy protein formulas not be used in the routine management of infantile colic.[38]

In several studies,[26,30] hydrolyzed casein formula was found to be more effective at reducing the symptoms of infantile colic than soy formula or cow's milk. Treem[7] suggests that a trial of hydrolyzed casein formula may be beneficial in 10% to 15% of infants with colic and a family history of allergy, asthma, or eczema. Jakobsson[39] does not recommend the use of casein hydrolysate in infant formulas, as its effects on gut closure and the release of gut hormones are speculative.

Pinyerd[3] suggests that the elimination of chocolate, eggs, milk and milk products, caffeine, and aromatic foods from the mother's diet may be beneficial in reducing the symptoms of colic in infants. Also, placing the infant in a more vertical position during breastfeeding or bottle feeding may reduce gas formation and reflux. Noting the benefits of high-calorie hindmilk, Kerner[12] advises mothers to avoid switching to a second breast during feeding.

As stated previously, there may be a transmission of tension from mother to infant, which could be an etiologic factor in colic.[20] Lehtonen and coworkers[40] also suggest that the perception of difficult temperament in colicky infants may be related to a dysfunctional mother-infant interaction. Additionally, mothers of infants with colic had multidimensional psychological distress and greater mood disturbance than mothers with infants without colic.[41] However, many of the studies examining mother-infant dynamics have methodological limitations.[4]

The counseling techniques of Taubman[22] focus on the parent's response to the infant. The following approach is suggested:

- Never let your baby cry.
- Consider hunger, the desire to suck, the need to be held, boredom, and fatigue as possible causes and make an appropriate response.
- If the crying continues more than 5 minutes, try another response.
- Do not be concerned about overfeeding.
- Do not be concerned about spoiling the baby.

Most parents will be reassured by a brief explanation of the normal developmental pattern of infant crying,[7] and Cervisi and colleagues[17] suggests that office management focus on guidance and parent education.

A number of investigators have explored the use of external stimulation to calm colicky infants. Belly massage and whole body massage, recordings of womb or heartbeat sounds, nursery songs or lullabies, machinery or vacuum noise, and background music may be helpful.[7,29,42] Larson and Ayllon[42] reported positive results following an operant conditioning program using differential reinforcement. The alert state was rewarded with music and parental attention, while crying resulted in a brief period of solitude. Rocking devices may also quiet an infant,[7,29] though Geertsma and Hyams[10] note that such devices have not been proven to be consistently effective.

There are countless anecdotes relating the beneficial outcomes of chiropractic manipulation for infants with colic. Unfortunately, very few published studies exist and high-quality research is lacking. In 1985, Nilsson[43] reported satisfactory results from chiropractic treatment in 91% of infants with colic, but the manipulative procedures used were not indicated in the article. In a retrospective, uncontrolled study of 316 infants with colic, Klougart and colleagues[44] found similar results. Fifty-three percent of the infants received only upper cervical (C0–1, C1–2) manipulation, 41% received both upper cervical and mid thoracic (T4–5 to T8–9) manipulation, and 6% received manipulation of areas of the spine other than the upper cervicals. Overall, 94% of the infants in this study showed satisfactory results.

A case study by Pluhar and Schobert,[45] published in 1991, details the treatment of a 3-month-old female diagnosed with infantile colic. The course of treatment consisted of spinal adjustments to the atlas using an Activator instrument and to T-7 using a double thumb contact. Each treatment was followed by a two-week interval of no treatment. The authors noted relief of the infant's symptoms within a "relatively short period of time," although they do not specify how short, nor indicate the length of time that the relief lasted. Algorithm 1 identifies care issues for infantile colic.

CONCLUSION

Infantile colic is a condition that plagues many families in the United States. It is truly a family condition, because not only is the infant inconsolable, but, as a consequence of the crying, the family undergoes mental and psychological distress. Infantile colic is hard to define. The etiology for this condition is also in question. Some researchers believe there are biomedical reasons for its existence, others believe it is more of a normal variant of crying, and others believe the etiology involves psychosocial factors. It is imperative that an accurate diagnosis be made, because the signs and symptoms associated with colic mimic those of a variety of conditions. There are multiple methods for managing colic, ranging from drug therapy and counseling for the parents to infant massage and chiropractic manipulation. All of these methods have had a degree of success, and it is up to the clinician to ascertain which method is best for the particular infant and family.

REFERENCES

1. Partridge E. *Origins: A Short Etymological Dictionary of Modern English*. New York, NY: MacMillian; 1958.
2. Pinyerd BJ, Zipf WB. Colic: idiopathic, excessive, infant crying. *J Pediatr Nurs*. 1989;4(3):147–161.
3. Pinyerd BJ. Strategies for consoling the infant with colic: fact or fiction? *J Pediatr Nurs*. 1992;7(6):403–411.
4. Miller AR, Barr RG. Infantile colic: is it a gut issue? *Pediatr Clin North Am*. 1991;38(6):1407–1423.
5. Larsen J. Infants' colic and belly massage. *Practitioner*. 1990;234:396–397.
6. Wessel MA, Cobb JC, Jackson EB, et al. Paroxysmal fussing in infancy, sometimes called colic. *Pediatrics*. 1954;14:421–434.
7. Treem WR. Infant colic: a pediatric gastroenterologist's perspective. *Pediatr Clin North Am*. 1994;41(5):1121–1138.
8. Brazelton TB. Crying in infancy. *Pediatrics*. 1987;29:579–588.
9. St. James-Roberts I. Persistent infant crying. *Arch Dis Child*. 1991;66:653–655.
10. Geertsma MA, Hyams JS. Colic: a pain syndrome of infancy? *Pediatr Clin North Am*. 1989;36(4):905–919.
11. Lester BM, Cucca J, Andreozzi L, et al. Possible association between fluoxetine hydrochloride and colic in an infant. *J Am Acad Child Adolesc Psychiatry*. 1993;32(6):1253–1255.
12. Kerner JA. Formula allergy and intolerance. *Gastroenterol Clin North Am*. 1995;24(1):1–25.
13. Weissbluth L, Weissbluth M. The photo-biochemical basis of infant colic: pineal intracellular calcium concentrations controlled by light, melatonin, and serotonin. *Med Hypotheses*. 1993;40:158–164.
14. Carey WB. Clinical application of infant temperament measurements. *J Pediatr*. 1972;81:823–828.
15. Farran C. *Infantile Colic: What It Is and What You Can Do about It*. New York: Scribners; 1983.
16. Hunziker UA, Barr RG. Increased carrying reduces infant crying: a randomized controlled trial. *Pediatrics*. 1986;77:646–648.
17. Cervisi J, Chapman M, Niklas B, Yamaoka C. Office management of the infant with colic. *J Pediatr Health Care*. 1991;5(4):184–190.
18. Barr RG. The normal crying curve: what do we really know? *Dev Med Child Neurol*. 1990;32:368–371.
19. St. James-Roberts I. Persistent crying in infancy. *J Child Psychol Psychiatry*. 1989;30:189–193.
20. Spock B. Etiological factors in the hypertrophic stenosis and infantile colic. *Psychosom Med*. 1944;6:162–165.
21. Stewart AH, Weiland IH, Leider AB, et al. Excessive infant crying (colic) in relation to parent behavior. *Am J Psychiatry*. 1954;110:687–694.
22. Taubman B. Clinical trial of the treatment of colic by modification of parent-infant interaction. *Pediatrics*. 1984;74:998–1003.
23. Hide D, Guyer B. Prevalence of infant colic. *Arch Dis Child*. 1982;57:559–560.
24. Rubin SP, Prendergast N. Infantile colic: incidence and treatment in a Norfolk community. *Child Care Health Dev*. 1984;10:219–226.
25. Lehtonen L, Korvenranta H. Infantile colic seasonal incidence and crying profiles. *Arch Pediatr Adolesc Med*. 1995;149:533–536.
26. Forsythe BW. Colic and the effect of change in formulas: a double-blind multiple-crossover study. *J Pediatr*. 1989;115:521–526.
27. Paradise JL. Maternal and other factors in the etiology of infantile colic. *JAMA*. 1966;197:191–199.
28. Weizman Z, Alkrinawi S, Goldfarb D, et al. Correspondence. *J Pediatr*. 1993;123(4):670–671.

29. Gurry D. Infantile colic. *Aust Fam Physician.* 1994;23(3):337–346.
30. Oggero R, Garbo G, Savino F, Mostert M. Dietary modifications versus dicyclomine hydrochloride in the treatment of severe infantile colic. *Acta Paediatr.* 1994;83:222–225.
31. Sethi KS, Sethi JK. Simethicone in the management of infant colic. *Practitioner.* 1988;232:508.
32. Metcalf TJ, Irons TG, Sher LD, Young PC. Simethicone in the treatment of infant colic: a randomized, placebo-controlled, multi center trial. *Pediatrics.* 1994;94(1):29–34.
33. Weizman Z, Alkrinawi S, Goldfarb D, Bitran C. Efficacy of herbal tea preparation in infantile colic. *J Pediatr.* 1993;122(4):650–652.
34. Sampson HA, Scanlon SM. Natural history of food hypersensitivity in children with atopic dermatitis. *J Pediatr.* 1989;115:23–27.
35. Lothe L, Lindberg T. Cow's milk whey protein elicits symptoms of infant colic in colicky formula-fed infants: a double blind crossover study. *Pediatrics.* 1989;83:262–266.
36. Iacono G, Carroccio A, Montalto G, et al. Severe infantile colic and food intolerance: a long-term prospective study. *J Pediatr Gastroenterol Nutr.* 1991;12:332–335.
37. Businco L, Bruno G, Giampietro PG, et al. Allergenicity and nutritional adequacy of soy protein formulas. *J Pediatr.* 1992;121:521–528.
38. American Academy of Pediatrics, Committee on Nutrition. Soy protein formulas: recommendations for use in infant feeding. *Pediatrics.* 1983;72:359–363.
39. Jakobsson I. Intestinal permeability in children of different ages and with different gastrointestinal diseases. *Pediatr Allergy Immunol.* 1993;4(suppl 3):33–39.
40. Lehtonen L, Korhonen T, Korvenranta H. Temperament and sleeping patterns in colicky infants during the first year of life. *J Dev Behav Pediatr.* 1994;15(6):416–420.
41. Pinyerd BJ. Infant colic and maternal mental health: nursing research and practice concerns. *Issues Comp Pediatr Nurs.* 1992;15:155–167.
42. Larson K, Ayllon T. The effects of contingent music and differential reinforcement on infantile colic. *Behav Res Ther.* 1990;28:119–123.
43. Nilsson N. Infant colic and chiropractic. *Eur J Chiro.* 1985;33:264–265.
44. Klougart N, Nilsson N, Jacobsen J. Infantile colic treated by chiropractors: a prospective study of 316 cases. *J Manipulative Physiol Ther.* 1989;12(4):281–288.
45. Pluhar GR, Schobert PD. Vertebral subluxation and colic: a case study. *J Chiro Res Clin Invest.* 1991;7(3):75–76.

Algorithm 1

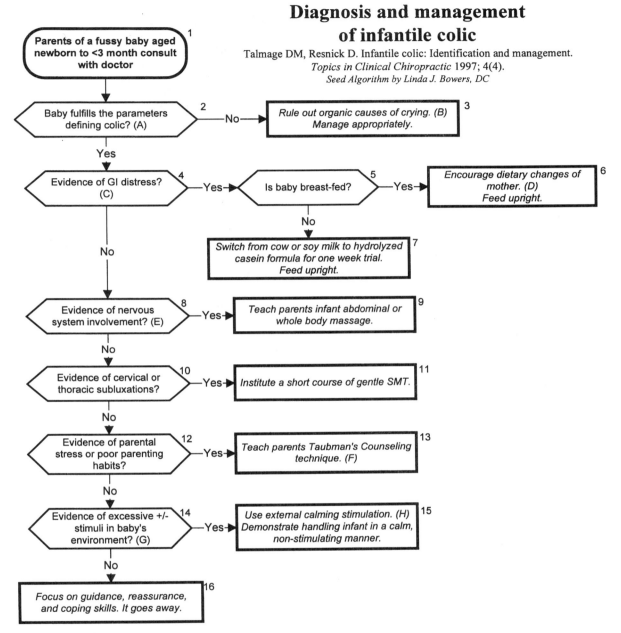

Diagnosis and management of infantile colic

Talmage DM, Resnick D. Infantile colic: Identification and management.
Topics in Clinical Chiropractic 1997; 4(4).
Seed Algorithm by Linda J. Bowers, DC

Annotations:
(A) Abnormal crying that lasts > 3 hours for at least 3 times per week.
(B) e.g., meningitis, sepsis, strangulated hernia, occult fractures.
(C) e.g., abdominal distention, cramps, excessive gas, drawing up of legs.
(D) e.g., eliminate chocolate, eggs, milk and milk products, caffeine, aromatic foods.
(E) e.g., fist clenching, back arching, inconsolable crying.
(F) Never let your baby cry, consider hunger, the desire to suck, need to be held, boredom, and fatigue as possible causes and give appropriate response; if crying continues more than 5 minutes, try another response; don't be concerned about overfeeding; don't be concerned about spoiling the baby.
(G) *Negative stimuli*: hunger, gas pains, temperature differences, fatigue; *Positive stimuli*: musical toys, television, voices, lights, faces, excessive handling, playing catch using the baby.
(H) e.g., white noise, car rides, rocking, womb/heartbeat recordings, music, abdominal and whole body massage.

7

Understanding Childhood Cancer: Keys for the Chiropractor

Tracy Barnes

"Onion skin reaction" was all I could think of when I first met Eddie. Like Pavlov's dog, when the bell rang "Ewing's sarcoma," I went to this classic radiographic finding. The problem was that this label said virtually nothing about the 15-year-old boy who stood in front of me with a slightly edematous face and not a hair on his head. Eddie was so much more than the spiculating frays of bone I remembered from school. I met Eddie during my first summer as a volunteer counselor for Sky High Hope Camp—a special camp for children affected by cancer.

Sky High, and other camps like it, did not exist 20 years ago. That is because most of the campers would not have survived long enough to come to camp in those days. Since that time, however, treatment advances have increased the overall cure rate for a child with leukemia to 75%.[1] Today, campers at Sky High come with a variety of cancer diagnoses such as acute lymphocytic leukemia, Wilm's tumor, astrocytoma, and osteosarcoma. Camp is the one place where many of these children can lead "normal" lives. They get a chance to ride a horse, paddle a canoe, cook over a campfire, and just plain get dirty.

These children, however, do not come only to Sky High Hope Camp. They can walk into our offices any day of the week. As primary care physicians, chiropractors must be acutely aware of the need to detect childhood cancers. Our often unique relationship with patients allows us the opportunity to be on the front line of diagnosis. We may see the child more frequently than any other care provider. Many of the signs and symptoms of childhood cancer are those that commonly bring children to a chiropractor's office. These significant signs include back and leg pains, stiff necks, persistent headaches, and gait abnormalities.[2,3] Table 1 presents a list of red flags for childhood cancer.

This chapter examines the top five pediatric cancers; alerts the chiropractor to diagnostic red flags for each condition; describes appropriate treatment and referral, and provides resources for gathering more information. Seventy percent of children who are diagnosed with cancer have a variety of solid tumors such as those of the central nervous system (CNS).[3] The remaining 30% are affected by acute leukemia.[3] The five principal cancers of childhood are leukemia, CNS tumor, bone cancer, neuroblastoma, and lymphoma.[3–5] Between 1989 and 1991 the three most common types of infant cancers were neuroblastoma, CNS tumor, and leukemia.[6] By the time 80% of pediatric cases are diagnosed, the child already has advanced stage disease.[4] The most favorable treatment outcomes occur in children who are diagnosed early and referred to a pediatric oncology center. These special centers have teams of professionals with specific expertise in dealing with pediatric oncology.[1]

A GLOBAL VIEW OF CANCER IN CHILDREN

Childhood cancer is the second leading cause of death in American children from 1 to 14 years of age. Only accidents are responsible for more pediatric fatalities. It is estimated that by the year 2000, 1 in 1,000 adults in the United States will be a survivor of childhood cancer.[3,6] Worldwide rates of childhood cancers are increasing. While many developing countries have high rates of death due to infectious disease and malnutrition, the rate of pediatric neoplasm is also on the rise. It is estimated that many cases of cancer, especially brain tumors, are substantially underreported in the developing world.[5]

Adult cancers are primarily those of lung, colon, breast, prostate, and pancreas. In contrast, childhood cancers com-

---

Adapted from *Top Clin Chiro* 1999; 6(1): 56–36
© 1999 Aspen Publishers, Inc.

Table 1. Red flags of pediatric cancers

- Hard, nonmobile, non-tender lymph nodes (Mobile, tender, firm, or fluctuant nodes are more likely to represent infection.)
- Bone pain, especially when accompanied by recurrent fever
- Recurrent headaches, especially those that wake a child from sleep or are accompanied by vomiting
- Unexplained weight loss in a child
- Abdominal masses, especially those accompanied by blood in the urine
- Occult blood in stool or urine
- Cervical lymphadenopathy, especially those that are antibiotic resistant

monly attack blood, brain, and bone cells and lymphatic systems. Cancer in adults generally stems from years of lifestyle factors such as smoking, improper diet, environmental and occupational exposure to carcinogens, and sexual practices. Table 2 compares adult and pediatric cancer.

The cause of most cases of pediatric tumor is unknown. Certain hereditary and environmental factors may play a role in some children. Children who have been exposed to radiation have a significantly higher risk for cancer. For example, an increased incidence of acute leukemia was found in children exposed to radiation following atomic bomb blasts in Japan and after the Chernobyl accident.[3-6] Other risk factors for childhood cancer are listed in Table 3.

Table 2. A comparison of adult and pediatric cancer

	Adult	Pediatric
Causes	Smoking	Genetic predisposition
	Diet	Environmental exposure
	Occupation	Exposure to carcinogens
Median age at diagnosis	67 years	6 years
Areas affected	Lung	White blood cells
	Colon	Brain
	Breast	Bone
	Prostate	Lymphatic system
	Pancreas	Tumors of muscle, kidney, and nervous system
Stage at initial diagnosis	20% have advanced stage	80% have advanced stage

LEUKEMIA

Overall acute lymphoblastic leukemia (ALL) is the most common malignancy in children. It is diagnosed in approximately 3,000 children per year, and it accounts for one third of all pediatric cancer cases. The highest incidence of leukemia occurs in children between age 2 and 10, with peak onset at age 4. The overall cure rate for childhood leukemia has increased dramatically in the last 20 years, particularly for children diagnosed with ALL. This success is largely due to advances in early detection and vastly improved treatment protocols.[1-3] Children with acute myelogenous leukemia (AML) have a lower cure rate than those with ALL. Without treatment, children with acute leukemia have an average survival of 3 to 5 months.[2]

Although viruses cause several forms of leukemia in animals, the cause of pediatric ALL is undetermined. Exposure to ionizing radiation and certain chemicals such as benzene

Table 3. Possible risk factors for childhood cancer[36-43]

Risk factor	Type of cancer
Radiation exposure	Leukemia
Neurofibromatosis or tuberous sclerosis	Astrocytoma
Cryptorchidism (undescended testicle)	Testicular cancer
Children who do not have an iris	Wilm's tumor
Family members with neuroblastoma	Neuroblastoma
Maternal consumption of cured meats	Pediatric brain tumors
Maternal exposure to flea/tick products	Pediatric brain tumors
Parental daily tobacco consumption	All childhood cancers
Magnetic field exposure	All childhood cancers
Home pesticides	
Pest strips	Leukemia
Yard treatments for pests	Soft tissue sarcomas
Siblings of Hodgkin's lymphoma patients	Hodgkin's lymphoma
Exposure to chemicals (phenoxzacetic acids, chlorophenols, dioxins)	Non-Hodgkin's lymphoma
Exposure to organic solvents (benzene, polychlorinated biphenyls, clorophenols)	Non-Hodgkin's lymphoma
Prior use of immunosuppressive drugs	Non-Hodgkin's lymphoma
Exposure to motor vehicle exhaust	Leukemia, central nervous system tumors

and antineoplastics is associated with increased risk of leukemia.[2,3] Genetic factors such as Down syndrome and Fanconi's anemia appear to predispose some children.[4-6] ALL results from a rapid, uncontrolled proliferation of immature lymphocytes. A single lymphoid cell undergoes malignant transformation and then replicates endlessly. These leukemic cells replace normal bone marrow cells resulting in anemia, thrombocytopenia, and infections. Definitive diagnosis of ALL is made by bone marrow aspiration identifying the presence of more than 25% malignant hematopoietic cells or blasts.[2] Cells may spread to the liver, spleen, lymph nodes, CNS, kidney, and gonads. Organ infiltration can cause hepatosplenomegaly and lymphadenopathy, but it may not cause any disruption of normal organ function. When leukemic cells infiltrate the CNS and bone marrow, symptoms of stiff neck, headache, vomiting, and bone pain may occur. If the leukemic cells destroy the satiety center of the hypothalamus, the child may present with an increased appetite and immense weight gain or insatiable thirst.[1]

Signs and symptoms

A child with leukemia may simply feel ill. He or she may appear pale, flushed, or lethargic and complain of a chronic cough. Commonly, the child with leukemia will have ashen, sunken eyes that signal a serious chronic illness. Although the child's appearance may trigger an alarm reaction for the doctor, those who see the child on a daily basis, such as the parent, may not notice these gradually appearing changes. Rapid expansion of leukemic cells within the marrow space may have caused bone pain, and the child may present with a limp. Additional symptoms include a "rash" of small pinpoint red spots all over the body and an unexplained fever. Vital signs will likely be normal with the exception of a possible fever or tachycardia if the child has become anemic or is febrile. Unilateral or asymmetric enlargement of palatine tonsils may suggest leukemic cell infiltration but may more likely be non-Hodgkin's lymphoma.[1,7]

The symptoms of leukemia can be quite nonspecific and often resemble other conditions such as a mild infection or flu. However, should any of these signs appear repeatedly or with no apparent etiology, the clinician should stay alert for the possibility of leukemia.

Laboratory tests and special studies

A complete blood count (CBC) with differential is the most useful initial laboratory test for diagnosing leukemia. Although the total white blood cell (WBC) count is normal in up to half of all children with ALL, 90% of patients have a decrease in at least one cell type (neutropenia, thrombocytopenia, or anemia).[1] A child whose CBC reveals a WBC count of more than 50,000 should be referred immediately for medical attention.[1] Definitive diagnosis of leukemia is made by bone marrow aspiration and biopsy.[1,3]

A chest radiograph is helpful to ascertain the possibility of a mediastinal mass, which is present in 5% to 10% of patients with ALL. Spinal and long bone radiographs may show decreased mineralization and vertebral body compression.[7-9]

Treatment

Early diagnosis and initiation of treatment are essential for the survival of a child with leukemia. Multiple drug regimens and systemic chemotherapy are generally the treatments of choice. Adjunct use of radiation to treat local accumulations of leukemic cells also may be employed. Bone marrow transplantation is used in some cases, but it is rarely used in the initial treatment phase. Most patients are treated according to protocols designed by the National Children's Cancer Group or Pediatric Oncology Group. These protocols are planned to increase the long-term survival rate while decreasing the threat of treatment toxicity.[1]

The initial goal of treatment is to induce a state of remission. Remission is indicated by the absence of leukemic cells and restoration of normal hematopoiesis. Remission is usually established in the first month of care. It is followed by a period of consolidation chemotherapy that lasts approximately 2 months and is designed to maintain the remission phase and prevent disease in other sites. During this period, medications are administered to deter manifestations of the disease in the CNS and prolong remission. Interim maintenance and delayed intensive therapies follow. These therapies generally involve the use of various chemotherapeutic agents. Less intensive drug therapies follow for a period of 2 to 3 years with boys receiving therapy for a longer period of time as their chance of relapse is greater. The probability of cure decreases each time a child relapses.[10]

The burden of treatment for a child with leukemia often falls heavily on the shoulders of the parent. Many are required to administer oral and intravenous (IV) medications, tend to catheters, transport the child to and from frequent hospital visits, and vigilantly be on the alert for signs of infection. This at-home care, along with the monumental stress of watching their child suffer, can be overwhelming. The doctor of chiropractic who cares for such a family can aid by not only providing hands-on care to the parents, but also referring them for emotional support. Cancer is a "family disease" that affects the entire family unit as well as the sick child. For this reason, both parents and siblings benefit from continuous support from a network of individuals. The clinician may serve as a resource for local agencies, support groups, and so forth.

The family chiropractor also can aid in watching for many of the late effects of treatment that plague some children with leukemia well after their initial treatment is completed. These delayed effects include scoliosis, significant weight changes, avascular necrosis, edema, bone asymmetries, thyroid dysfunction, hearing loss, and neuropathy. Learning disabilities and psychosocial difficulties also may be part of the child's treatment sequelae.[4,7] Table 4 presents an overview of key factors related to leukemia and Algorithm 1 examines the clinical manifestations.

Prognosis

Favorable indicators for cure in a child with leukemia include a total WBC count of <25,000/`µL and no manifestation of CNS disease at the time of diagnosis. Children between the age of 3 and 7 years have the best prognosis of all age groups.[1,3] Although the likelihood of initial remission for all children with ALL is at or above 90%, the overall disease cure rate is 75%.[1,3,4] Some lower risk groups actually have a 95% long-term survival rate.[1,3] The long-term outcome is better for girls than boys.[1,10]

BRAIN TUMOR

Tumors of the brain and spinal cord are the most common type of solid tumors in children. They account for 20% of all childhood cancer diagnoses and are second only to leukemia in childhood cancer incidence.[11] Pediatric brain tumors often are misdiagnosed or diagnosed in late stage due to their ability to grow rapidly as well as mimic other conditions. Early diagnosis is mandatory for good prognosis. Only half of all children diagnosed with brain tumors will live more than 5 years past diagnosis.[11]

Primary intracranial neoplasms can be divided into six classes to include tumors of the skull, meninges, cranial nerves, neuroglia, pituitary or pineal body, and those of congenital origin. Metastases can involve the skull or any other intracranial structure but will rarely spread outside the CNS. Brain tumors in infants and children most often arise from central neuroepithelial tissue, whereas most adult brain tumors come from CNS coverings such as a meningioma or adjacent tissue such as pituitary adenoma.[2,3,12]

Risk factors

Although the majority of childhood brain tumors are idiopathic in nature, recent studies have shed light on several risk factors. The mothers of 540 children under age 20 who had a primary brain tumor diagnosis were found to have a significantly higher dietary consumption of cured meats.[8] An increase of CNS tumors has been noted in the offspring of mice fed with nitrosamine precursors such as sodium nitrite and alkylamide.[8] They are the same compounds found in the majority of processed meats. Children of mothers who took a daily prenatal vitamin had a decreased risk of brain tumors, despite high nitrosamine consumption. Vitamins C and E appear to block the endogenous formation of nitroso compounds and carry a protective effect to both the mother and her offspring.[8]

The use of household flea and tick products also has shown strong correlation with the development of pediatric brain tumors. This correlate is highest in children who are less than 5 years old at the time of diagnosis and for pregnant females who had an increased exposure in preparing, applying, or cleaning up these products. The sprays and fogging type applications were the only products with significant associated risks. Elevated risks were not found with the use of products to control termite, louse, or snail populations.[13] Other studies[14,15] have noted a genetic predisposition to develop pediatric brain tumors.

Table 4. Leukemia at a glance

Incidence
- Most common malignancy in children
- More common in boys than girls (1.2 to 1) and in whites than blacks (1.8 to 1)
- Siblings of children with leukemia are two to four times more likely to develop the disease than the general population

Age of onset
- 2 to 10 years
- Peak onset at 4 years

Signs and symptoms
- Fever
- Pallor
- Bleeding
  - Easy bruising
  - Petechiae or purpura
  - Mucous membrane hemorrhage such as epistaxis
- Bone pain, especially in the pelvis, vertebral bodies, and legs
- Fatigue
- Exercise intolerance
- Pharyngitis
- Antibiotic-resistant infection such as otitis media or sinusitis
- Swollen gums
- Lymphadenopathy
- Hepatosplenomegaly (present in over 60% of patients)
- Testicular enlargement

Radiographic findings
- Diffuse osteopenia
- Radiolucent metaphyseal bands
- Periosteal new bone formation
- Bone destruction
- Osteosclerosis
- Mixed osteolysis and sclerosis
- Growth arrest lines
- Soft tissue swelling

Signs and symptoms

A child with an undiagnosed brain tumor may present to a chiropractor's office complaining of persistent headache and nausea. He or she may have had an episode of vomiting or even a seizure. A seizure is a common initial event. Other common events are a change of personality and persistent recurrent torticollis. The parents may report an increase in the child's irritability or a concern that the child is "failing to thrive."[3,4] Observation may reveal a child with unsteady gait and difficulty with coordination. Vision and speech problems also may be noted. A complete neurologic examination including a thorough investigation of cranial nerve function is essential. Decreased dermatomal sensations may be found. Any patient with a suspected brain tumor should be referred immediately for advanced imaging such as computed tomography (CT) or magnetic resonance imaging (MRI) and additional referral made to a pediatric oncologist. Bone scans and bone marrow examinations also may be performed to assess the possibility of medulloblastoma. Definitive diagnosis is made by tumor visualization on CT or MRI scan.[4,9]

Approximately one half of all pediatric brain tumors occur above the tentorium. The other half occur in the posterior fossa.[11] Tumors of the posterior fossa invariably affect the ability to gaze upward and cause a loss of the corneal reflex. They are very important red flags on examination. Astrocytomas are the most common types of brain tumors in childhood.[4,11] Most are low-grade tumors found in the posterior fossa. Surgical excision provides a 10-year survival rate of approximately 80%.[11]

Treatment

Treatment for this type of childhood cancer has not yielded the gains in cure rate achieved in childhood leukemia. The best prognosis belongs to the children who are diagnosed and treated in an early stage. Most children with tumors of the CNS are treated with a multimodal package of surgery, radiation, and/or chemotherapy. Gene therapy also has shown promise in recent trials.[12,14,15] Treatment prognosis varies depending on location and growth of the tumor. Central astrocytomas grow very rapidly and carry a less than 25% 2-year survival rate while optic tract gliomas are slow growing and have a better than 75% 5-year survival rate.[4,11] Table 5 summarizes key aspects of pediatric brain tumors.

BONE TUMORS

While the incidence of primary bone tumors in children is relatively rare, it is one of prime importance for the chiropractor to watch for as its cardinal sign—bone pain—may be a likely "chiropractic problem." Osteogenic sarcoma (osteosarcoma) and Ewing's sarcoma are the most common

Table 5. Brain tumors at a glance

Incidence
- Most common solid tumor of childhood
- Account for 1,500 to 2,000 new malignancies each year in the United States
- 25% to 30% of all childhood cancers are those of the central nervous system

Age of onset
- Peak incidence is between 5 and 10 years

Signs and symptoms
- Headache, especially progressively worsening morning headaches
- Vomiting
- Nausea
- Personality change (eg, increased irritability)
- Seizure
- Blurred vision, diplopia
- Failure to thrive
- Precocious or delayed puberty
- Cranial nerve palsies
- Dysarthria
- Ataxia
- Hemiplegia
- Papilledema
- Hyperreflexia
- Macrocephaly, hydrocephaly

---

types of pediatric bone tumors.[16,17] Other less common tumors of the bone seen in children include chondrosarcoma, fibrosarcoma, and synovial sarcoma. Adolescents and young adults ages 10 to 25 years are the most likely candidates for diagnosis with a 2:1 male predominance noted.[4] The median age for diagnosis of osteosarcoma is 18 years for males and 17 years for females.[16] Approximately 900 new cases of osteosarcoma are diagnosed each year in the United States.[4,16]

The etiology for pediatric bone tumors is not known. However, individuals who have a history of treatment for previous cancer have an increased risk for osteosarcoma.[17] In addition, children who experience rapid bone growth appear at greater risk for tumor formation.[17] Patients with osteosarcoma have been noted to be significantly taller than their peers, although this finding has never been clearly understood.[16,17]

Signs and symptoms

Most cases of osteosarcoma initially involve the distal femur or the proximal humerus. While 58% of all osteosarcomas occur around the knee, the disease also can present in the sacrum, pelvis, rib, hand, tibia, calcaneus, and spine.[3] Ewing's sarcoma is most commonly found in the rib, femur, and pelvis. A child with a bone tumor will most likely complain of pain and swelling at the site of the tumor. The pain may initially be insidious and transitory with a progression toward severe and unrelenting pain. Key initial signs include limping and being awakened at night by fever or sweating. Some cases of osteosarcoma are discovered after trauma to the area of lesion reveals the malignancy. Fractures can commonly occur through a region of cortical bone destruction. Metastases to the lungs, other bones, and kidneys can occur as sequelae to primary osteosarcoma.[2-4]

Laboratory tests and special studies

An elevation of the alkaline phosphatase enzyme level may be the only abnormal laboratory finding. A child with chronic widespread metastatic disease also may show anemia. On radiograph, the most likely finding is a "permeative" or "ivory" medullary lesion in the metaphysis of a long bone. Another radiographic finding is the "sunburst" periosteal reaction of osteosarcoma and the "onion skin or peel" appearance of Ewing's sarcoma. A soft tissue mass also is commonly seen in osteosarcoma. Chest radiograph may reveal lung metastasis. CT scans, MRI, radionuclide bone scan, and biopsy are all used for definitive diagnosis of both osteosarcoma and Ewing's sarcoma.[3,9]

Treatment and prognosis

The 5-year disease-free survival rate is approximately 60% to 80% for patients with osteosarcoma and about 35% to 50% for those with Ewing's sarcoma.[2,3] Treatment for both forms of pediatric bone tumors includes radiation, chemotherapy, and amputation. Limb-salvage or limb-preservation procedures are possible in some cases of primary bone tumor. One procedure is a surgical technique involving tumor resection and limb reconstruction. Complete amputation is not required. A prosthesis can often be attached either externally or surgically to replace the bone that is removed. Patients with pelvic sarcomas and those whose bone tumors have metastasized have a poor prognosis. In addition, Ewing's sarcoma tumors can relapse many years after the initial treatment phase is completed. Table 6 presents a summary of bone tumors.

NEUROBLASTOMA

Neuroblastoma is a highly malignant tumor that is found in infants and young children. Approximately one third of neuroblastomas arise from medullary cells in the adrenal glands, another third begin in the neural crest tissue of abdominal sympathetic ganglia, and the remaining cases start in the sympathetic ganglia of the chest, pelvis, and neck.[18] Neuroblastomas are the most common solid tumors found in children outside of the CNS.[3] Fifty percent of neuroblastomas are diagnosed in the first 2 years of life.[4] There are approximately 550 new cases of neuroblastoma diagnosed each year in the United States.[18] Global statistics for neuroblastoma frequency are similar.[4,6]

A familial form of neuroblastoma exists and can increase a child's risk for developing the disease. The average age at diagnosis for familial neuroblastoma is 9 months. This figure is in contrast to noninherited or sporadic neuroblastoma, which carries a 22-month average age at diagnosis.[4,18] Children with familial neuroblastoma are more likely to develop multiple tumors in different organ systems than those with sporadic neuroblastoma.[3]

Signs and symptoms

All infants and young children who are seen in a chiropractic office should be watched for signs of neuroblastoma. Warning signs include bone and abdominal pain, fever, weight loss, failure to thrive, pallor, and irritability. Specific

Table 6. Bone tumors at a glance

Incidence
- Osteosarcoma is the sixth most common malignancy in childhood.
- Ewing's sarcoma is the second most common malignant bone tumor.
- Males are more commonly affected than females.

Age of onset
- Adolescents and young adults are most affected.
- Peak occurrence happens during the adolescent growth spurt.

Signs and symptoms
- Persistent pain and swelling occur at the tumor site.
- Most common tumor site is above or below the knee, hip, or proximal arm.
- Systemic signs of infection possible (mild fever, anemia, leukocytosis, increased erythrocyte sedimentation rate), especially with Ewing's sarcoma.
- An elevated serum alkaline phosphatase level is possible with osteosarcoma.

Radiographic findings: Osteosarcoma
- "Permeative" or "ivory" medullary lesion in metaphysis of long bone
- "Sunburst" or "sunray" periosteal reaction with lytic and blastic elements
- Cortical disruption with soft tissue mass formation
- "Cumulus cloud" appearance
- "Cannonball metastases" and pneumothorax with lung metastases

Radiographic findings: Ewing's sarcoma
- Moth-eaten and lytic tumor
- "Onion skin" (elevation of the periosteum) periosteal reaction
- "Groomed" or "trimmed whiskers" effect
- Cortical "saucerization"
- Pathologic fracture (evident in 5% of cases)

symptoms vary according to the primary site of disease. Cervical neuroblastoma presents with a mass in the neck that is often misdiagnosed as infection. Horner's syndrome (constricted pupil, ptosis, facial anhidrosis) may occur with involvement of cervicothoracic ganglia. Patients who present with paresis, paralysis, or a change in bowel or bladder habits may be suffering from paraspinal neuroblastoma tumors causing compression on the cord. Opsoclonus-myoclonus ("dancing eyes and dancing feet") is another possible manifestation. Masses can be found on the skull (particularly on the sphenoid) and can cause both periorbital ecchymosis and proptosis.

Bluish subcutaneous nodules may indicate neuroblastoma, especially those with an erythematous flush that blanch when compressed. Hepatomegaly may be evident, especially in the affected infant. Chronic, watery diarrhea is likely due to tumor secretion of vasoactive intestinal peptides. Posterior thoracic tumors may present with respiratory symptoms such as cough, croup, dysphagia, and fatigue. A sign of neuroblastoma often first noticed by a parent while bathing the baby is a lateral asymmetry in the abdomen associated with a palpable abdominal mass. A neuroblastoma may be found on routine abdominal examination in a child free of symptoms.

Laboratory tests and special studies

Anemia is found in 60% of children with neuroblastoma, and it is often due to chronic disease, hemorrhage into tumor, or marrow infiltration.[19] Thrombocytosis also is common. Elevated urinary catecholamine levels are present in 90% of patients at initial diagnosis.[2–4,19]

Radiographic signs of neuroblastoma include multiple destructive bone lesions with "moth-eaten" appearance. The spine, pelvis, skull, and ends of long bones are common sites of involvement. Pathologic fractures, periosteal reactions, and stippled calcifications also may be noted on plain film. Sunburst spiculations of the skull with gross widening of the sutures are classic signs of metastatic neuroblastoma.[4,9]

A retroperitoneal mass that displaces adjacent organs may be seen on plain film. Primary adrenal tumors generally displace the kidney inferolaterally. CT scan or MRI is necessary to ascertain extent of tumor growth and evaluate the presence of spinal cord involvement. Radionuclide bone scans often are used to assess for bone metastases.[4,12] Bilateral bone marrow studies and biopsies are essential for determining the stage of metastatic disease and for differentiating neuroblastoma from ALL.

Prognosis

The overall survival rate for children with neuroblastoma has changed little in the last 20 years, despite advances in understanding the tumor. Prognosis varies depending on age and stage of disease at initial diagnosis.[4] Treatment is generally a multimodal approach involving surgery, radiation therapy, and chemotherapy. Infants with neuroblastoma have a greater prognosis than older children. This finding may be due to the fact that often younger children have less disseminated disease than older children. Children diagnosed at less than 1 year of age have an approximate 80% survival rate while those older than 2 years at the time of diagnosis have about a 25% survival rate.[19] There is often a spontaneous remission in those under 1 year of age. Children with an advanced stage IV disease have been shown to have only a 10% survival rate.[18–20] Table 7 provides a concise review of neuroblastoma.

HODGKIN'S LYMPHOMA

Hodgkin's lymphoma was the first malignancy of the lymphoid system to be described. The first cases were reported in 1832 by British physician Thomas Hodgkin.[3] Today, the disease is a relatively uncommon malignancy that accounts for 6% of new cancer diagnoses each year in the United

---

Table 7. Neuroblastoma at a glance

Incidence
- Accounts for 7% to 10% of all pediatric malignancies
- Most common solid neoplasm outside the central nervous system

Age of onset
- 50% are diagnosed before age 2 years
- 90% are diagnosed before age 5 years

Signs and symptoms
- Bone and abdominal pain
- Fever
- Weight loss
- Failure to thrive
- Pallor
- Irritability
- Cervical masses
- Paresis
- Paralysis
- Bowel or bladder dysfunction
- Opsoclonus-myoclonus
- Periorbital ecchymosis
- Proptosis
- Bluish subcutaneous nodules
- Hepatomegaly may be evident
- Chronic, watery diarrhea

Radiographic findings
- Widened skull sutures (ie, "sunburst" spiculations)
- Soft tissue mass
- Multiple, diffuse, symmetric, osteolytic lesions

States.[4] Hodgkin's disease does, however, account for 50% of the lymphomas of childhood with children between the ages of 10 and 16 years at highest risk.[3,4]

Signs and symptoms

A child with undiagnosed Hodgkin's lymphoma might present to a chiropractor's office complaining of feeling tired, feverish, coughing, itching, and experiencing night sweats. He or she also may have recently begun to lose weight without dieting. On examination, painless cervical or supraclavicular nodes, which are firm and enlarged, may be noted. The growth of these lymph nodes is variable, and involved nodes may change over weeks to months. Should the clinician position the child on a high-low table and recline him or her to a supine position, a facial color change or a difficulty for the child to breathe (due to a mediastinal mass) may be noticed. The child may confide that alcohol consumption increases their pain level.

Laboratory tests and radiographic findings

A chest radiograph should be taken of any child suspected of having Hodgkin's lymphoma in order to determine the presence of a mediastinal mass. This mass is present in half of the patients diagnosed with Hodgkin's lymphoma.[3,4] It may be asymptomatic unless the growth has compressed vital thoracic structures. Skeletal radiographs also may reveal Hodgkin's lymphoma lesions of the bone, although this finding is generally a secondary manifestation of systemic disease that occurs in approximately 10% to 20% of those diagnosed.[2,4]

Hodgkin's disease is unique in that the tumors contain a majority of normal cells and very few cancer cells. The presence of the malignant Reed-Sternberg cells are pathognomonic for Hodgkin's lymphoma. The origin of this malignant cell is currently unknown. A CBC is likely to be normal, although there is the possibility of anemia, neutrophilia, eosinophilia, and thrombocytosis. The erythrocyte sedimentation rate (ESR) also can be elevated. Clinical staging of the disease is made using the Ann Arbor classification system that defines advancing stage based on the number of anatomic sites involved.[2] For example, stage I disease represents involvement of a single lymph node region or localized involvement of a singe organ, whereas stage IV disease is characterized by widespread involvement of one or more extra lymphatic organs with or without associated lymph node involvement. Staging is accomplished by CT scan and lymphangiography procedures. Bone marrow aspirates and biopsies also are used to assess disease progression. Radiation therapy and combination chemotherapy are the current medical treatments, especially in stage III and stage IV disease.[2,4]

Prognosis

Prognosis for children with Hodgkin's disease is largely dependent on the stage of initial disease. Children with stage I or II have an approximate 85% to 90% rate of 5-year survival.[3,4] Ranges drop from 80% to 50% for those with stage III and stage IV at initial diagnosis.[2-4] Table 8 presents a synopsis of Hodgkin's lymphoma.

NON-HODGKIN'S LYMPHOMA

Hodgkin's lymphoma behaves in a very predictable way with tumor progression moving from one site to another in an expected pattern. There are other malignant lymphomas, however, that do not behave in such a foreseeable fashion. These forms are grouped together as non-Hodgkin's lymphomas and include B and T cell lymphomas and Burkitt's tumor (African lymphoma), among others. In the United States non-Hodgkin's lymphomas account for 7% to 13% of all malignancies in children less than 15 years of age.[21] In contrast, 50% of the children of Africa who have cancer are affected by some form of non-Hodgkin's lymphoma.[3,21] There is an estimated 3 to 1 male:female ratio of the disease, with approximately 390 new cases diagnosed each year in the United States.[3,21]

Table 8. Hodgkin's lymphoma at a glance

Incidence
- Hodgkin's lymphoma accounts for 6% of new cancer diagnoses each year in the United States.
- Behaves in a more predictable manner than non-Hodgkin's lymphomas

Age of onset
- 60% are ages 10 to 16 years at initial diagnosis

Signs and symptoms
- Fatigue
- Fever
- Chronic cough
- Night sweats
- Pain worsened by alcohol ingestion
- Painless cervical or supraclavicular adenopathy
- Mediastinal mass
- Anorexia
- Weight loss
- Pruritis

Radiographic findings
- Osteolytic, sclerotic, and mixed destructive lesions most commonly in vertebral bodies
- "Ivory" vertebrae
- Periosteal reaction is possible

Signs and symptoms

Generally all forms of childhood non-Hodgkin's lymphoma have a tendency for rapid proliferation with diffuse malignancies arising from extra nodal tissue. These aggressive tumors can affect any site of lymphoid tissue as well as the thymus, liver, spleen, Peyer's patches, and Waldeyer's ring. Other common sites of extra lymphatic involvement include bone, bone marrow, CNS, skin, and testes. Because of this wide range of tissue involvement, children with undiagnosed non-Hodgkin's disease can present with a host of symptoms depending on the location of their lesion and the degree of dissemination.

The symptom presentation may occur very rapidly in a period of days to a few weeks. The nonspecific symptoms of the disease are shared with other forms of childhood cancer and include fatigue, fevers, chills, night sweats, decreased appetite, and weight loss. Other possible symptoms include shortness of breath, cough, abdominal pain, headache, changes in vision, seizure, and change in bowel habits. If the disease is present in the child's sinus, upper airway, or throat, he or she may present with nasal stuffiness, sore throat, or difficulty swallowing.

The physical examination may reveal enlarged cervical, axillary, or femoral lymph nodes; pleural effusion; facial edema; hepatomegaly or splenomegaly; abdominal mass; and tonsilar swelling. If the disease is present in the bone (also known as reticulum cell sarcoma of bone), the child may complain of pain in the femur, tibia, or humerus, which are the most common sites of osseous involvement.[2-4]

Laboratory tests and special studies

The diagnosis of non-Hodgkin's lymphoma is made by biopsy with histology, immunophenotyping, and cytogenetic studies. The CBC will likely be normal unless widespread disease and marrow infiltration have occurred. Serum uric acid and LDH levels may be elevated.

A chest radiograph should be taken to determine the presence of a mediastinal mass. Radiographs of the area of bone pain are also needed. Analysis may show a permeative medullary lesion in the diaphysis or metaphysis of any long tubular bone. A well-defined soft tissue mass also may be noted. Pathologic fracture is a common finding. Radionuclide bone scan, abdominal ultrasound, CT scan, and bone marrow studies are used to assess tumor burden.

Table 9. Non-Hodgkin's lymphoma at a glance

Incidence
- Includes B and T cell lymphomas and Burkitt's tumor
- Accounts for 7% to 13% of all malignancies in children less than age 15 years in the United States

Age of onset
- Most commonly seen in children 15 years of age or older
- Uncommon in children under 5 years of age

Signs and symptoms
- Fatigue
- Fever
- Chills
- Night sweats
- Decreased appetite
- Weight loss
- Facial edema
- Constipation
- Shortness of breath
- Cough
- Abdominal pain
- Headache
- Changes in vision
- Lymphadenopathy
- Mediastinal or abdominal mass
- Hepatosplenomegaly

Radiographic findings
- Permeative medullary destruction
- Pathologic fracture
- Periosteal reaction is possible
- Well-defined soft tissue mass

Table 10. What the chiropractor can do to help a child with cancer

- Continue to provide quality care to both the child and his or her family.
- Become a member of the bone marrow transplant registry. Let patients know where to sign up for this simple blood test.
- Find out if any of your patients are childhood cancer survivors. Ask them to tell you their story. Be alert to the signs of late effects of cancer.
- Encourage monthly breast self-examinations, especially in those patients who have a history of childhood cancer.
- Locate the nearest Ronald McDonald House. Volunteer time, money, or supplies.
- Establish a relationship with an oncologist in the area. Find the location of the closest pediatric cancer treatment center.
- Get to know a child with cancer.
- Pay special attention to the sibling of a child with cancer. They suffer too and need your support.
- Take time to listen to a parent of a child with cancer.
- Share this information with patients and staff. Stay alert for red flags of childhood cancer.

Table 11. Suggested reading on childhood cancer

Jill Krementz. *How It Feels To Fight for Your Life.* Boston: Little, Brown and Co; 1989.

Erma Bombeck. *I Want To Grow Hair, I Want To Grow Up, I Want To Go to Boise.* MassMarket Paperback, Harper Prism; 1990.

David Walter Adams and Eleanor J. Deveau. *Coping with Childhood Cancer: Where Do We Go from Here.* Reston, Va: Reston Publishing Co; 1984.

Barbara Hoffman, ed. *A Cancer Survivor's Almanac: Charting Your Journey.* National Coalition for Cancer Survivorship. Minnetonka, Minn: Chronimed Publishing; 1996.

Arthur R. Ablin. *Supportive Care of Children with Cancer.* Baltimore: Johns Hopkins University Press; 1993.

Lisa J. Bain. *A Parent's Guide to Childhood Cancer.* New York: Dell Trade Paperbacks; 1995.

David J. Bearson. *They Never Want To Tell You: Children Talk about Cancer.* Cambridge, Mass: Harvard University Press; 1991.

David R. Tomal and Annette Tomal. *Every Parent's Nightmare: A Young Family's Triumph over Their Son's Critical Illness.* Grand Rapids, Mich: Zondervan Publishing House; 1993.

Joan Taska Rolsky. *Your Child Has Cancer: A Guide to Coping.* Philadephia: Committee to Benefit the Children, St. Christopher's Hospital for Children; 1992.

Prognosis

Chemotherapy is the standard treatment for the child with non-Hodgkin's lymphoma. Prognosis for this disease is akin to other childhood diseases in that it is largely dependent on stage of progression at initial diagnosis. If only localized disease is present, the child can expect a 90% long-term disease-free survival.[4] A poorer prognosis exists for those with advanced disease on both sides of the diaphragm or with CNS or bone marrow involvement.[3,22] Table 9 contains a review of non-Hodgkin's lymphoma.

LIFE AFTER CHILDHOOD CANCER

The numbers of children who have survived childhood cancer have markedly increased in the past 15 years. For many of these children, the health problems associated with childhood cancer do not end with their final treatment. The treatments that saved their life in the time of crisis may leave them with a host of physical and psychological stresses. Childhood cancer survivors who received radiation therapy or chemotherapy are at greater risk than their peers of developing secondary malignancy neoplasms, heart disease, osteoporosis, dental disease, infertility, and impaired bone growth.[23–29]

Female survivors of Hodgkin's lymphoma who were treated with radiation have an increased risk for developing solid tumors later in life.[30,31] Children whose cancers were treated with cranial irradiation suffer alterations to the hypothalamus, pituitary, and adrenal glands. These alterations make them likely candidates for growth hormone deficiency and primary hypothyroidism later in life.[24,29]

Legal and societal implications also exist for the childhood cancer survivor. Employment and health insurance discrimination are certainly possibilities for which the child must be prepared. In addition, those survivors who bear physical reminders of previous treatment face psychological strains associated with poor self-esteem and self-image.[32]

Table 12. Pediatric cancer vignettes

Case 1. 10-year-old James is the star quarterback on his team and a straight A student. His aunt notices a slight swelling around his left knee. He states that the knee was initially mildly painful, but is getting worse. He has no history of recent trauma outside of what he describes as his "usual activities." The knee pain is constant throughout all ranges of active and passive motion. He has no fever.

Case 2. 7-year-old Crystal complains of increasing periods of "tiredness" and "strange little bruises on her arms and legs." She states that she's been so tired that she has had to miss her last three soccer games. Her mother notes that she has recently been complaining of "growing pains" in both legs. She appears pale and listless. Vital signs are normal, but she has lost 6 lb since last month's adjustment. On oral examination, one tonsil is slightly swollen, and her supraclavicular lymph nodes are enlarged.

Case 3. 2-year-old Courtney presents with a 3-month history of vomiting and coughing spells. Her mother wonders if this is "some kind of virus." Courtney also has difficulty swallowing and "has been falling a lot." She has had several headaches in the last month including three that have awakened her from sleep. Her recent visit to the eye doctor revealed a normal check-up although she's been complaining that she sees "two Barneys on television." She has no fever and no history of seizure.

Case 4. 14-year-old Sally presents with a complaint of right arm pain that she says has been there for approximately 1 month. She thinks she was bitten by a spider. She says she feels as if her right breast has become "much larger than the left." She also complains of being short of breath and "sweating at night." When reclined on a high-low table, her face turns a striking purple. This facial color change is reproducible. Chest radiographics reveal a large mass in the mediastinum.

Case 1 = Osteosarcoma
Case 2 = Acute lymphocytic leukemia
Case 3 = Central nervous system tumor
Case 4 = Non-Hodgkin's lymphoma

The doctor of chiropractic can play a key role in educating childhood cancer survivors on the essentials of maintaining healthy lifestyle habits such as proper diet and exercise. Encouragement also can be given to avoid cancer-promoting behaviors such as smoking and high dietary fat consumption. Table 10 presents ways that the family chiropractor may help these children and their families. Table 11 gives a list of suggested reading for understanding more about childhood cancer, and Table 12 presents pediatric cancer vignettes.

NUTRITIONAL AND PSYCHOSOCIAL ASPECTS OF PEDIATRIC CANCER

While a full discussion of nutritional therapy for children with cancer is outside the scope of this article, it is clear that the doctor of chiropractic can be an important resource for information for families whose children have been diagnosed with cancer. A nutritional approach can play an important supportive role during and after traditional medical treatment.[33] The goals of a supportive nutrition plan for a child with cancer include maintaining adequate food intake and hydration, supporting the immune system, providing adequate antioxidants, and supporting detoxification pathways in the liver.[34]

One study[35] at the University of Cleveland showed positive effects from the use of a ketogenic diet in the care of two female pediatric patients with advanced stage malignant astrocytoma tumors. The diet was shown on positron emission tomography (PET) scan analysis to decrease glucose uptake by an average of 21.8% at the tumor sites in both cases. More research is needed in this promising area of nutritional intervention.

CONCLUSION

Childhood cancer is not an easy subject to broach. It brings visions of children without hair and with missing limbs. It makes one question the fairness of life and pulls at the heart strings of all those who encounter it. It is, however, a condition of utmost importance for the doctor of chiropractic to understand and stay alert for. Chiropractic care cannot cure children with cancer. Nevertheless, the chiropractic physician who cares for a child with cancer can be a vital link in his or her health care chain.

REFERENCES

1. Friebert S, Shurin S. Acute lymphoblastic leukemia: diagnosis and outlook. *Contemp Pediatr.* February 1998:118.
2. Dollinger M, Rosenbaum E, Cable G. *Everyone's Guide to Cancer Therapy.* Kansas City, KS: Somerville House Books Ltd; 1997.
3. Hay WW, Groothuis JR, Hayward AR, Levin MJ. *Current Pediatric Diagnosis and Treatment.* Stamford, CT: Appleton & Lange; 1997.
4. Merenstein GB, Kaplan DW, Rosenberg AA. *Handbook of Pediatrics.* Norwalk, CT: Appleton & Lange; 1994.
5. Barr RD. The challenge of childhood cancer in the developing world. *East Afr Med J.* April 1994:223–225.
6. Kenney LB, Miller BA, Ries LA, et al. Increased incidence of cancer in infants in the United States: 1980–1998. *Cancer.* April 1998:1396–1400.
7. Gallageher DJ, Phillips DJ, Heinrich SD. Orthopedic manifestations of acute pediatric leukemia. *Orthop Clin North Am.* July 1996:634–644.
8. Preston-Martin S, Pogoda JM, Mueller BA, et al. Maternal consumption of cured meats and vitamins in relation to pediatric brain tumors. *Cancer Epidem—Biomarkers Prev.* August 1996:599–605.
9. Yochum TR, Rowe LJ. *Essentials of Skeletal Radiology.* Baltimore: Williams & Wilkins; 1987.
10. Friebert SE, Shrun SB. ALL: treatment and beyond. *Contemp Pediatr.* March 1998:39–54.
11. Shiminski-Maher T, Shields M. Pediatric brain tumors: diagnosis and management. *J Pediatr Oncol Nurs.* October 1995:188–198.
12. Maria BL, Friedman T. Gene therapy for pediatric brain tumors. *Neuro Semin Pediatr.* December 1997:333–339.
13. Pogoda JM, Preston-Martin S. Household pesticides and risk of pediatric brain tumors. *Environ Health Perspect.* November 1997:1214–1220.
14. Orellana C, Hernandez-Mart'i M, Mart'inez F, et al. Pediatric brain tumors: loss of heterozygosity at 17p and TP53 gene mutations. *Cancer Genet Cytogenet.* April 1998:93–99.
15. Agamanolis DP, Malone JM. Chromosomal abnormalities in 47 pediatric bone tumors. *Cancer Genet Cytogenet.* June 1995:125–134.
16. Moss ME, Kanarek MS, Anderson HA, et al. Osteosarcoma, seasonality, and environmental factors in Wisconsin, 1979–1989. *Arch Environ Health.* May–June 1995:235–242.
17. Gelberg KH, Fitzgerald EF, Hwang S. Growth and development and other risk factors for osteosarcoma in children and young adults. *Int J Epidemiol.* April 1997:272–278.
18. Suita S, Zaizen Y, Sera Y, et al. Neuroblastoma in infants aged less than 6 months: is more aggressive treatment necessary? *J Pediatr Surg.* May 1995:715–721.
19. Tasdemiroglu E, Patchell RA. Neurologic complications of the primary pediatric extracranial neuroblastomas. *Neurol Res.* February 1997:45–50.
20. Russo C, Cohn S, Petruzzi M, deAlarcon P. Long-term neurologic outcome in children with opsoclonus-myoclonus associated with neuroblastoma: a report from the Pediatric Oncology Group. *Med Pediatr Oncol.* April 1997:284–288.
21. Hardell L, et al. Some aspects of the etiology of non-Hodgkin's lymphoma. *Environ Health Perspect.* April 1998:679–681.
22. Cerhan JR. New epidemiologic leads in the etiology of non-Hodgkin's lymphoma in the elderly: the role of blood transfusion and diet. *Biomed Pharmacother.* 1997;51(5):200–207.
23. Hawkins MH. Radiotherapy, alkylating agents and risk of bone cancer after childhood cancer. *J Natl Cancer Inst.* March 1996:270–278.
24. Oberfield SE. Endocrine late effects of childhood cancers. *J Pediatr.* July 1997:S37–S41.
25. Marina N. Long-term survivors of childhood cancer. The medical consequences of cure. *Pediatr Clin North Am.* August 1997:1021–1042.
26. Duggal MS. Dental parameters in the long-term survivors of childhood cancers compared with siblings. *Oral Oncol.* September 1997:348–353.

27. Aisenberg J, Hsieh K, Kalaitzoglou G, et al. Bone mineral density in young adult survivors of childhood cancer. *J Pediatr Hematol Oncol.* May–June 1998:241–245.
28. Fochtman D. Follow-up care for survivors of childhood cancer. *Nurs Pract Forum.* December 1995:194–200.
29. Talvensaari KK, Lanning M, Tapanainen P, et al. Long-term survivors of childhood cancer have an increased risk of manifesting the metabolic syndrome. *J Clin Endocrinol Metab.* August 1996:3051–3055.
30. Bhatia S, Robison LL, Oberlin O, et al. Breast cancer and other second neoplasms after childhood Hodgkin's disease. *New Engl J Med.* March 1996:745–751.
31. Kaste SC, Hudson MM, Jones DJ, et al. Breast masses in women treated for childhood cancer: incidence and screening guidelines. *Cancer.* February 1998:784–792.
32. Monaco GP, Fiduccia D, Smith G. Legal and societal issues facing survivors of childhood cancer. *Pediatr Clin North Am.* August 1997:1043–1058.
33. Andrawwy RJ, Chwals WJ. Nutritional support of the pediatric oncology patient. *Nutrition.* January 1998:124–129.
34. Conable K. Cancer-supportive nutrition. Pediatric nutrition from stages to specifics. October 1996.
35. Nebeling LC, Miraldi F, Shurin SB, et al. Effects of a ketogenic diet on tumor metabolism and nutritional status in pediatric oncology patients: two case reports. *J Am Coll Nutr.* April 1995:202–208.
36. Sorahan T, Lancashire RJ, Hult'en MA, et al. Childhood cancer and parental use of tobacco: deaths from 1953 to1955. *Br J Cancer.* AV4 1997:134–138.
37. Leiss JK, Savitz DA. Home pesticide use and childhood cancer: a case-control study. *Am J Public Health.* February 1995:249–252.
38. Wertheimer N, Savitz DA, Leeper E. Childhood cancer in relation to indicators of magnetic fields from ground current sources. *Bioelectromagnetics.* 1995;16(2):86–92.
39. Wakeford R. The risk of childhood cancer from intrauterine and preconceptional exposure to ionizing radiation. *Environ Health Perspect.* November 1995:1018–1025.
40. Feychting M. Magnetic fields and childhood cancer—a pooled analysis of two Scandinavian studies. *Eur J Cancer.* November 1995:2035–2039.
41. Ji BT, Shu XO, Linet MS, et al. Paternal cigarette smoking and the risk of childhood cancer among offspring of nonsmoking mothers. *J Natl Cancer Inst.* February 1997:238–244.
42. Daniels JL, Olshan AF, Savitz DA. Pesticides and childhood cancers. *Environ Health Perspect.* October 1997:1068–1077.
43. Feychting M, Svensson D, Ahlbom A. Exposure to motor vehicle exhaust and childhood cancer. *Scan J Work Environ Health.* February 1998:8–11.

Algorithm 1

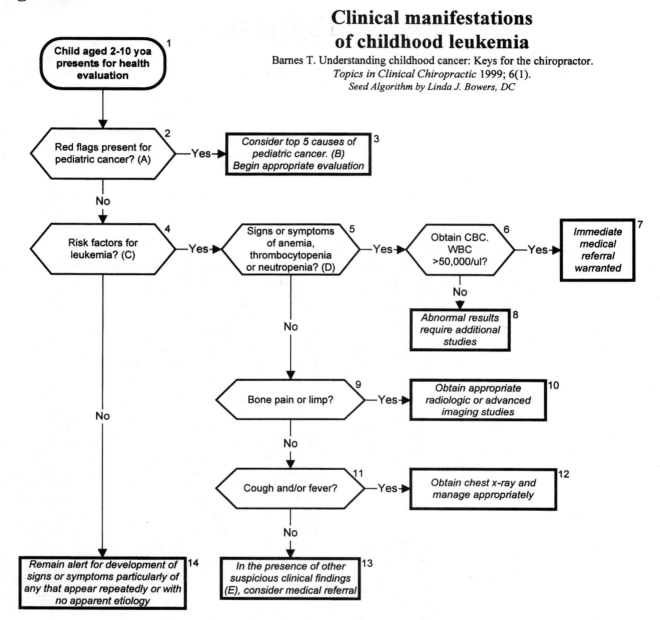

Annotations:
- (A) e.g., hard, non-mobile, non-tender lymph nodes; bone pain, especially when accompanied by recurrent fever; recurrent headaches, especially those that wake a child from sleep and/or those accompanied by vomiting
- (B) Leukemia, solid tumors of the CNS, bone cancer, neuroblastoma, lymphoma
- (C) e.g., exposure to ionizing radiation and certain chemicals such as benzene and antineoplastics; genetic factors such as Down's syndrome and Fanconi's anemia
- (D) e.g., anemia (pallor, fatigue, weakness); thrombocytopenia (epistaxis, bleeding gums, easy bruising); neutropenia (recurrent bacterial infections)
- (E) e.g., organ infiltration (splenomegaly, hepatomegaly); CNS infiltration (stiff neck, headache, vomiting); hypothalamus destruction (insatiable thirst or hunger); miscellaneous findings (ill feeling, rash, unilateral or asymmetric enlargements of palatine tonsils)

8

Adjusting the Pediatric Spine

Gregory Plaugher and Joel Alcantara

The subject of chiropractic care of children must by necessity include a discussion of the various techniques chiropractors use to address a subluxation.[1,2] The act of introducing a force into a spinal joint in an effort to restore mobility or alignment is termed an *adjustment*. This chapter discusses the technical aspects of adjusting the pediatric spine (ie, occiput to pelvis). Adjustment of the cranial bones and extremity articulations is not covered. The reader is referred to other resources for a discussion of these topics.[3–6]

Although rare, vertebrobasilar injury and stroke can occur following rotational motions of the neck, including those sustained during a rotational–thrust type of adjustive technique.[7] This subject is discussed along with recommendations for technique application in children.

SUBLUXATION

Although it is obvious to practicing chiropractors and their patients, the outside observer may not be aware of the clinical necessity of the spinal adjustment, since few may understand the "why" of this form of therapy. Basically, chiropractors adjust the vertebrae of the spine because signs of articular dysfunction (eg, restricted mobility, abnormal alignment, or inflammation) are present. This "dysfunction" is termed *subluxation*.

Subluxation, or sprain of a joint,[1] occurs when excessive loads are placed on the spinal column that exceed the elastic limits of the articulation. If the load that is applied is resisted by the individual within his or her normal range of motion, then injury is unlikely. If, instead, the motion segment is moved into the plastic zone, two changes occur simultaneously. First, trauma to the soft tissue–restraining elements (eg, annulus fibrosis or interspinous ligament) can occur, and second, there may be abnormal displacement of the motion segment, but usually less than that seen in a dislocation. Excessive loads can also occur due to compression trauma, leading to damage of the hyaline cartilage end plate[8] or fracture of the bony elements. Fracture–subluxations and subluxations combined with additional dislocations can also occur.[9,10]

In utero constraint,[11] birth trauma,[12] and a child's everyday activities or specific types of sports or recreational injuries can all potentially lead to damage of the spinal joints. The specific signs associated with spinal subluxation can include pain, limitation of motion, point tenderness, edema, redness, and neurologic changes (eg, altered joint proprioception, nerve irritation, and asymmetric skin temperature). These physical manifestations can vary somewhat in the newborn compared to an adult or adolescent. The positional displacement of the spinal segment can be assessed radiographically, and altered patterns of movement, fixation dysfunction, and hypermobility or instability are further assessed with radiographs taken at the end ranges of movement (eg, flexion-extension). Gross changes in spinal position can often be detected posturally (eg, structural scoliosis).

In some newborn patients the normal elasticity of the neonatal spine exceeds that of the stretch of the spinal cord, leading to severe injury. This can occur in the absence of significant radiographic alterations and is referred to as *spinal cord injury without radiographic abnormality* (SCIWORA).

Reprinted from *Top Clin Chiro* 1997; 4(4): 59–69
© 1997 Aspen Publishers, Inc.

The authors wish to thank Dr. Claudia, Dr. Ernst, Dr. Daniel, and Dr. Susi Anrig for providing the illustrations used in this chapter.

SUBLUXATION PATHOLOGY AND BACK PAIN IN CHILDREN AND ADOLESCENTS

Clinical research has shown that a variety of pathologic alterations can occur at spinal joints in adolescents. Erkintalo and colleagues[13] studied the development of degenerative changes in lumbar intervertebral discs. In this prospective randomized study, 31 subjects with back pain and 31 subjects without this complaint were sequestered from an original cohort of 1,503 14-year-old school children. The authors concluded that degenerative changes of the spine, including dehydration of the disc (ie, the nucleus pulposus), protrusion, and Scheuermann's changes emerge rapidly following the adolescent growth spurt. The degenerative process occurred in many asymptomatic as well as symptomatic patients. However, the signs associated with degeneration appeared more commonly in children with back pain and also occurred at an earlier age. These changes, including those ascribed to the Danish physician Scheuermann, are believed to be related to spinal trauma,[14] although genetic factors do play a role.

A study of 640 14-year-old children followed from 1965 through 1990 attempted to determine risk factors for the development of low back pain in adulthood.[15] Low back pain occurring during the growth period and family history were both associated with an increased risk. The lifetime prevalence for back pain was 84% for this cohort. Radiologic findings of lumbar or thoracic Scheuermann's disease were also evaluated and occurred in 13% of subjects. Irregular end plates occurred in 11% in subjects and disc degeneration was detected in 12%. Four subjects had spondylolisthesis, one subject had a structural scoliosis combined with Scheuermann's changes, and one had a congenital block formation between T-7 and T-8. The proportion of subjects having radiographic abnormalities was 36%. The studied radiographic changes were not associated with an increased incidence of back pain in adulthood. Interestingly, the investigators also found that there was a higher frequency of mental problems (eg, fear or depression) in the group of patients with radiographic changes in the T11–L2 area.

Taimela and colleagues[16] studied the prevalence of low back pain among children and adolescents in a nationwide, cohort-based survey in Finland. The subjects were 594 girls and 577 boys from 45 different schools. The questionnaire included items that investigated the subjects' past and current history of low back pain. Low back pain was classified based on its timing, duration, and location. Subjects with pain in the low back area that interfered with schoolwork or leisure activities during the preceding 12 months were defined as having back pain. Seven-year-olds had a low prevalence of back pain (1%), but 6% of 10-year-olds reported the problem. Eighteen percent of 14- to 16-year-olds had back pain. Overall, 26% of boys and 33% of girls reported chronic pain. The authors concluded that low back pain is a relatively common complaint during adolescence. By 14 years of age, a significant percentage of children report chronic and recurrent conditions.

Trauma to the intervertebral disc from excessive loading resulting in pain may first be noticed by the patient during adolescence, but many injuries cause only minimal symptoms or perhaps none at all. Salminen and colleagues[17] studied the association of disc abnormalities and low back pain in adolescents. Subjects were followed for 3 years. Nineteen percent of 15-year-olds without back pain had degenerated discs. This rose to 26% in the asymptomatic group by age 18. In subjects with back pain, 42% had degenerated discs at age 15, a percentage that rose to 58% by age 18. Disc protrusions had a similar pattern. No subject without back pain had a disc protrusion at age 15. By age 18, however, 16% of asymptomatic patients had signs of disc protrusion. Disc protrusion occurred in 65% of the 15-year-olds with back pain. Twenty-six percent of 18-year-olds with back pain had disc protrusions.

Ebrall[18] investigated the epidemiology of male adolescent low back pain in 610 12- to 19-year-old males from north suburban Melbourne, Australia. Point prevalence was 16.7%. A history of back pain at some point in the subjects' lives was reported by 57%. Most subjects with pain reported chronic problems, a few days at a time for several times a month, confirming results seen in other longitudinal studies.

Osteopaths[19] and European manual medicine physicians[20] have also discussed "somatic dysfunction" and "blockages" of the spinal articulations. Helig[19] noted that the longer the duration of osseous development during which asymmetric forces are acting, the greater the occurrence, duration, and extent of spinal damage. He also stated that if aberrant spinal function could be recognized and improved early on, there was a greater likelihood that normal developmental patterns would be established. Addressing the osteopathic profession, Helig appealed to his colleagues to consider spinal manipulation for children, since developmental changes can be most easily affected at an early age.

The studies cited above provide compelling evidence of motion segment injury in adolescents. How these variables relate to misalignment of the motion segment or motion dysfunction (eg, fixation) is presently unknown. In addition, the proportion of adolescents or other children who show alterations in cervical lordosis, retrolisthetic segments, or malpositions in lateral flexion or other directions of displacement is also unknown and deserves further study. Even in adults, this type of epidemiologic information is sorely lacking. Hopefully, spinal findings relating to childhood sports injuries (eg, gymnastics)[21] will provide the impetus for further work in this area. Unfortunately, many physicians as well as parents believe that the child's spine is nearly impervious to trauma, and only severe injuries (often neurologic), including motion segment dislocation, deserve clinical attention.

Biedermann,[22] a manual medicine practitioner, studied biomechanical problems (ie, subluxation) of the upper cervical spine in newborns. One hundred thirty-five infants who were available for follow-up were reviewed in this case series report. The infants were referred to the author because of asymmetric posture, and the case histories included tilt posture of the head or torticollis, head tilt in flexion, uniform sleeping patterns, crying when the mother tried to change the child's position, fixation of the sacroiliac joints, extreme sensitivity of the neck to palpation, and loss of appetite. Biedermann stated that if motor asymmetries, sleeping alterations, or facial scoliosis are present, then suboccipital articulations should be evaluated for blockages (ie, fixation dysfunction or subluxation). He also advocated the use of plain film radiographs for determining malalignment of the suboccipital region and for determining the appropriate direction for the force (ie, adjustment). The radiograph is also used for the detection of anomalies. Most patients in the series required one to three adjustments before returning to normal. The effects of chiropractic care on the newborn with suboccipital subluxation needs to be addressed in prospective randomized or comparison investigations.

Back pain is a highly prevalent condition in children. A large-scale survey[23] of 1,178 schoolchildren found that the cumulative prevalence of back pain was 51.2%. Lumbar, leg, and thoracic pain were the most common forms. Multivariate analysis showed that age, previous back injury, volleyball playing, female sex, and time spent watching television were positively correlated with the presence of back pain. Findings of a significant impact on low back pain among adolescent schoolchildren have been confirmed by other researchers.[24,25]

Low back pain is even more common among adolescent athletes. The excessive spinal loading that accompanies many sporting activities (eg, gymnastics and ice hockey) involves additional risk for acute low back injuries during the growth spurt and is harmful to the lower back.[26]

Manga and colleagues report on several independent evaluations of the effectiveness of chiropractic care in the management of adult patients with low back pain.[27] With regard to pain reduction, lost time from work, and patient satisfaction, chiropractic methods have continually been shown to be of greater benefit to patients than medical or physiotherapeutic treatments.[27–29] Children with these disorders have yet to be studied in large-scale investigations. However, the basic biologic nature of the lesion and therapeutics is likely to be similar in children and adults. Evidence of chronic problems developing in juveniles and adolescents and continuing into adulthood is provided above. This information provides further support for the clinical necessity of chiropractic care in children, despite the lack of specific clinical trial data in younger populations. Although studies of adult patients with back pain and the effects of chiropractic adjustments may be compelling, the specific issues surrounding the care of individual patients remains largely clinician driven, owing largely to the lack of substantive research on which to base clinical decision making. This is even more true in the pediatric population.

ADJUSTIVE TECHNIQUE MODIFICATIONS IN CHILDREN

Compared to adjusting the adult spine, adjusting the pediatric spine requires a number of modifications depending on the age and clinical presentation of the patient. These changes can be made readily by the seasoned clinician familiar with differing strategies for the adjustment. For example, a 6-foot, 200-pound man will be adjusted somewhat differently than a 5-foot, 100-pound woman. Although treating children may not be a large portion of practice for the average chiropractor, the fact that adjustments are modified constantly in adults should provide some assurance that both similar and unfamiliar modifications can be made in children, producing a safe and efficacious clinical encounter.

Age-related changes

The age and size of the patient should help guide the application of force. Older adolescents are adjusted similar to young adults. In the juvenile, however, one must consider some force modification, table positioning, and clinician contact points. The amount of force needed to produce the desired movement and positioning of the segment is less in smaller patients. These are, of course, generalizations, and a patient in acute pain with muscle spasm may need to be adjusted with a force similar to that used in a much older patient with substantially greater muscle mass, but not necessarily spasm.

The needs of young toddlers are quite substantial in comparison with those of other patient groups. The patient is beginning to demonstrate more muscle control, combined with an equally robust will. When these factors are combined, along with perhaps an ineffective understanding of the clinicians's needs in terms of patient relaxation and clinical presentation (eg, an acute asthma attack), one has a rather complex adjusting situation. It is not recommended that one try to surmount these challenges by treating the patient with less care or specificity or by forcing something on the patient that he or she does not wish to receive. Communication appears to be the only reasonable way of surmounting these difficulties. Communication can happen in a number of ways beyond the usual verbal (eg, affect–body language or demonstrations). If children are familiar with the protocol when their parents are being adjusted, then they may be more receptive to participate in the process once their turn comes. On the other hand, some clinicians generally avoid demonstrating the procedure prior to performing it, since some adjustments may appear more forceful and perhaps uncomfortable than the adjustment required by the patient. An element of surprise may also be helpful in executing the initial thrust, especially when the patient has a more serious disorder, and this cannot be discounted. If the patient can understand instructions, then in general the element of surprise should be used less. Ultimately, the patient may be under care for a long period of time, and almost always for more than one visit, so a patient who is trying to understand the procedures and cooperate with the clnician is favored over the patient who succumbs to a "surprise attack." Sometimes a combination of the two approaches can be made—perhaps an element of less education and surprise for the first adjustment, followed by gradually more patient information in order to make the encounter more similar to that of the older child. One of the authors' preferences is to provide minimal information except regarding how the adjustment may feel (eg, audible aspects) and how it will help the patient at the initial encounter, especially if the patient is acutely ill. The child–patient also should not watch the parent's care if such care is being provided at the same visit. If required, the parent is adjusted after the child. For infants, an explanation of the adjustment process is provided only to the parent.

Specificity of contact points

Because of the smaller dimensions of the child's spine, specificity of segmental contact points is necessary to avoid introducing forces into adjacent normal or hypermobile motion segments. In some instances smaller digits will have to be used in combination to achieve the desired level of specificity (Fig 1). The lack of specificity seen in double-thenar contacts (Fig 2) or the anterior dorsal adjustment (Fig 3) makes them unsuitable for the small child's spine.

Adjusting apparatus and positioning options for the child patient

Adjustments can be performed with the patient prone, seated, or in the lateral recumbent or supine positions. Several types of modifications of adjustive technique are available depending on the size and age of the patient and the segment to be adjusted.

The cervical spine can be adjusted in the prone position with a double-thumb contact (Fig 4). This type of contact enhances specificity on the small cervical spinous processes, and this type of adjustment with primarily a posterior to anterior (ie, flexion) pattern of thrust would be appropriate for a segment in an extended position.

If the clinician's hand is small enough and the patient is older, then the pisiform contact can be used (Fig 5). If specificity cannot be achieved, then the procedure is contraindicated.

Adjustment of the atlas in an infant, with the thumb used as the clinician's contact point, is shown in Fig 6. The patient

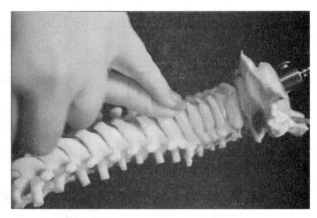

Fig 1. Digit-on-digit contact to enhance specificity on the spinous process of C-6. The pattern of thrust demonstrated is superior to inferior and posterior to anterior and is used to reduce a hyperextension subluxation of C-6 on C-7.

can be seated on a parent's or an assistant's lap. The cervical chair can also be used if the child is large enough (Fig 7).

The occiput can be adjusted in the supine position. Fig 8 shows an adjustment for an anterosuperior condyle subluxation (ie, hyperextension). The small-sized condyle block is used to support the posterior ring of the atlas and the subjacent cervical segments, and the thrust is made through the glabella to achieve flexion of the C0–C1 motion segment.

Thoracic adjustments can be performed in the prone position. In the case of the newborn, the patient can be positioned on the clinician's lap (Fig 9). The knee–chest table's headpiece can also be used for prone adjustments of the newborn (Fig 10). In the juvenile and adolescent, the knee–chest table

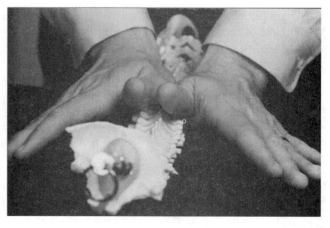

Fig 2. Double-thenar contact lacks specificity for the child's small spine.

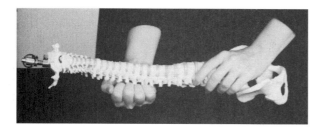

Fig 3. Anterior dorsal adjustment with contact on a child's spine. Five to six motion segments may be contacted depending on the size of the clinician's hand.

can also be used for specific adjustments. The knee–chest table can be modified to the small child's dimensions.[30] Fig 11 shows the knee–chest table being used in an adolescent and configured to the adult sizing position. By using the double-thumb contact, specificity is combined with the ability to generate sufficient force to move the segment (Fig 12). Similar positioning can be attained on the hi-lo table with a slackening of the tension of the abdominal section. However, the smaller child usually does not adapt well to the adult lengths of the various head, abdominal, and pelvic sections. The pelvic bench usually has a breathing/nose vent at one end and is acceptable for prone adjustments, especially those of the upper thoracic/lower cervical region.

Lumbar adjustments are accomplished with similar positions as in the adult. Adjustments can be made prone or in side posture. The side posture position for the adjustment, especially in the case of the acute injury, tends to be more comfortable for the patient. Clinician contact points should reflect the size of the patient's processes. Finger contact points are preferred over broad thenar contacts. In the infant

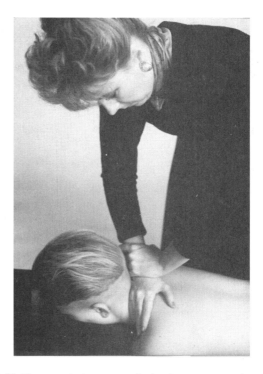

Fig 5. Pisiform contact on a cervical spinous process in a larger child.

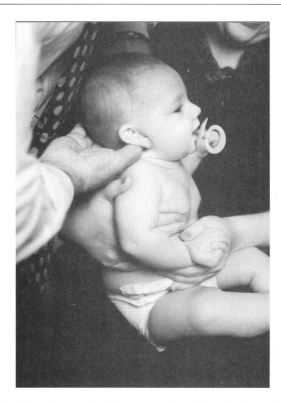

Fig 6. Atlas adjustment with the patient seated on the lap and supported.

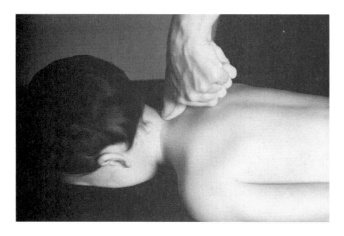

Fig 4. Double-thumb contact on a cervical spinous process.

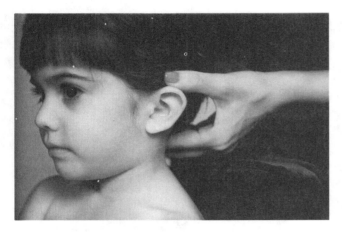

Fig 7. Cervical adjustment with the contact made at the distal lateral and palmar portion of the first index finger. The thrust is made inferior to superior and posterior to anterior to follow the pattern of motion of the segment in the sagittal plane.

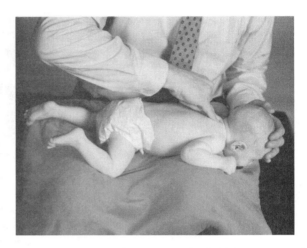

Fig 9. Prone adjustment of T-2 using a single-digit contact. Notice the towel placed under the child.

Thrust characteristics

With high-velocity–low-amplitude thrust techniques, substantial alterations can be made in the pediatric spine when compared to the adult spine, especially in toddlers and infants. In order to bring the motion segment "to tension," or preload, the pediatric spine usually requires a greater amount of displacement forward (ie, posterior to anterior). This ex-

the prone position can be used to adjust the lower lumbar vertebrae, as well as sacral segments (Fig 13). The infant can also be adjusted in the side posture position for both lumbar and sacral subluxations (Fig 14). The clinician should avoid excessive Y-axis torsion. Preload is applied at the level of the segment rather than attempting to achieve tension by winding up the spine from the top down (Fig 15).

The ilium can also be adjusted in the side posture and prone positions (Figs 16 and 17). The different force vectors that are applied are dependent on the specific findings of the patient.

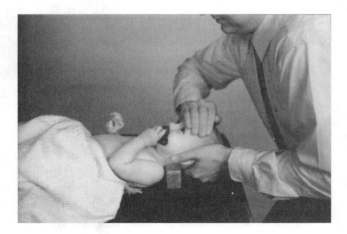

Fig 8. Anterosuperior condyle subluxation adjustment in the supine position.

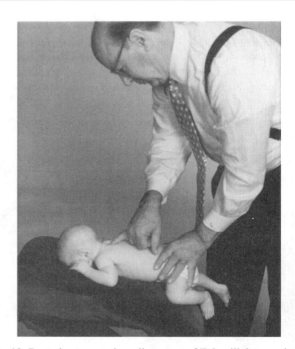

Fig 10. Posterior-to-anterior adjustment of T-2 utilizing a spinous process contact. The single fifth digit contact is appropriate for the large-fingered clinician.

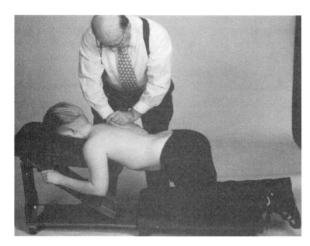

Fig 11. Knee–chest table thoracic adjustment using a transverse process–pisiform contact.

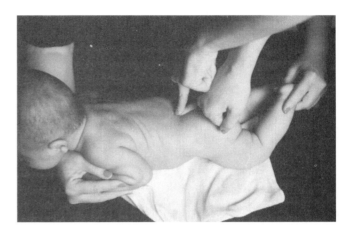

Fig 13. Prone digit-on-digit L-5 adjustment.

cursion of the articulation is essentially work (ie, force × distance). The increased range of motion in flexion–extension necessitates the increased preload. If the patient is agitated by the contact or loading provided by the clinician, then alterations and accommodations must be made. Only in rare circumstances should the thrust be made as the patient resists the force. The segment should be moved with as gentle a force as possible. Taking into account the different planes of the facet joints and the disc angles should result in a minimal amount of force being imparted to the patient.

In addition to enhanced preload, the high-velocity thrust will generally require an increased distance over the application (ie, work) owing to the greater flexibility in the child's spine. Although increased "depth" of the thrust may be required, the clinician should be aware that the thrust (the load) should be ceased immediately following the movement of the segment (usually combined with cavitation and an audible). The high-velocity loading should be decreased much more than what is usually performed in an adult. In the adult, a set-hold procedure, is usually well tolerated. The patient in essence can "stop" the thrust of the clinician. Therefore, "follow-through" is very important to achieving the desired movement. However, in the small child's spine, the follow-through is eliminated. Due to the potential danger of imparting too much force after joint cavitation, loading should be ceased immediately following cavitation of the articulation.

Increased acceleration during the thrust is generally required in the smaller spine. The infant or newborn is especially demanding in this regard. Little preload can be applied in many circumstances, necessitating that the clinician over-

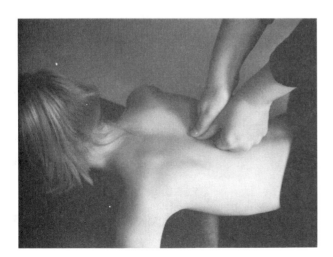

Fig 12. Double-thumb adjustment on the spinous process in the knee–chest position.

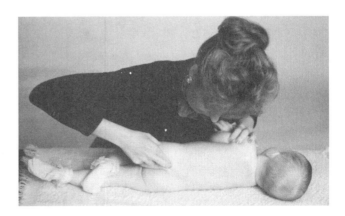

Fig 14. Side posture S-2 adjustment.

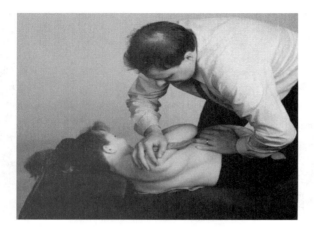

Fig 15. Incorrect side posture technique with excessive Y-axis torsion applied to the spinal column.

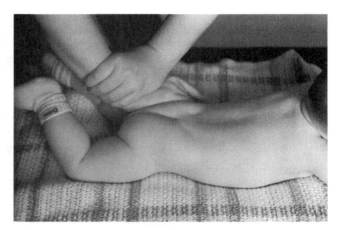

Fig 17. Prone anterosuperior ilium adjustment. The sprain is at the inferior aspect of the sacroiliac articulation, and the clinician's contact is with the pisiform on the rim of the acetabulum.

come the inertia of the segment in a more neutral position. This requires greater acceleration (high velocity) to accomplish the desired joint movement with cavitation. The cavitation may be very small, especially in the infant. It can be considered a benign by-product of the adjustment. The clinician should be focused instead on the extent of movement detected by his or her contact point. This important feedback provides information about the health of the articulation and how the adjustment can be accomplished in the future. Each adjusting encounter can be used by the clinician to "perfect" his or her technique with the individual patient. If the clinician gives some attention to these matters, then the patient receives a more safe and comfortable adjustment. Adjustment's should never be traumatic or cause inflammation. Inflammation associated with the delivery of the adjustment may further prolong the recovery from the sprain. Pain at a segment following an adjustment should be regarded as a contraindication for further treatment until a more thorough assessment can be made of the patient. The longer lasting the pain, the more serious the clinician's concern should be.

VERTEBROBASILAR STROKE IN CHILDREN

Incidence and mechanism of injury

Stroke in children is a very uncommon event, with an incidence estimated at about 2.52 cases per 1,000 per year in all

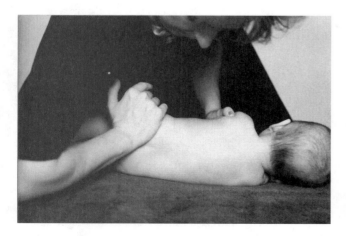

Fig 16. Side posture "internal" ilium adjustment. The PSIS is contacted by the pisiform on its medial aspect. The thrust is made posterior to anterior and medial to lateral.

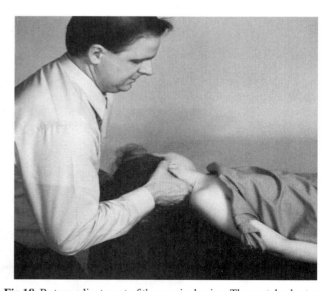

Fig 18. Rotary adjustment of the cervical spine. The vertebral artery is stretched in this maneuver. Cervical trauma or rotational thrust techniques can, in extremely rare instances, lead to a vertebrobasilar stroke.

racial and ethnic groups.[31] The mechanism of ischemic injury to the brain may be similar in children and adults (ie, embolism, thrombosis, or decreased systemic blood supply), but the causes of such injury differ. Adults are largely predisposed due to hypertension or atherosclerosis, whereas strokes in children are due in a large part to congenital heart disease (eg, heart valve stenosis, ventricular septal defects, or air and fat embolus), infection (eg, viral infection), metabolic disorders (eg, Ehlers-Danlos Syndrome, homocystinuria, and Fabry disease), hematologic diatheses (eg, protein S and C deficiency), and vasculopathy (eg, sickle cell disease or trauma).[32] Our discussion will focus mainly on traumatic cervical vascular injury.

Injuries to the carotid arteries may occur following traumatic insults to the neck and head due to motor vehicle and bicycle accidents, athletic injuries, falls, diving, or fights. Injury may also result intraorally, such as in a child who falls with a penetrating object (ie, a pencil) in his or her mouth. If the injury is to the common carotid arteries, hemiparesis is a common presentation. Angiographic studies show that injury is most common at the level of the carotid bifurcation. Pathologic findings may range from an intimal tear with a resulting thrombus to luminal obstruction from arterial dissection.

Injuries to the vertebral arteries may also occur due to trauma, as described above. However, traction injuries of the neck appear to especially cause injuries to the blood vessels, particularly at the atlanto-axial segment. Garg and colleagues[33] described three cases of children suffering from stroke due to trauma to the vertebral artery. They also described 16 other cases in the literature of children who had strokes due to pathologic abnormality in the vertebral arteries. In a majority of the cases, the significant damage was at the C1–C2 level. One case reported involved a 7-year-old boy who sustained a left vertebral artery occlusion at the C2 level after a chiropractic adjustment. Reported patient signs involved recurrent headaches, vomiting, left face weakness, ataxia, diplopia, and dysarthria manipulation.[33,34] In the upper cervical spine, the vertebral artery traverses superiorly in a posterolateral direction from the axis to the atlas. It is here that the vertebral artery is most vulnerable to compression and stretching, as well as forced lateral flexion, during head rotation.[35] Garg and Edwards-Brown[36] reported the case of a 21-month-old girl who suffered a thalamic stroke due to vertebral artery compression as a result of head turning. The child did not have vertebral anomalies such as spondylosis or osteophytes. The caveat regarding rotary adjustments—particularly excessive rotation and lateral flexion to achieve "tension"—must be kept in mind. The resultant injuries occur at the vertebrobasilar portion of the circulation. The central nervous system structures possibly affected are the brain stem, cerebellum, thalamus, and occipital and temporal lobes.[37] Symptoms of ischemic injury may include ataxia, facial paresis, tinnitus, vertigo, anisocoria, eye muscle palsies, dysmetria, dysesthesia, cortical blindness, difficulty swallowing, and changes in mental status, as well as general sensory-motor deficits.[38] Diagnosis relies heavily on recognition of the various signs of focal cerebral injury, as well as on familiarity with disorders mimicking cerebral infarction (eg, acute hemiplegia due to epileptic seizure). The chiropractor must obtain an accurate history and perform a complete physical examination.

The prognosis for the cases described by Garg and colleagues[33] was quite good. The reasons for better outcome in children are not clear but may be due in part to younger age and the state of the arteries. For example, there is a greater amount of vascular collateral reserve in the young brain, as well as greater scope for functional recovery (ie, brain plasticity). Also, children may have less exposure to risk factors such as hypertension, diabetes, smoking, and atherosclerosis.[33,39]

Rotational adjustments of the cervical spine

Although stroke following rotational spinal manipulation (Fig 18) is rare (1 per 1.46 million manipulations),[40] the results of such injuries can often be catastrophic (eg, lifetime disability or death). Screening procedures are very ineffective in identifying those patients at increased risk,[7] necessitating the use of nonrotational methods for this reason alone.

For biomechanical reasons, purely rotational forces directed at motion segments that normally exhibit primarily flexion–extension motion (eg, C0–C1, C2–L5) are unlikely to change fixation or altered position (eg, retrolisthesis) in this sagittal plane dimension.

In the upper cervical spine (eg, atlas) the neutral zone or "free play" of the C1–C2 motion segment is approximately 30° in the adult.[41] Rotational thrust techniques must move into this zone of movement and beyond in order to bring the joint to tension. The rotational thrust is intended to move the joint to its end range, approximately 40°, without exceeding the anatomic limits. These are generalities, and the individual patient's characteristics and the extent of any joint fixation can alter these values. A purely rotational method of achieving tension, combined with a thrust in Y-axis rotation, can stretch the vertebral artery. The ipsilateral artery on the side of rotation becomes kinked at approximately 30° and the contralateral vessel at 40°. Fortunately, the arteries are quite resilient to rotational forces. After all, humans were meant to turn their head. However, in a very small percentage of patients, the rotational thrust can cause an injury where none was previously present or aggravate an arterial injury already in progress from the patient's initial trauma.

Rotational adjustments of the cervical spine remain a part of the collection of various techniques a practitioner may use, but their use seems to be on the decline, at least in Perth,

Australia,[42] along with, apparently, a commensurate reduction in stroke injuries.[43] In the adult, these types of procedures should be avoided in preference to adjustments that are associated with less risk of injury.[7,44] It appears reasonable that their use as first-line treatment in children should not be recommended.

REFERENCES

1. *Oxford Dictionary of the English Language.* Oxford University Press; 1990.
2. Gatterman MI, Hansen DT. Development of chiropractic nomenclature through consensus. *J Manipulative Physiol Ther.* 1994;17:302–309.
3. Upledger JE, Vredevoogd JD. *Craniosacral Therapy.* Seattle, Wash: Eastland Press; 1983.
4. Upledger JE. *Craniosacral Therapy II: Beyond the Dura.* Seattle, Wash: Eastland Press; 1987.
5. Phillips C. Craniosacral therapy. In: Anrig CA, Plaugher G, eds. *Pediatric Chiropractic.* Baltimore, Md: Williams & Wilkins; 1998.
6. Collins SL, Sill MS, Ginsberg DA. Extravertebral disorders: Upper and lower extremities. In: Plaugher G, ed. *Textbook of Clinical Chiropractic: A Specific Biomechanical Approach.* Baltimore, Md: Williams & Wilkins; 1993.
7. Terrett AGJ. *Vertebrobasilar Stroke Following Spinal Manipulation.* Des Moines, Iowa: National Chiropractic Mutual Insurance Co; 1995.
8. Farfan HF. Biomechanics of the lumbar spine. In: Kirkaldy-Willis WH, ed. *Managing Low Back Pain.* New York, NY: Churchill Livingstone; 1983.
9. Plaugher G, Alcantara J, Hart CR. Management of the patient with a Chance fracture of the lumbar spine and concomitant subluxation. *J Manipulative Physiol Ther.* 1996;19:539–551.
10. Alcantara J, Plaugher G, Abblett D. Chiropractic management of a patient with a C6 lamina fracture and concomitant subluxation. *J Manipulative Physiol Ther.* 1997;20:113–123.
11. Dunne KB, Clarren SK. The origin of prenatal and postnatal deformities. *Pediatr Clin North Am.* 1986;33:1,277–1,297.
12. Gottlieb M. Neglected spinal cord, brain stem and musculoskeletal injuries stemming from birth trauma: Review of the literature. *J Manipulative Physiol Ther.* 1993;16:537–543.
13. Erkintalo MO, Salminen JJ, Alanen AM, Paajanen HEK, Kormano MJ. Development of degenerative changes in the lumbar intervertebral disk: Results of a prospective MR imaging study in adolescents with and without low-back pain. *Radiology.* 1995;196:529-533.
14. Ascani E, La Rosa G. Scheuermann's kyphosis. In: Weinstein SL, ed. *The Pediatric Spine: Principles and Practice.* New York, NY: Raven Press; 1994.
15. Harreby M, Neergaard K, Hesselsoe G, Kjer J. Are radiologic changes in the thoracic and lumbar spine of adolescents risk factors for low back pain in adults. A 25-year prospective cohort study of 640 school children. *Spine.* 1995;20:2,298–2,302.
16. Taimela S, Kujala UM, Salminen JJ, Viljanen T. The prevalence of low back pain among children and adolescents. A nationwide, cohort-based questionnaire survey in Finland. *Spine.* 1997;22:1,132–1,136.
17. Salminen JJ, Erkintalo M, Laine ML, Pentti J. Low back in the young. *Spine.* 1995;20:2,101–2,108.
18. Ebrall PS. The epidemiology of male adolescent low back pain in a north suburban population of Melbourne, Australia. *J Manipulative Physiol Ther.* 1994;17:447–453.
19. Helig D. Osteopathic pediatric care in prevention of structural abnormalities. *J Am Osteopath Assoc.* 1949;48:478–481.
20. Lewit K. *Manipulative Therapy in Rehabilitation of the Locomotor System.* London, England: Butterworth & Co; 1985.
21. Hager HJ. *Junghans' Clinical Implications of Normal Biomechanical Stresses on Spinal Function.* Rockville, Md: Aspen Publishers; 1990.
22. Biedermann H. Kinematic imbalances due to suboccipital strain in newborns. *J Manual Med.* 1992;6:151–156.
23. Troussier B, Davoine P, deGaudemaris R, Fauconnier J, Phelip X. Back pain in school children. A study among 1178 pupils. *Scand J Rehabil Med.* 1994;26:143–146.
24. Olsen TL, Anderson RL, Dearwater SR, et al. The epidemiology of low back pain in an adolescent population. *Am J Public Health.* 1992;82:606–608.
25. Balague F, Dutoit G, Waldburger M. Low back pain in school children. *Scand J Rehabil Med.* 1988;20:175–179.
26. Kujala UM, Taimela S, Erkintalo M, Salminen JJ, Kaprio J. Low back pain in adolescent athletes. *Med Sci Sports Exerc.* 1996;28:165–170.
27. Manga P, Angus D, Papadopoulos C, Swan W. *The Effectiveness and Cost-Effectiveness of Chiropractic Management of Low-Back Pain.* Ottawa, Ontario, Canada: Pran Manga & Associates; 1993.
28. *Clinical Practice Guidelines for Acute Low Back Problems in Adults.* Washington, DC: Agency for Health Care Policy and Research, US Public Health Service; 1994.
29. Shekelle PG, Adams AH, Chassin MR, Hurwitz EL, Brook RH. Spinal manipulation for low-back pain. *Ann Intern Med.* 1992;117:590–598.
30. Plaugher G, Lopes MA. The knee chest table: Indications and contraindications. *Chiro Tech.* 1990;2:163–167.
31. Schoenberg BS, Mellinger JF, Schoenberg DG. Cerebrovascular disease in infants and children: A study of incidence, clinical features and survival. *Neurology.* 1978;28:763–768.
32. Rivkin MJ, Volpe JJ. Strokes in children. *Pediatr Rev.* 1996;17:265–278.
33. Garg BP, Ottingger CJ, Smith RR, Fishman MA. Strokes in children due to vertebral artery trauma. *Neurology.* 1993;43:2,555–2,558.
34. Zimmerman AW, Kumar AJ, Gadoth N, Hodges FJ III. Traumatic vertebrobasilar occlusive disease in childhood. *Neurology.* 1978;28:185–188.
35. Frisoni GB, Anzola GP. Vertebral basilar ischemia after neck motion. *Stroke.* 1991;22:1,452–1,460.
36. Garg BP, Edwards-Brown MK. Vertebral artery compression due to head rotation in thalamic stroke. *Pediatr Neurol.* 1995;12:162–164.
37. Martin JH. *Neuroanatomy, Text and Atlas.* 2nd ed. Norwalk, Conn: Appleton & Lange; 1996.
38. Waxman SG, deGroot J. *Correlative Neuroanatomy.* 22nd ed. Norwalk, Conn: Appleton & Lange, 1995.
39. Martin PJ, Enevoldson TP, Humphrey PRD. Cause of ischaemic stroke in the young. *Postgrad Med J.* 1997;73:8–16.

40. Coulter ID, Hurwitz EL, Adams AH, et al. *The Appropriateness of Manipulation and Mobilization of the Cervical Spine.* Santa Monica, Calif: RAND; 1996.
41. White AA, Panjabi MM. *Clinical Biomechanics of the Spine.* 2nd ed. Philadelphia, Pa: JB Lippincott; 1990.
42. Haynes MJ. Stroke following cervical manipulation in Perth. *Chiro J Aust.* 1994;24:42–46.
43. Haynes MJ. Cervical spinal adjustments by Perth chiropractors and post-manipulation stroke: Has a change occurred?. *Chiro J Aust.* 1996;26:43–46.
44. Klougart N, Leboeuf-Yde C, Rasmussen LR. Safety in chiropractic practice. Part 1: The occurrence of cerebrovascular accidents after manipulation to the neck in Denmark from 1978–1988. *J Manipulative Physiol Ther.* 1996;19:371–377.

Appendix I–A

The Periodic Health Examination: Birth to 18 Months
(Schedule: 2, 4, 6, 15, 18 Months)*†

Leading Causes of Death

Conditions originating in perinatal period
Congenital anomalies
Heart disease
Injuries (nonmotor vehicle)
Pneumonia/influenza

Screening	Parent Counseling	Immunizations and Chemoprophylaxis
Height and weight	*Diet*	Diphtheria-tetanus-pertussis (DTP) vaccine[3]
Hemoglobin and hematocrit[1]	Breast feeding	Oral poliovirus vaccine (OPV)[4]
High Risk Groups	Nutrition intake, especially iron-rich foods	Measles-mumps-rubella (MMR) vaccine[5]
Hearing[2] (HR1)	*Injury Prevention*	*Haemophilus influenzae* type b (hib)
Erythrocyte protoporphyrin (HR2)	Child safety seats	**High-Risk Groups**
	Smoke detector	Fluoride supplements (HR3)
Remain Alert For	Hot water heater temperature	**First Week**
Ocular misalignment	Stairway gates, window guards, pool fence	Ophthalmic antibiotics[7]
Tooth decay		Hemoglobin electrophoresis (HR4)[7]
Signs of child abuse or neglect	Storage of drugs and toxic chemicals	T4/TSH[8]
	Syrup of ipecac, poison control telephone number	Phenylalanine[8]
	Dental Health	Hearing (HR1)
	Baby bottle tooth decay	
	Other Primary Preventive Measures	
	Effects of passive smoking	

High-Risk Categories

HR1 Infants with a family history of childhood hearing impairment or a personal history of congenital perinatal infection with herpes, syphilis, rubella, cytomegalovirus, or toxoplasmosis; malformations involving the head or neck (eg, dysmorphic and syndromal abnormalities, cleft palate, abnormal pinna); birth weight below 1500 g; bacterial meningitis; hyperbilirubinemia requiring exchange transfusion; or severe perinatal asphyxia (APGAR scores of 0–3, absence of spontaneous respirations for 10 min, or hypotonia at 2 hr of age). **HR2** Infants who live in or frequently visit housing built before 1950 that is dilapidated or undergoing renovation; who come in contact with other children with known lead toxicity; who live near lead processing plants or whose parents or household members work in lead-related occupation; or who live near busy highways or hazardous waste sites. **HR3** Infants living in areas with inadequate water fluoridation (less than 0.7 parts per million). **HR4** Newborns of Caribbean, Latin American, Asian, Mediterranean, or African descent.

*Five visits are required for immunizations. Because of lack of data and differing patient risk profiles, the scheduling of additional visits and the frequency of the individual preventive services listed in this table are left to clinical discretion (except as indicated in other footnotes).
†This list of preventive services is not exhaustive. It reflects only those topics reviewed by the US Preventive Services Task Force. Clinicians may wish to add other preventive services on a routine basis, and after considering the patient's medical history and other individual circumstances. Examples of target conditions not specifically examined by the Task Force include developmental disorders; musculoskeletal malformations; cardiac anomalies; genitourinary disorders; metabolic disorders; speech problems; behavioral disorders; parent/family dysfunction.
[1]Once during infancy.
[2]At age 18-month visit, if not tested earlier.
[3]At ages 2, 4, 6, and 15 months.
[4]At ages 2, 4, and 15 months.
[5]At age 15 months.
[6]At age 18 months.
[7]At birth.
[8]Days 3 to 6 preferred for testing.
Source: Reprinted with permission from *Report of the US Preventive Services Task Force: Guide to Clinical Preventive Services.* © 1989, Lippincott Williams & Wilkins.

The Periodic Health Examination: Ages 2–6 (Schedule)*†

Leading Causes of Death
Injuries (nonmotor vehicle)
Motor vehicle crashes
Congenital anomalies
Homicide
Heart disease

Screening	Patient and Parent Counseling	Immunizations and Chemoprophylaxis
Height and weight Blood pressure Eye examination for amblyopia and strabismus[1] Urinalysis for bacteriuria **High-Risk Groups** Erythrocyte protoporphyrin[2] (HR1) Tuberculin skin test (PPD) (HR2) Hearing[3] (HR3) **Remain Alert For** Vision disorders Dental decay, malalignment, premature loss of teeth, mouth breathing Signs of child abuse or neglect Abnormal bereavement	***Diet and Exercise*** Sweets and between-meal snacks, iron-enriched foods, sodium Caloric balance Selection of exercise program ***Injury Prevention*** Safety belts Smoke detector Hot water heater temperature Window guards and pool fence Bicycle safety helmets Storage of drugs, toxic chemicals, matches, and firearms Syrup of ipecac, poison control telephone number ***Dental Health*** Tooth brushing and dental visits ***Other Primary Preventive Measures*** Effects of passive smoking ***High-Risk Groups*** Skin protection from ultraviolet light (HR4)	Diphtheria-tetanus-pertussis (DTP)vaccine[4] Oral poliovirus vaccine (OPV)[4] ***High Risk Groups*** Fluoride supplements (HR5)

High-Risk Categories

HR1 Children who live in or frequently visit housing built before 1950 that is dilapidated or undergoing renovation; who come in contact with other children with known lead toxicity; who live near lead processing plants or whose parents or household members work in lead-related occupation; or who live near busy highways or hazardous waste sites. **HR2** Household members of persons with tuberculosis or others at risk for close contact with the disease; recent immigrants or refugees from countries in which tuberculosis is common (eg, Asia, Africa, Central and South America, Pacific Islands); family members of migrant workers; residents of homeless shelters; or persons with certain underlying medical disorders. **HR3** Children with a family history of childhood hearing impairment or a personal history of congenital perinatal infection with herpes, syphilis, rubella, cytomegalovirus, or toxoplasmosis; malformations involving the head or neck (eg, dysmorphic and syndromal abnormalities, cleft palate, abnormal pinna); birthweight below 1500 g; bacterial meningitis; hyperbilirubinemia requiring exchange transfusion; or severe perinatal asphyxia (APGAR scores of 0–3, absence of spontaneous respirations for 10 min, or hypotonia at 2 hr of age). **HR4** Children with increased exposure to sunlight. **HR5** Children living in areas with inadequate water fluoridation (less than 0.7 parts per million).

*One visit is required for immunizations. Because of lack of data and differing patient risk profiles, the scheduling of additional visits and the frequency of the individual preventive services listed in this table are left to clinical discretion (except as indicated in other footnotes).
†This list of preventive services is not exhaustive. It reflects only those topics reviewed by the US Preventive Services Task Force. Clinicians may wish to add other preventive services on a routine basis, and after considering the patient's medical history and other individual circumstances. Examples of target conditions not specifically examined by the Task Force include developmental disorders; speech problems; behavioral and learning disorders; parent/family dysfunction.
[1]Age 3–4.
[2]Annually.
[3]Before age 3, if not tested earlier.
[4]Once between ages 4 and 6.
Source: Reprinted with permission from *Report of the U.S. Preventive Services Task Force: Guide to Clinical Preventive Services.* © 1989, Baltimore, Lippincott Williams & Wilkins.

The Periodic Health Examination: Ages 7–12 (Schedule)*†

Leading Causes of Death

Motor vehicle crashes
Injuries (nonmotor vehicle)
Congenital anomalies
Leukemia
Homicide
Heart disease

Screening	Patient and Parent Counseling	Chemoprophylaxis
Height and weight	*Diet and Exercise*	*High-Risk Groups*
Blood pressure	Fat (especially saturated fat), cholesterol, sweets and between-meal snacks, sodium	Fluoride supplements (HR3)
High-Risk Groups		
Tuberculin skin test (PPD) (HR1)	Caloric balance	
	Selection of exercise program	
Remain Alert For	*Injury Prevention*	
Vision disorders	Safety belts	
Diminished hearing	Smoke detector	
Dental decay, malalignment, mouth breathing	Storage of firearms, drugs, toxic chemicals, matches	
Signs of child abuse or neglect	Bicycle safety helmets	
Abnormal bereavement	*Dental Health*	
	Regular tooth brushing and dental visits	
	Other Primary Preventive Measures	
	High-Risk Groups	
	Skin protection from ultraviolet light (HR2)	

High-Risk Categories

HR1 Household members of persons with tuberculosis or others at risk for close contact with the disease; recent immigrants or refugees from countries in which tuberculosis is common (eg, Asia, Africa, Central and South America, Pacific Islands); family members of migrant workers; residents of homeless shelters; or persons with certain underlying medical disorders. **HR2** Children with increased exposure to sunlight. **HR3** Children living in areas with inadequate water fluoridation (less than 0.7 parts per million).

*Because of lack of data and differing patient risk profiles, the scheduling of visits and the frequency of the individual preventive services listed in this table are left to clinical discretion.
†This list of preventive services is not exhaustive. It reflects only those topics reviewed by the US Preventive Services Task Force. Clinicians may wish to add other preventive services on a routine basis, and after considering the patient's medical history and other individual circumstances. Examples of target conditions not specifically examined by the Task Force include developmental disorders; scoliosis; behavioral and learning disorders; parent/family dysfunction.
Source: Reprinted with permission from *Report of the U.S. Preventive Services Task Force: Guide to Clinical Preventive Services.* © 1989, Baltimore, Lippincott Williams & Wilkins.

# The Periodic Health Examination: Ages 13–18 (Schedule)*†

Leading Causes of Death

Motor vehicle crashes
Homicide
Suicide
Injuries (nonmotor vehicle)
Heart disease

Screening	Counseling	Immunizations and Chemoprophylaxis
History	***Diet and Exercise***	Tetanus-diphtheria (Td) booster[5]
Dietary intake	Fat (especially saturated fat), cholesterol, sodium, iron,[2] calcium[2]	***High-Risk Groups***
Physical activity	Caloric balance	Fluoride supplements (HR15)
Tobacco/alcohol/drug use	Selection of exercise program	
Sexual practices	***Substance Use***	
Physical Examination	Tobacco: cessation/primary prevention	
Height and weight	Alcohol and other drugs: cessation/primary prevention	
Blood pressure	Driving/other dangerous activities while under the influence	
High-Risk Group	Treatment for abuse	
Complete skin examination (HR1)	***High-Risk Groups***	
Clinical testicular examination (HR2)	Sharing/using unsterilized needles and syringes (HR12)	
Laboratory Diagnostic Procedures	***Sexual Practices***	
High-Risk Groups	Sexual development and behavior[3]	
Rubella antibodies (HR3)	Sexually transmitted diseases: partner selection, condoms	
VDRL/RPR (HR4)	Unintended pregnancy and contraceptive options	
Chlamydial testing (HR5)	***Injury Prevention***	***Remain Alert For***
Gonorrhea culture (HR6)	Safety belts	Depressive symptoms
Counseling and testing for HIV (HR7)	Safety helmets	Suicide risk factors (HR11)
Tuberculin skin test (PPD) (HR8)	Violent behavior[4]	Abnormal bereavement
Hearing (HR9)	Firearms[4]	Tooth decay, malalignment, gingivitis
Papanicolaou smear (HR10)[1]	Smoke detector	Signs of child abuse and neglect
	Dental Health	
	Regular tooth brushing, flossing, dental visits	
	Other Primary Preventive Measures	
	High-Risk Groups	
	Discussion of hemoglobin testing (HR13)	
	Skin protection from ultraviolet light (HR14)	

High-Risk Categories

HR1 Persons with increased recreational or occupational exposure to sunlight, a family or personal history of skin cancer, or clinical evidence of precursor lesions (eg, dysplastic nevi, certain congenital nevi). **HR2** Males with a history of cryptorchidism, orchiopexy, or testicular atrophy. **HR3** Females of childbearing age lacking evidence of immunity. **HR4** Persons who engage in sex with multiple partners in areas in which syphilis is prevalent, prostitutes, or contacts of persons with active syphilis. **HR5** Persons who attend clinics for sexually transmitted diseases; attend other high-risk health care facilities (eg, adolescent and family planning clinics); or have other risk factors for chlamydial infection (eg, multiple sexual partners or a sexual partner with multiple sexual contacts). **HR6** Persons with multiple sexual partners or a sexual partner with multiple contacts, sexual contacts of persons with culture-proven gonorrhea, or persons with a history of repeated episodes of gonorrhea. **HR7** Persons seeking treatment for sexually transmitted diseases; homosexual and bisexual men; past or present IV drug users; persons with a history of prostitution or multiple sexual partners; women whose past or present sexual partners were HIV-infected, bisexual, or IV drug users; persons with long-term residence or birth in an area with high prevalence of HIV infection; or persons with a history of transfusion between 1978 and 1985. **HR8** Household members of persons with tuberculosis or others at risk for close contact with the disease; recent immigrants or refugees from countries in which tuberculosis is common (eg, Asia, Africa, Central and South America, Pacific Islands); migrant workers; residents of correctional institutions or homeless shelters; or persons with certain underlying medical disorders. **HR9** Persons exposed regularly to excessive noise in recreational or other settings. **HR10** Females who are sexually active or (if the sexual history is thought to be unreliable) aged 18 or older. **HR11** Recent divorce, separation, unemployment, depression, alcohol or other drug abuse, serious medical illnesses, living alone, or recent bereavement. **HR12** IV drug users. **HR13** Persons of Caribbean, Latin American, Asian, Mediterranean, or African descent. **HR14** Persons with increased exposure to sunlight. **HR15** Persons living in areas with inadequate water fluoridation (less than 0.7 parts per million).

*One visit is required for immunizations. Because of lack of data and differing patient risk profiles, the scheduling of additional visits and the frequency of the individual preventive services listed in this table are left to clinical discretion (except as indicated in other footnotes.)
†This list of preventive services is not exhaustive. It reflects only those topics reviewed by the U.S. Preventive Services Task Force. Clinicians may wish to add other preventive services on a routine basis, and after considering the patient's medical history and other individual circumstances. Examples of target conditions not specifically examined by the Task Force include developmental disorders; scoliosis; behavioral and learning disorders; parent/family dysfunction.
¹Every 1–3 years.
²For females.
³Often best performed early in adolescence and with the involvement of parents.
⁴Especially for males.
⁵Once between ages 14 and 16.
Source: Reprinted with permission from *Report of the U.S. Preventive Services Task Force: Guide to Clinical Preventive Services.* © 1989, Baltimore, Lippincott Williams & Wilkins.

APPENDIX I–B

Adolescent Health: On-line and Text Resources

Below are listed a number of resources for adolescents and practitioners on the Internet as well as several major texts recommended for further reading.

Texts
Adolescent Medicine. 2nd ed. Adele D Hofmann and Donald E Greydanus, eds. Norwalk, Conn: Appleton & Lange; 1989. ISBN 0-8385-0075-7.
Adolescent Medicine: A Practical Guide. Victor C Strasburger and Robert T Brown. Boston: Little, Brown; 1991. ISBN 0-316-81872-0.
Comprehensive Adolescent Health Care. Stanford B Friedman, ed. St Louis: Quality Medical Publishing; 1992. ISBN 0-942219-14-7.

Internet Resources for Practitioners
Centre for Adolescent Health home page at http://www.rch.unimelb.edu.au/adolescent/
Cooperative State Research, Education and Extension Service at http://www.agnr.umd.edu/users/nnfr/evaluation.html
National Clearing House for Youth Studies at http://131.217.45.44/ncys/home.htm
SHARK-Net Systems Helping At-Risk Kids at http://www.uq.edu.au/sharknet/
Youth Affairs Research Network (YARN) at http://yarn.edfac.unimelb.edu.au/
Youth Research Centre at http://yarn.edfac.unimelb.edu.au/yarn/yrc-home.html

Internet Resources for Adolescents
Caper at http://www.caper.com.au/ (for younger adolescents)
Lawstuff at http://www.lawstuff.org.au/
TeenNet at http://www.cyberisle.org/teennet/index.html

Appendix I–C

Children's Health Internet Sites

American Academy of Pediatric Dentistry	aapd.org/TOPICS.html
American Academy of Pediatrics	www.aap.org
Bright Futures	www.brightfutures.org
Canadian Paediatric Society	www.cps.ca/
Children and Medicine from US Pharmacopeia	www.usp.org/did/children
Children's Defense Fund	www.childrensdefense.org/
Consumer Products Safety Commission	cpsc.gov/
International Pediatric Association	www.urmc.rochester.edu/IPA/welcome.htm
iPeds, The Interactive Journal of Pediatrics	www.medconnect.com/finalhtm/journals/ipedsmain.htm
National Maternal and Child Health Clearinghouse	www.nmhc.org/
Pediatric Database (PEDBASE)	www.icondata.com/health/pedbase/index.htm
Pedatrics Journal	www.pediatrics.org/
Physician's Desk Reference	www.pdr.net/
United States Preventive Service Task Force 2nd Edition	158.72.20.10/pubs/guidecps/

Part II

Women's Health

9

Heart Disease in Women

Jennifer R. Jamison

Coronary heart disease (CHD) remains a major cause of death in developed countries. Although ischemic heart disease is a more prevalent cause of death among men and much of the information on this condition has been derived from male-dominated studies, a substantial body of specific evidence is emerging with respect to the prevalence, pathogenesis, presentation, and prognosis of this condition in women. CHD is responsible for the death of approximately 250,000 American women each year, affecting some 10.4 million American women.[1,2] It is the leading cause of death in American women over the age of 50 and the second most common cause of death in white females between the ages of 35 and 39.[1,2] Mortality rates among women in the United States declined after 1968 but then leveled off in 1976. In contrast, death rates in white males continued to decline during the 1968 to 1985 period. More recent studies[3] including North, South, and Central America suggest a relatively greater decline among women when mortality attributable to all cardiovascular diseases is the end point.[3]

CHARACTERISTICS

When compared with men,[1,2] CHD in women is more age dependent. Older women are at far greater risk than young women. CHD presents most often as angina pectoris. Angina attributable to coronary artery spasm rather than atherosclerosis is also more common in women. A study comparing unstable angina in men and women under the age of 60 years found that women were, on average, almost 2 years younger than the males, had a higher serum cholesterol level, were more likely to be hypertensive, and less likely to be lifetime smokers.[4] Women are less prone to present with myocardial infarction or sudden death than men.

CHD in women is associated with a higher proportion of unrecognized myocardial infarcts and a poorer initial survival rate after infarction. Women are more likely to die within the first year after infarction and are more likely to have a reinfarction in the first 10 years after the initial event than men. Female gender is an independent and significant risk factor for mortality following acute myocardial infarction.

CHD in women is more difficult to diagnose by noninvasive means. Except for women over the age of 70 with angina, history provides, at best, a moderate guide to diagnosis. History and noninvasive tests are far less conclusive in women than in men. Exercise electrocardiography (ECG) in women, although useful for assessing fitness and prognosis after myocardial infarction, fails to evaluate the presence of disease. Rest and exercise radionuclide ventriculography are relatively inaccurate, and the results of thallium 201 perfusion imaging are compromised by overlying breast tissue. Cardiac fluoroscopy used to detect calcification of coronary arteries has greater specificity than exercise ECGs in women, yet a disproportionate number of women with unstable angina have normal coronary arteries. The prevalence of calcium in coronary arteries in asymptomatic individuals is half that in men until women reach 60 years of age.[5,6] Therefore, diagnosis in women requires coronary angiography.

It is often less aggressively treated,[7] and interventions are often less effective in women than men. Women have an unfavorable prognosis following myocardial infarction. The importance of preventing infarction therefore becomes a major goal in management of this condition. While primary prevention of CHD should remain the major strategy, as women who have angina have a more favorable prognosis than men, intervention at this level constitutes a viable de-

Adapted from *Top Clin Chiro* 1997; 4(3): 21–29
© 1997 Aspen Publishers, Inc.

fault option. In both instances the dominant thrust of intervention is to identify and correct modifiable risk factors.

PATHOGENESIS

Angina and myocardial infarction represent varying degrees of cardiac ischemia attributable to structural or functional obstruction of the coronary arteries. The clinical presentation varies depending on the completeness of the occlusion, the distribution of the affected artery, and the collateral circulation of the involved area. It is generally accepted that coronary disease may become symptomatic once more than half the lumen is lost. Intervention during this asymptomatic period focuses on the early detection and correction of various risk factors. In general risk factors fall into two groups: those responsible for the generation of the atheromatous plaque and those precipitating the critical event.

The initial arterial lesion is a fatty streak resulting from the accumulation of droplets of fat in the endothelial and smooth muscle cells of the arterial wall. The consequence of macrophage ingestion of low density lipoprotein-cholesterol (LDL-C) is the formation of foam cells. The presence of oxidized LDL enhances foam cell formation, inhibits macrophage migration, and attracts circulating monocytes to the evolving lesion. The resultant inflammatory lesion proliferates and ultimately bulges into the arterial lumen. The precipitating or critical event occurs when the vessel is occluded either due to thrombus formation or vasospasm. Ulceration of the lesion provides a focus for thrombosis. Lesion ulceration also sheds atheromatous debris that may occlude the vessel distally.

Risk factors have been linked both with atherosclerosis and the critical event. The critical event may be precipitated by thrombosis or vasospasm. Although particular risk factors may have a stronger impact at one level, many risk factors have a dual action. Smoking and the more recently recognized risk of low serum vitamin E levels have been clearly implicated in the pathogenesis of coronary artery disease at both the level of atherosclerosis and thrombosis. The potential for smoking to enhance a hypercoagulable state and facilitate vasospasm links it more closely to the critical event. In contrast, the concentration and nature of serum cholesterol levels have been strongly implicated in atherosclerosis. Of all risk factors, it has been estimated that hypercholesterolemia accounts for 30% to 40% of all coronary disease, hypertension for 20% to 25%, and smoking for 15%.[8] Diabetes mellitus and obesity also have been recognized as risk factors for coronary artery disease. Diabetes mellitus and left ventricular hypertrophy appear to be particularly important risk factors for CHD in older women.[2]

While it may be argued that some of these risk factors are more important in men, their role in the pathogenesis of female coronary artery disease is not disputed. Indeed, while smoking and hypercholesterolemia are more prevalent in young men than young women, this relationship is reversed in the older age groups.[9] The prevalence of hypertension is similar or actually favors women. An additional, well established risk factor unique to women is menopause with its resultant drop in estrogen levels. Other risk factors more tenuously linked with an increased risk of coronary artery disease in women have been studied. Objective monotonous work conditions, especially when involving short cycle hectic repetitive work, are consistently related to CHD risk factors in women.[10] Repetitive work appears to be positively associated with blood pressure and serum lipid levels in women.

Studies[11] suggest that 6 years or more of shift work may increase the risk of CHD in women. Women with parents who have had higher education have lower levels of cholesterol, triglycerides, and apolipoprotein-B, and higher levels of apolipoprotein A-1 (good cholesterol) than those whose parents were not well-educated persons.[12] As the female group in this study was limited to 47 subjects, these results need further investigation. In any event, no similar association was found in men.[13] Low socioeconomic status in childhood was associated with a modest increase in the risk of nonfatal myocardial infarction and cardiovascular disease in women in a 14-year prospective study of approximately 117,000 registered female nurses in the United States.[14]

The risk of atherosclerosis is a function of genetic composition and environmental exposure. Individuals with apoprotein E4 alleles are at increased risk of developing increased serum cholesterol levels, enhanced cholesterol absorption, and demonstrable failure to control cholesterol metabolism metabolically. Despite such genetic susceptibility, modifying the cellular environment may reduce the likelihood of coronary artery disease. The magnitude of risk reduction depends on the underlying genetic risk, and the combined impact of each beneficial lifestyle choice and patient compliance with management recommendations. Algorithm 1 details risk factor considerations.

HYPERTENSION

The ideal target for blood pressure is less than 140/90 mm Hg. Current explanations linking hypertension and atherosclerosis suggest three important variables that deserve consideration.[14] First, the endothelium is a metabolically active secretory organ that secretes a potent vasoconstrictor, endothelin, and a powerful vasodilator, nitric oxide. Like other vasoactive agents, these chemicals affect vascular proliferation. Vasoconstrictors promote cellular growth, whereas vasodilators inhibit growth. Endothelial endocrine function responds to changes in shear stress imposed on cells by adjacent blood flow characteristics. Therefore, changes in blood flow and viscosity may affect vasoactive secretions.

Second, the renin-angiotensin system is found throughout the arterial tree and is principally located in the medial layer of arteries. A potent vasoconstrictor and cellular growth promoting system is consequently located close to the potential site for atheroma formation. Inhibition of the renin-angiotensin system may reduce formation of atherogenic LDL-C fragments and antagonizes trophic and growth effects exerted on small muscle cells and macrophages during atherogenesis.

Last, hypertension is one component of the genetically linked insulin-resistant syndrome. This syndrome, characterized by central/abdominal obesity, hypertriglyceridemia, low high density lipoprotein cholesterol (HDL-C), hypertension, and impaired glucose tolerance has been associated with an increased risk of coronary artery disease.

Whatever the mechanism, it has been suggested that should the population decrease its systolic blood pressure by an average of 2 mm Hg, a 4% reduction in CHD will result.[15] Greater reductions in systolic hypertension are postulated to achieve even greater reductions in deaths attributable to CHD. Based on 1985 figures, it was suggested that a systolic reduction of 2 mm Hg to 5 mm Hg would save 11,800 lives and 27,600 lives, respectively, in the 45 to 64 age group.[15] Blood pressure reductions of this amplitude are possible using non-drug measures such as lifestyle modifications. A reduction of sodium intake from 170 to 70 µmol is predicted to reduce systolic blood pressure by 2 mm Hg; reduction of the body mass index (BMI) from 25 to 23 can reduce blood pressure by 1.55 mm Hg; and reduction of alcohol intake may achieve a fall in systolic blood pressure of even greater magnitude (2.8 mm Hg).[15]

The major non-drug measures are to reduce sodium intake, to limit alcohol consumption, and to achieve an ideal body weight.[15] Regular consumption of 30 g to 40 g of alcohol has a pressor effect. More than three drinks (3 oz of alcohol) a day is regarded as excessive. The pressor effect of alcohol plateaus at a daily consumption of about 80 g. A useful lay guideline is that for every one alcoholic drink consumed each day systolic blood pressure rises 1 mm Hg. The hypertensive effect of alcohol is probably reversed in 7 to 28 days.[15] Blood pressure medication is not as effective in heavy drinkers as in light drinkers, and "binge" drinkers are at increased risk of having a stroke.

Although body weight and alcohol intake are more important predictors of hypertension than sodium intake, sodium reduction remains a viable strategy, particularly in salt-sensitive persons. A rise in systolic blood pressure of 2.2 to 4.5 mm Hg is predicted for each 100 µmol of sodium intake. Furthermore, the rise in blood pressure with age appears to be sodium dependent. At least 5 weeks of reduced intake is required before the effects of sodium reduction are detectable. About 10% of sodium intake is from natural sources, 15% from salt added during home cooking, and 75% from manufactured foods. Dietary measures that achieve an intake of around 70 µmol (1.5 g) of sodium per day are listed in Table 1.[16]

Care should be taken to read labels. "Reduced sodium" indicates that at least 25% less sodium is present than in the product being replaced. Low sodium and very low sodium labels indicate the presence of no more than 140 mg and 35 mg, respectively, of sodium per serving. A sodium free label indicates that one serving contains no more than 5 mg of sodium. An awareness that table salt is not the only vehicle for dietary sodium ingestion is also necessary.

As the sodium:potassium (Na:K) ratio appears a better predictor of blood pressure than either sodium or potassium alone, a diet rich in fruit and vegetables is desirable. A change in the Na:K ratio from 3.09 to 1.0 is anticipated to cause a 1.55 mm Hg reduction in systolic blood pressure.[15] A Na:K ratio of less than 1.0 is recommended for optimum health.

The vegetarian diet combines a number of factors associated with lower blood pressure. Its beneficial effect may be related to the favorable effect on blood glucose levels from a diet high in complex carbohydrates; increased dietary potassium, magnesium, fiber, and decreased fat; unidentified substances in fruit and vegetables; and the lower BMI of vegetarians.

In all cases, dietary changes should be accompanied by exercise advice. A high level of physical fitness has been associated with a lower subsequent risk of developing hypertension in women, and moderate intensity aerobic exercise is able to reduce blood pressure in hypertensive women. Female cardiorespiratory fitness is construed as a useful strategy for reducing the risk of coronary events.[17]

Exercise equivalent to brisk walking (60% to 70% of maximum work capacity) for 30 min on 3 days of the week is recommended. There seems to be little gain from increasing exercise sessions beyond three times per week in the management of hypertension. The benefits associated with exercise have been found to persist in those who continue to train (study undertaken over a 12-month period).[18] The benefits of exercise are demonstrable within 1 week of initiating the exercise program.[18]

Table 1. Dietary measures to decrease salt consumption

- Never add salt to prepared food.
- Do not add salt to food during its preparation.
- Avoid all visibly or heavily salted foods.
- Avoid most processed foods such as bacon, peanut butter, and corned beef.
- Replace salted sauces with "low" or "no" salt varieties.

Source: Data from Jamison Health Promotion for Chiropractic Practice, p. 199.

CHOLESTEROL

Low blood cholesterol levels are a major target for the prevention of atherosclerosis. At levels of over 6.5 µmol/L (251 mg/dL), each 0.5 µmol/L (19 mg/dL) rise of cholesterol doubles the risk of CHD.[19] An increase of 0.5 µmol/L of total cholesterol corresponds to a 12% increase in death from CHD.[20]

The total serum cholesterol level is, however, a composite figure that reflects different indices with diverse implications. Total cholesterol measures both LDL-C of which high levels are associated with a increased risk of CHD, and HDL-C, which is inversely proportional to the risk of CHD. The risk of CHD increases progressively as the LDL-C level rises above 3.0 µmol/L.[19] CHD risk increases 2% to 3% for every 1% drop in HDL-C. The prevalence of low HDL levels is 17 times greater in women with coronary artery disease.[21] A low HDL-C level predicts coronary artery disease at all levels of total cholesterol.[22]

Hypertriglyceridemia (>2.3 µmol/L) becomes a risk factor in those patients who have a reduced HDL. Triglycerides and HDL-C levels are inversely proportional. As triglycerides increase, HDL-C levels decrease. Patients with this lipid pattern have a pattern of LDL particles that are smaller, more dense, and more readily oxidized.[21] Ideal blood lipid profiles are listed in Table 2.

Although the excess risk of fatal and nonfatal coronary heart events correlates more directly with total cholesterol and LDL levels in men under 65 years of age, this parameter is relevant to older men and women.[23] As there is no threshold level for blood cholesterol, and reduction of high serum cholesterol correlates with a decreased risk of CHD in men and women, monitoring and modifying blood cholesterol remain relevant for both sexes.

Dietary measures to reduce the risks of hypercholesterolemia include increasing HDL levels and reducing LDL and triglyceride levels. Various authors[22,24] have proposed lifestyle modifications that may increase HDL-C. Table 3 indicates measures that may raise HDL-C. HDL levels are also reduced by certain noncardioselective beta-blockers and diuretics (thiazides). Use of these agents should therefore be avoided if possible when treating hypertension in women with other coronary risk factors. Table 4 reflects methods of reducing LDL-C.

Triglyceride levels are reduced by achieving and maintaining an ideal body weight. Weight loss, in addition to normalizing triglycerides, affects cholesterol levels. Excess weight has been found to correlate with an increased cardiovascular risk in Caucasian American women. Total cholesterol levels are higher, and HDL levels are significantly lower in overweight persons.[25]

Contemporary thinking suggests that the major cholesterol risk may arise, not from native, but from oxidized cholesterol. Oxidized LDL is not recognized by the LDL receptor and is instead taken up by scavenger receptors found on macrophages. Oxidized LDL, when taken up by subendothelial macrophages, initiates their transformation into foam cells. Oxidized LDL appears to be cytotoxic to endothelial cells and may enhance arterial vasoconstriction. There are several means to minimize oxidation of LDL-C.[26–29] These techniques are listed in Table 5.

Ingesting 800 IU of vitamin E halves the rate of oxidation of LDL. While no threshold level has been identified, 300 IU of vitamin E decreases the oxidation rate of LDL while less than 100 IU appears not to be effective. The body tends to utilize more of each milligram of natural alpha-tocopherol

Table 2. Desirable blood lipid profiles

Ideal targets for blood lipids are:
- Total cholesterol <5.5 µmol/L
- HDL cholesterol >1.0 µmol/L
- Triglyceride <2.0 µmol/L
- Cholesterol: HDL <4.5 females, <5.0 males

Source: Data from Jamison Health Promotion for Chiropractic Practice, p. 199.

Table 3. Factors that increase HDL-cholesterol

- Regular aerobic exercise
- Smoking cessation
- Maintaining an ideal body weight
- Supplementing with beta-carotene
- Increasing dietary monounsaturated fatty acids (olive oil, canola oil, peanut oil)
- Supplementing with nicotinic acid
- Light alcohol consumption (1 oz/day)

Source: Data from Jamison Health Promotion for Chiropractic Practice, p. 199.

Table 4. Factors that lower LDL-cholesterol

- Increase dietary soluble fiber 25 g/day (oats, barley, lentils, legumes, fruit).
- Eat monounsaturated fatty acids.
- Avoid saturated fats.
- Avoid trans fatty acids (eg, processed vegetable oils).
- Avoid foods rich in preformed cholesterol (eg, brains, shellfish).
- Avoid palm kernel oil and coconut oil.

Source: Data from Jamison Health Promotion for Chiropractic Practice, p. 199.

Table 5. Minimizing oxidation of LDL-cholesterol

- Supplement with beta-carotene 6–20 mg/day.
- Supplement with vitamin E.
- Drink red wine (1 oz alcohol [8 oz wine]).
- Take garlic tablets (300 mg three times a day).
- Cease smoking.

Source: Data from Jamison Health Promotion for Chiropractic Practice, p. 199.

---

than an equal amount of synthetic forms of vitamin E. However, the E in supplements is sold in international units (IU), which measure the vitamin activity in the body, not by weight. Therefore, 100 IU units of synthetic vitamin E is supposed to be as potent as 100 IU of natural vitamin E. As it is difficult to obtain this much vitamin E in the typical diet, supplementation is recommended.

Garlic deserves particular mention. It appears to benefit cardiovascular health through mechanisms that favorably influence serum lipid levels, lipid oxidation, platelet function, fibrinolysis, and blood pressure. Garlic reduces total cholesterol[30,31] and more specifically reduces LDL-C without affecting HDL-C.[32] In vivo tests have furthermore suggested that garlic may retard lipoprotein oxidation.[29] Encouraging patients to eat more garlic is prudent advice.

In addition to garlic and vitamin E, coronary artery disease risk appears to be reduced when plasma concentrations of the following vitamins meet the listed concentration per liter: >27.5 to 30.0 µmol vitamin D, 0.4 to 0.5 µmol carotene, 40 to 50 µmol vitamin C, and 2.2 to 2.8 µmol vitamin A.[33] The benefits of vitamins E and C and beta-carotene in women with preexisting cardiovascular disease are currently under investigation.[34]

MENOPAUSE

A particular risk factor that deserves consideration in any discussion of coronary artery disease in women is menopause. Estrogen is known to have a favorable effect on serum lipids, in particular HDL-C. In postmenopausal women this effect is achieved using estrogen replacement.[35,36] Prevention of CHD requires at least 10 years, and possibly lifelong, hormone replacement therapy (HRT). This strategy reduces the risk of heart disease in postmenopausal women by as much as 50%.[37,38]

HRT raises HDL-C and lowers LDL-C. Postmenopausal women, compared with premenopausal women, have significantly higher levels of total cholesterol, triacylglycerols, and LDL-C.[39] HRT lowers lipoprotein(a) levels by 35% as well as reducing total and LDL-C by 17%. Combined HRT lowers LDL-C by an average of 0.6 µmol/L. HRT should be regarded as the first line of drug therapy for postmenopausal women with hypercholesterolemia. In addition to its effects on blood lipids, estrogen relaxes the blood vessel wall and reduces anginal pain. The anti-anginal effects of estrogen are noted in women but not men.

In addition to its anti-atherogenic effect, HRT has an antithrombotic effect. There is an increase in the risk of thrombosis when serum levels of lipoprotein(a) exceed 18 mg/dL. Lipoprotein(a) contains a protein that impedes the dissolution of blood clots. HRT reduces lipoprotein(a) levels.

OBESITY

Body fat distribution is genetically determined. The biologic factors determining body fat distribution also seem to influence cardiovascular risk. Central body fat distribution is emerging as an important risk factor for atherosclerosis. Abdominal fat distribution appears to be associated with decreased insulin sensitivity, increased activity of hepatic lipase, and a shift to small dense LDL particles. The typical male pattern of body fat distribution (abdominal, android, or apple shape) differs from the typical female pattern of fat distribution (buttocks and hips, gynoid or pear shape). The male or abdominal rather than female distribution of body fat carries an increased risk of coronary artery disease. A report in the *Australian Doctor*[40] discusses an experimental group of 50 non-obese men and women who were put on a diet high in saturated fat and cholesterol. The result was an increased total cholesterol, LDL-C, and HDL-C in both groups. While LDL-C increased equally in both groups, there was a differential increase of HDL-C. HDL-C increased most in pears (female fat distribution) and least in apples (male fat distribution). Whether body fat distribution represents an index of the protective effects of estrogen is unknown.

In 1990 the United States modified its weight guidelines recommending a BMI of between 21 and 27 for women over the age of 35.[41] These changes increased the upper limit of desirable weights and suggested that weight gain of 4.5 to 6.8 kg was consistent with good health. These recommendations have been disputed.[41] In a longitudinal study of 115,818 women aged 30 to 55 years over a period of 14 years, Willett and co-workers[41] found that weight gain after 18 years of age remained a strong predictor of heart disease, even when such weight gain occurred within the 18 to 25 BMI range. High levels of body weight within the "normal" range as well as modest weight gains after the age of 18 years appear to increase the risk of coronary artery disease in middle-aged women. The lowest risk of coronary artery disease is found in women with a BMI less than 21 kg/m². BMI is calculated by dividing the weight in kilograms by the height in meters squared. In a study of

121,700 nurses in the United States, it was found that weight was inversely related to the risk of coronary artery disease.[42] The excess risk of diabetes mellitus with even modest weight gain is substantial.[43]

SMOKING

Cigarette smoking has also been found to be an independent, modifiable risk factor for non–insulin-dependent diabetes mellitus.[44] Nicotine and carbon monoxide adversely affect blood lipids, coagulation, and vascular stability. Smoking cessation may halve the risk from dying of CHD after 5 to 10 years.[45] Women who currently smoke are 3.5 times more likely than non-smokers to have a first myocardial infarct or fatal heart attack; men are 2.9 times as likely. Current smokers with hypertension are 4.5 (men) or 7.9 (women) times as likely to have an infarct than non-smokers.[45]

Women who stop smoking will reduce their excess risk of CHD by one quarter to one third within 2 years and approximate the risk of those who have never smoked in 10 to 14 years.[46] This pattern of reduced excess risk also applies to stroke and is consistent regardless of the number of cigarettes smoked, the age of starting, or the presence of other risk factors for stroke.[47] Passive smoking increases the risk of a myocardial infarct or death in both males and females. Increased fibrinogen levels have been found to be a marker for detecting the effect of passive smoking.[48]

Smoking also diminishes the beneficial effects of therapy in patients with coronary artery disease. The combination of smoking and oral contraceptive use is a major risk factor for women under 50 years of age.[49] Oral contraceptives aside, smoking appears to be a stronger risk factor for myocardial infarction in middle-aged women than in men.[50] Given the relatively greater susceptibility of women to cardiac ischemia in the absence of organic coronary lesions and the very strong association between cigarette smoking and coronary spasm in young women,[51] smoking cessation in women deserves particular consideration. Physicians should routinely discuss smoking cessation with their patients regardless of the patient's current health problem or complaint (eg, low back pain or headaches).

THROMBOGENIC RISK FACTORS

While serum cholesterol and HDL-C levels and systolic hypertension have long been regarded as highly significant predictors of heart disease in both sexes,[50] fibrinogen and vitamin E levels have more recently emerged as good indicators of CHD risk.[52] Eighteen months after menopause the fibrinogen level in women rises to a level at which it is considered a risk factor.[2]

While high blood levels of fibrinogen are hazardous, low serum levels of vitamin E correlate with increased risk. Cross-cultural comparisons of the mortality from ischemic heart disease and a case-control study of angina pectoris have revealed strong inverse correlations for low serum levels of vitamin E.[53] Among middle-aged women vitamin E supplementation is associated with a reduced risk of coronary artery disease. To achieve substantial antithrombotic benefit, vitamin E in doses of at least 100 IU needs to be consumed for more than 2 years.[54] Vitamin E in doses exceeding 100 IU/day has been angiographically demonstrated to reduce the progression of coronary artery lesions.[55]

While the antioxidant effect of vitamin E explains this finding, the antithrombotic effect of this vitamin also deserves consideration. Levels of 200 to 400 IU of vitamin E decrease platelet adhesiveness. After 2 weeks of supplementation with vitamin E, platelet adhesion was found to decrease by over 75%.[56]

The importance of platelet adhesiveness and aggregation is evidenced by a prospective study of US nurses, aged 34 to 65 years, without a history of diagnosed coronary artery disease. A reduction in myocardial infarction was demonstrated in those nurses who took one to six aspirin tablets per week. This effect was seen only in subjects over the age of 50 years.[57] The authors recommended 325 mg of aspirin every other day for women over the age of 50 years. As aspirin decreases platelet aggregation and vitamin E decreases adhesiveness, these agents may be combined to good effect.

Additional dietary options deserving special mention are garlic and deep, cold-water fish. Garlic, in addition to lowering LDL-C and reducing LDL oxidation, decreases platelet aggregation and stickiness and may also increase fibrinolysis.[58] Fish rich in omega-3 fatty acids reduce thrombosis by decreasing platelet aggregation, platelet thromboxane A2 (TXA2), and fibrinogen and by increasing bleeding time and vascular prostacyclin (PGI3).[59] Additional protective actions attributable to fish consumption are reductions in very low density lipoproteins, blood pressure, and triglyceride levels.[60] Because fish is an animal product, it contains cholesterol. At high doses fish may increase serum cholesterol, but this rise may involve some increase in HDL as well. Women should be advised to eat deep cold-water fish (ie, fish rich in omega-3 fatty acids) once or twice a week to obtain this protective effect.

In the short term (ie, within a 5-year period), fibrinogen levels are a better predictor of CHD than cholesterol levels.[61] High levels of fibrinogen have recently been recognized as a substantial risk factor. Variables associated with increased fibrinogen levels include smoking, oral contraceptive drug use, pregnancy, inactivity, adiposity, stress, and menopause.[62]

Behavioral choices associated with lower fibrinogen concentration are estrogen replacement therapy, regular physical activity, smoking cessation, and chronic light alcohol consumption. The cardioprotective effect of alcohol plateaus at one to two drinks per day.[63] While the beneficial effects of alcohol were once thought to be related to HDL-C levels, current thinking suggests the beneficial effects of alcohol are related to thrombogenecity. Persons consuming two or more drinks per day have higher levels of endogenous tissue-type plasminogen activator than alcohol abstainers.[64] Intermediate alcohol consumption was shown to be a factor that contributed to a low coronary risk lifestyle in both men and women, once an allowance was made for a lower alcohol consumption among female study participants. Wine drinkers of both sexes seemed to be at lower risk than beer drinkers.[65]

PLASMA HOMOCYSTEINE

In persons deficient in vitamin B_{12} and folic acid, methionine metabolism results in increased production of homocysteine, a toxic metabolite.[66] An increase of 5 μmol/L of plasma homocysteine increases the risk of CHD by as much as a 0.5 μmol/L increment in cholesterol. An increase in plasma homocysteine level of 5 μmol/L leads to a 1.8-fold increase in the risk of CHD in women. Increasing daily folic acid intake by 200 μg/day reduces plasma homocysteine levels by about 4 μmol/L. Moderately elevated plasma homocysteine levels were reduced by 54% in persons supplemented with 1 mg/day folic acid, 0.05 mg/day vitamin B_{12}, and 10 mg/day vitamin B_6.[67] Betaine supplements may also be helpful.

MANAGEMENT

Intervention for the prevention and management of coronary artery disease focuses initially on lifestyle, including dietary factors, smoking cessation, increasing physical activity, and controlling weight. Later, in symptomatic cases, intervention strategies expand to include pharmacologic therapy.

The conventional diet advocated by heart associations specifically mentions fat, carbohydrate, salt, and alcohol intake.[68] It is recommended that no more than 30% of daily energy intake should be derived from fat and of that no more, and preferably less, than one third of fat intake should be in the form of saturated fats. A daily intake of up to 250 or 300 mg of cholesterol is usually permitted. Sodium intake and alcohol intake are limited, and a high intake of complex carbohydrates is encouraged. Even adherence to such dietary recommendations may require regular review in women at risk. A 12-month lifestyle study using coronary angiography as its end point found progression of established atheroma in patients on a diet consistent with these recommendations.[69]

General dietary recommendations consistent with cardiovascular health include avoiding animal fats and processed vegetable oils and replacing red meat with fish at least three times a week. Good fish selections include mackerel, Atlantic herring, chinook salmon, and canned sardines. Patients should eat generous quantities of complex carbohydrates, especially those rich in soluble fiber such as oats, legumes, rye, raisins, and prunes. Patients should be encouraged to use garlic and olive and canola oils when cooking or preparing meals. Replacement of full cream with low-fat dairy products is obligatory. Last, consuming a daily glass or two of red wine has shown beneficial results.

Although more rigorous adherence has been advocated, nutritional advice for angina patients is similar to that for asymptomatic patients with coronary risk factors. Both the prevention and management of coronary artery disease focus on known risk factors and attempt to modify these factors so that the development of atheromatous plaques is interrupted, established plaques may regress, and the possibility of thrombotic episodes is diminished. In symptomatic individuals it is also necessary to pay attention to interventions that reduce the likelihood of a critical event. Use of vitamin E supplements, garlic, aspirin, and estrogen replacement; smoking cessation; and regular exercise should therefore be emphasized.

Pharmacologic intervention particularly suited to women with overt coronary artery problems includes those drugs that modify vascular tone and those with an anti-atherogenic effect. Glyceryl trinitrate is used to dilate coronary arteries and improve blood supply. Both calcium blockers and nitrates are particularly good drug choices in women due to their impact on vasomotor tone. Antihypertensive therapy using calcium antagonists and angiotensin-converting-enzyme inhibitors provides benefits that go beyond their antihypertensive effect.

CONCLUDING REMARKS

Although CHD presents a greater population-based problem among young to middle-aged men, it is a substantial cause of death in women of all ages. In view of the increased propensity of female coronary arteries toward vasospasm and the relative inaccuracy of nonintrusive diagnostic measures in women, diagnosis of CHD is more problematic in this group. As the prognosis for women with an infarction is relatively poor and the incidence of a second infarct is high, efforts to prevent coronary artery disease by vigorously modifying known risk factors are justified.

REFERENCES

1. Wingate S. Women and coronary heart disease. Implications for the critical care setting. *Focus Crit Care.* 1991;18(3):212–214, 216–218, 220.
2. Kitler ME. Coronary disease: are there gender differences? *Eur Heart J.* 1994;15(3):409–417.
3. Nicholls ES, Peruga A, Restrepo HE. Cardiovascular disease mortality in the Americas. *World Health Stat Q.* 1993;46(2):134–150.
4. Robinson K, Conroy RM, Mulcahy R, Hickey N. The 15-year prognosis of a first acute coronary episode in women. *Eur Heart J.* 1992;13(1):67–69.
5. Janowitz WR, Agatston AS, Kaplan G, Viamonte M. Differences in prevalence and extent of coronary artery calcium detected by ultrafast computed tomography in asymptomatic men and women. *Am J Cardiol.* 1993;72(3):247–254.
6. Kaufmann RB, Sheedy PF, Maher JE, et al. Quantity of coronary artery calcium detected by electron beam computed tomography in asymptomatic subjects and angiographically studied patients. *Mayo Clin Proc.* 1995;70(3):223–232.
7. Feinglass J, McDermott MM, Foroohar M, Pearce WH. Gender differences in interventional management of peripheral vascular disease: evidence from a blood flow laboratory population. *Ann Vasc Surg.* 1994;8(4):343–349.
8. Barter PJ. Management of low HDL cholesterol. *Aust Fam Physician.* 1995;24:2066–2074.
9. Williams EL, Winkleby MA, Fortmann SP. Changes in coronary heart disease risk factors in the 1980s: evidence of a male-female crossover effect with age. *Am J Epidemiol.* 1993;137(10):1056–1067.
10. Melamed S, Ben-Avi I, Luz J, Green MS. Repetitive work, work underload and coronary heart disease risk factors among blue-collar workers—the CORDIS study. *J Psychosom Res.* 1995;39(1):19–29.
11. Kawachi I, Colditz GA, Stampfer MJ, et al. Prospective study of shift work and risk of coronary heart disease in women. *Circulation.* 1995;92(11):3178–3182.
12. Unden AL, Krakau I, Hogbom M, Romanus-Egerborg I. Psychosocial and behavioral factors associated with serum lipids in university students. *Soc Sci Med.* 1995;41(7):915–922.
13. Gliksman MD, Kawachi I, Hunter D, et al. Childhood socioeconomic status and risk of cardiovascular disease in middle aged US women: a prospective study. *J Epidemiol Community Health.* 1995;49(1):10–15.
14. Macdonald G. Do antihypertensive agents affect atheroma formation? *Curr Ther Cardiol.* 1995;1:3–5.
15. Stamler J, Rose G, Stamler R, Elliot P, Dyer A, Marmot M. Intersalt study findings: public health and medical care implications. *Hypertension.* 1989;14:570–577.
16. Jamison JR. *Health Promotion for Chiropractic Practice.* Gaithersburg, Md: Aspen Publishers; 1990.
17. Marti B. Health effects of recreational running in women. Some epidemiological and preventive aspects. *Sports Med.* 1991;11(1):20–51.
18. Jennings Gl. The impact of exercise on hypertension. *Mod Med Aust.* 1993;36:103–106.
19. French JK, Eliot JM, Williams BF, et al. Association of angiographically detected coronary artery disease with low levels of high-density lipoprotein cholesterol and systemic hypertension. *Am J Cardiol.* 1993;71:505–510.
20. Verschuren WM, Jacobs DR, Bloemberg BPM, et al. Serum total cholesterol and long term coronary heart disease prevention in different cultures. *JAMA.* 1995;274:131–136.
21. Simons L. Cholesterol and triglycerides can overstay their welcome. *Aust Doct.* In publication.
22. Barter PJ. Management of low HDL cholesterol. *Aust Fam Physician.* 1995;24:2066–2074.
23. Montague T, Tsuyuki R, Burton J, Williams R, Dzavik V, Teo K. Prevention and regression of coronary atherosclerosis. Is it safe and efficacious therapy? *Chest.* 1994;105(3):718–726.
24. Squires RW, et al. Low dose, time release nicotinic acid. *Mayo Clin Proc.* 1992;67:855–860.
25. Denke MA, Sempos CT, Grundy SM. Excess body weight: an underrecognized contributor to high blood cholesterol levels in white American men. *Arch Intern Med.* 1993;153:1093–1103.
26. Ishwarlal J, Fuller CJ. Oxidized LDL. *Clin Cardiol.* 1993;16(suppl 1):6–9.
27. Dixon ZR, Burri BJ, Clifford A, et al. Effects of carotene deficient diet on measures of oxidative susceptibility and superoxide dismutase activity in adult women. *Free Radic Biol Med.* 1994;17:537–544.
28. Fuhrman B, Lavy A, Aviram M. Consumption of red wine with meals reduces the susceptibility of human plasma and low-density-lipoprotein to lipid peroxidation. *Am J Clin Nutr.* 1995;61:549–554.
29. Phelps S, Harris WS. Garlic supplementation and lipoprotein oxidation susceptibility. *Lipids.* 1993;28:275–277.
30. Warshafsky S, Kamer RS, Sivak SL. Effect of garlic on total serum cholesterol. A meta-analysis. *Ann Intern Med.* 1993;119:599–605.
31. Silagy C, Neil A. Garlic as a lipid lowering agent—a meta-analysis of randomized controlled clinical trials. *J R Coll Physicians Lond.* 1994;28:39–45.
32. Jain AK, Vargas R, Gotzkowsky K, Mc Mahon FG. Can garlic reduce levels of serum lipids? A controlled clinical study. *Am J Med.* 1993;94:632–634.
33. Gey KF, Moser UK, Joran P, Stahelin HB, Eichholzer M, Ludin E. Increased risk of cardiovascular disease at suboptimal plasma concentrations of essential antioxidants: an epidemiological update with special attention to carotene and vitamin C. *Am J Clin Nutr.* 1993;57(suppl):787S–797S.
34. Manson JE, Gaziano JM, Spelsberg A, et al. A secondary prevention trial of antioxidant vitamins and cardiovascular disease in women. Rationale, design, and methods. *Ann Epidemiol.* 1995;5(4):261–269.
35. Stampfer MJ, Colditz GA. Oestrogen replacement therapy and coronary artery disease: a quantitative assessment of epidemiological evidence. *Prev Med.* 1991;20:47–63.
36. Stampfer MJ, Colditz GA, Willett WC, et al. Postmenopausal estrogen therapy and cardiovascular disease. Ten-year follow-up from the nurses' health study. *N Engl J Med.* 1991;325(11):756–762.
37. Darling G, Davis S. Hormone replacement therapy: logical prescribing. *Mod Med Aust.* 1994;37:57–66.
38. Barrett-Connor E. Risks and benefits of replacement estrogen. *Annu Rev Med.* 1992;43:239–251.
39. Olferev AM, Volozh OI, Sokolova MA, et al. Characteristics of the blood serum lipoprotein pattern in female Tallinn residents aged 35–54 years. *Cor-Vasa.* 1991;33(6):472–479.
40. *Australian Doctor,* 1991: 6 November.
41. Willett WC, Manson JE, Stampfer J, et al. Weight, weight change, and coronary heart disease in women. Risk within the "normal" weight range. *JAMA.* 1995;273(6):461–465.

42. Rich-Edwards JW, Manson JE, Stampfer MJ, et al. Height and the risk of cardiovascular disease in women. *Am J Epidemiol.* 1995;142(9):909–917.
43. Colditz GA, Willett WC, Rotnitzky A, Manson JE. Weight gain as a risk factor for clinical diabetes mellitus in women. *Ann Intern Med.* 1995;122(7):481–486.
44. Rimm EB, Manson JE, Stampfer MJ, et al. Cigarette smoking and the risk of diabetes in women. *Am J Public Health.* 1993;83(2):211–214.
45. Chun BY, Dobson AJ, Heller RF. Smoking and the increase of coronary heart disease in an Australian population. *Med J Aust.* 1993;159:508–512.
46. Kawachi I, Colditz GA, Stampfer MJ, et al. Smoking cessation and time course of decreased risks of coronary heart disease in middle-aged women. *Arch Intern Med.* 1994;154(2):169–175.
47. Kawachi I, Colditz GA, Stampfer MJ, et al. Smoking cessation and decreased risk of stroke in women. *JAMA.* 1993;269(2):232–236.
48. Dobson AJ, Alexander HM, Heller RF, Lloyd DM. Passive smoking and the risk of heart attack or coronary death. *Med J Aust.* 1991;154(12):793–797.
49. Martys R. Adverse cardiac effects of smoking. *Wien Med Wochenschr.* 1994;144:556–560. Abstract.
50. Njolstad I, Arnesen E, Lund-Larsen PG. Smoking, serum lipids, blood pressure, and sex differences in myocardial infarction. A 12-year follow-up of the Finnmark study. *Circulation.* 1996;93(3):450–456.
51. Caralis DG, Deligonul U, Kern MJ, Cohen JD. Smoking is a risk factor for coronary spasm in young women. *Circulation.* 1992;85(3):905–909.
52. Gey KF, Puska P, Jordan P, Moser UK. Inverse correlation between plasma vitamin E and mortality from ischemic heart disease in cross-cultural epidemiology. *Am J Clin Nutr.* 1991;53(Suppl 1):326S–334S.
53. Gey KF, Stahelin HB, Eichholzer M. Poor plasma status of carotene and vitamin C is associated with higher mortality from ischemic heart disease and stroke: Basel prospective study. *Clin Invest.* 1993;71(1):3–6.
54. Stampfer MJ, Hennekens CH, Manson JF, Colditz GA, Rosner B, Willett W. Vitamin E consumption and the risk of coronary disease in women. *New Engl J Med.* 1993;328:1444–1449.
55. Hodis HN, Mack WJ, LaBree L, et al. Serial coronary angiographic evidence that antioxidant vitamin intake reduces progression of coronary artery atherosclerosis. *JAMA.* 1995;273:1849–1854.
56. Jandak J, Steiner M, Richardson PD. a-Tocopherol, an effective inhibitor of platelet adhesion. *Blood.* 1989;73:141–149.
57. Dalen JE, Goldberg RJ. Prophylactic aspirin and the elderly population. *Clin Geriatr Med.* 1992;8(1):119–126.
58. Kiesewetter H, Jung F, Jung EM, Mroweitz C, Koscielny J, Wenzel E. Effect of garlic on platelet aggregation in patients with increased risk of juvenile ischaemic attack. *Eur J Clin Pharmacol.* 1993;45:333–336.
59. Saynor R, Gillott T. Changes in blood lipids and fibrinogen with a note on safety in a long-term study on the effects of n-3 fatty acids in subjects receiving fish oil supplements and followed for seven years. *Lipids.* 1992;27:533–538.
60. Leaf A, Weber PC. Cardiovascular effects of n-3 fatty acids. *New Engl J Med.* 1988;318(9):549–556.
61. Ernst E, Resch KL. Fibrinogen as a cardiovascular risk factor: a meta-analysis and review of the literature. *Ann Intern Med.* 1993;118:956–963.
62. de la Serna G. Fibrinogen: a new major risk factor for cardiovascular disease. *J Fam Pract.* 1994;39:468–477.
63. Criqui MH, Ringel BL. Does diet or alcohol explain the French paradox? *Lancet.* 1994;344:1719–1723.
64. Ridker R, Vaughan DR, Stampfer MJ, Glynn RJ, Hennekens CH. Association of moderate alcohol consumption and plasma concentration of endogenous tissue plasminogen activator. *JAMA.* 1994;272:929–933.
65. Woodward M, Tunstall Pedoe H. Alcohol consumption, diet, coronary risk factors, and prevalent coronary heart disease in men and women in the Scottish heart health study. *J Epidemiol Community Health.* 1995;49(4):354–362.
66. Robinson K, Mayer EL, Miller DP, et al. Hyperhomocysteinemia and low pyridoxal phosphate. Common and reversible risk factors for coronary artery disease. *Circulation.* 1995;92:2825–2830.
67. Ubbink JB, van der Merwe A, Vermaak WJ, Delport R. Hyperhomocysteinemia and the response of vitamin supplementation. *Clin Invest.* 1993;71:993–998.
68. American Heart Association. Position statement of the American Heart Association. Dietary guidelines for healthy American adults. *Circulation.* 1988;77(3):721a–724a.
69. Ornish D, Brown SE, Scherwitz LW, et al. Can lifestyle changes reverse coronary disease? *Lancet.* 1990;336:129–133.

Algorithm 1

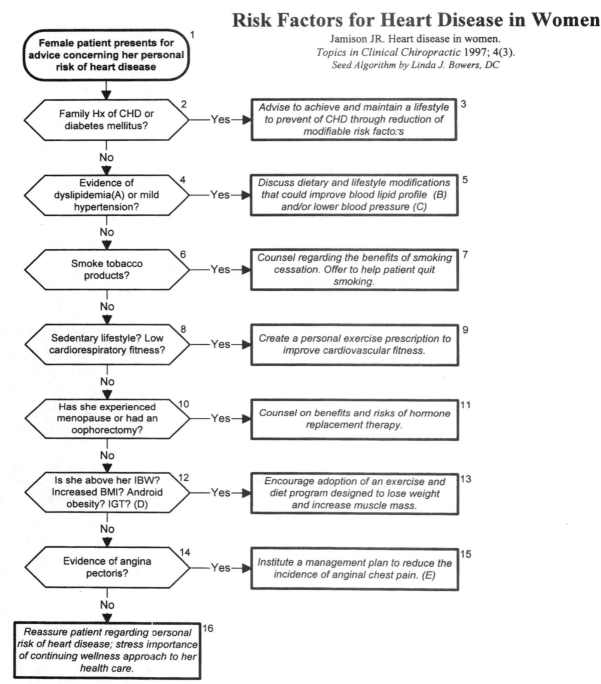

Risk Factors for Heart Disease in Women

Jamison JR. Heart disease in women.
Topics in Clinical Chiropractic 1997; 4(3).
Seed Algorithm by Linda J. Bowers, DC

Annotations:
(A) e.g., increased total blood cholesterol, LDLc, hypertriglyceridemia, or low HDLc levels.
(B) e.g., decrease saturated fat and cholesterol intake, increase fiber and antioxidant intake, exercise, lose weight, increase dietary monounsaturated fatty acids, light alcohol consumption, increase fish consumption.
(C) e.g., decrease sodium and alcohol intake, increase fruits and vegetables, achieve ideal body weight, exercise.
(D) IBW-ideal body weight; BMI-body mass index; IGT-impaired glucose tolerance; Android obesity-central distribution of fat.
(E) e.g., hormone replacement therapy, exercise, improve dietary habits, smoking cessation, weight loss, and if over 50 years of age, 325 mg aspirin every other day.

10

Osteoporosis: Assessment and Treatment Options

Donna M. Mannello

Osteoporosis is a common metabolic disease characterized by low bone mass with simultaneous microarchitectural deterioration of bone tissue leading to an increase in fracture risk.[1] This condition affects approximately 25 million Americans, particularly women over the age of 45, or at least one third of all postmenopausal women.[2-4] It is responsible for 1.5 million fractures annually.[2,5,6] Evidence[7-9] suggests that by the age of 70, over 40% of women will have experienced at least one fracture.

The risk of fracture increases as bone mass reaches a critical depletion level, decreasing the ability of the bone to withstand trauma and lessening the force required to cause a fracture.[10] The World Health Organization defines *osteopenia* (low bone mass) as bone density levels less than 1 standard deviation (SD) below the mean of normal healthy young adults and *osteoporosis* as bone density levels less than 2.5 SD.[4] The normative value is dependent on the assessment technique utilized with a twofold increased risk of fracture for each SD below the norm.[10-13]

Differences in the rate of fracture occurrence have been demonstrated between skeletal sites, genders, and within age groups. Variations in bony shape and size; composition of the bone, specifically cortical thickness and trabecular bone density; and load bearing properties are directly related to the incidence of fractures at a particular location. For example, axial loading of the spine, combined with considerable trabecular bone loss occurring at the time of menopause, is responsible for the increased vertebral fracture incidence in women. In contrast, the proximal femur, especially the cortical bone, is affected by age related osteoporosis as well as hormonal decline.[14-16]

Of the approximately 1.5 million osteoporosis-related fractures sustained each year, 250,000 involve the hip and 250,000 involve the wrist.[9,10] Though it is difficult to know exactly how many vertebral fractures occur annually due to the variability in pain and radiographic presentation, estimates of vertebral fractures are in excess of half a million.[9,10]

Approximately 260,000 patients with vertebral fractures are sufficiently symptomatic to seek a physician's care, and an additional 650,000 fractures are demonstrated on radiographs as subacute or chronic deformities.[10,17,18] Unlike wrist and hip fractures that most often occur with a fall, vertebral fractures are often induced by minimal axial loading or no specific trauma.

The number of deaths associated with osteoporosis-related fractures and the complications involved are astounding. Fractures of the hip are associated with more deaths, permanent disabilities, and costs than all other osteoporotic fractures combined.[9,18] Mortality in the first 6 months post hip fracture is as high as 20%, as compared with the expected mortality in the general population. Death is estimated to occur every 20 min due to pulmonary embolism and other complications of forced inactivity.[8,10,14] More devastating is the fact that over one half of those who survive a hip fracture suffer a decline in physical function and often are permanently disabled resulting in a 20% to 30% institutionalized rate.[9-11,19]

Trauma is the other factor associated with an increased risk of fracture. Unfortunately, the majority of osteoporotic patients are at increased risk for sustaining a fall. Table 1 provides the relevant risk factors.[10,19,20]

The expense associated with osteoporosis is approaching $20 billion per year.[4-6] More alarming is the fact that the number of older Americans is growing as well. In 1980, only 11% of the population was over the age of 65. By the year 2050, this percentage is expected to double.[4,19,21] Undoubtedly, so will the financial burden unless better methods of

Adapted from *Top Clin Chiro* 1997; 4(3): 30–43
© 1997 Aspen Publishers, Inc.

Table 1. Risk factors associated with falling

Muscle weakness
Impaired balance or weakness
Sensory loss
Various medical conditions (arthritis, poor vision, cerebral vascular disease, Parkinson's disease)
Environmental hazards
Use of sedatives, tranquilizers
Cognitive impairment

---

dealing with this disease are found and implemented. Physicians must have a basic understanding of the pathogenesis, risk factors, evaluation procedures, and treatment options to provide proper intervention and prevention.

PATHOGENESIS OF OSTEOPOROSIS

As with most other tissues in the body, bone is in a constant state of growth and repair. This process is termed *remodeling,* and it relies on the coupling mechanism between osteoblasts, the bone building cells, and osteoclasts, the bone resorbing cells.[3,22] The osteoclastic phase hones out resorption cavities, and, when completed, the osteoblasts repair or fill in the cavity with new bony material. Optimal bone strength and integrity rely on achieving a balance between bone resorption and bone tissue formation. Many variables are involved in the balance between these two cell types and subsequent amount and strength of bone mass. Genetics has the most influence on bone programming, accounting for 80% of the bone mass variance. Lifestyle factors such as nutrition, physical and social activities, hormone levels, and general health determine the other 20%.[14,23,24]

Peak bone mass is attained between 20 and 30 years of age, at which time a balance is reached between the bone formation and resorption.[7,10,15,22–27] At peak bone mass density (BMD) the long bones of the extremities are approximately 80% cortical and 20% trabecular bone; the vertebral bodies and pelvis approximate 50% trabecular and cortical bone each.[22] Unfortunately, this state of equilibrium is short lived with an imbalance occurring in about the fourth decade of life.

With aging there is an increase in osteoclastic activity resulting in an increase in bone resorption. The osteoblasts fail to replace the resorbed bone completely, which leads to areas of bony interruption and weakened architectural structure. This mechanism of suboptimal remodeling results in a slow loss of bone mass that continues throughout life and is considered to be, to some degree, a part of the natural process of aging.[7,10,15,22,23,26,28] In both males and females, a decrease in trabecular bone density begins in early adulthood, and decreased cortical bone density begins slightly later.

The discrepancy that exists between the genders relative to the incidence and area of fractures is related to initial bone mass and hormonal influences. Trabecular bone, which is metabolically more active and has a greater surface area, is rapidly lost in women during the early postmenopausal phase, approximating 15% or more in this first decade.[7,25,27] Cortical bone loss is influenced by aging and approximates 3% per decade in men and 6% per decade in women.[27] This difference is again due to the effects of estrogen deficiency.

BMD is also approximately 30% greater in men than women, at least in the fourth decade and has been demonstrated to be greater from ages 15 through 80.[27] Thus progressive decrease in bone density is more pronounced and accelerated in women.[7,27]

Based on the etiologic mechanisms, the National Osteoporosis Foundation classifies osteoporosis as primary and secondary. Primary osteoporosis is further divided into type I, type II, and idiopathic categories.[29,30]

Postmenopausal (type I) osteoporosis is the most common form of this condition, and it affects the entire skeleton. As noted, a period of rapid reduction of bone mass begins with the onset of menopause. This reduction is directly linked to the depletion of estrogen. It appears that this hormonal decrease leads to an increase in osteoclastic activity with shorter osteoblastic phases. There is also an excessive loss of horizontal cross-bracing trabeculae that considerably weakens the structural architecture.[11,15,18,31]

In the early postmenopausal years, bone loss can vary from 1% to more than 5% per year.[23] The rate of diminishment slows, eventually becoming indistinguishable from age-related bone loss (type II).[7,30] Unfortunately, by this time significant damage has occurred to the bony structural integrity. This period of increased cellular turnover and depth of bony erosion affects women in their late fifties to mid sixties (within 10 years of the onset of menopause), with vertebral crush fractures the most common sequelae. The resultant peak incidence of fractures occurs in the late sixties to mid seventies when the cortex becomes weakened.[22] A gender ratio of 6:1(female:male) exists for vertebral osteoporosis and fracture ratio.[11,22,29,30] Although estrogen deficiency is considered to be the predominant etiology for this accelerated bone loss, depletion in calcium and vitamin D absorption, as well as increases in parathyroid hormone, are also implicated.[15,22]

Type II or senile osteoporosis affects both genders with a female:male ratio of 2:1. It manifests in the age groups of the mid seventies and beyond. Type II osteoporosis is viewed as an exaggeration of the physiologic process of skeletal aging and may also be associated with changes in calcium and parathyroid hormone levels and vitamin D metabolism. Osteoblastic activity is decreased while osteoclastic activity may be increased or normal. Thinning of the cortex is demonstrated with continued trabecular perforations occurring, leading to increased weakness and subsequent fractures in the predominant cortical-containing bones such as the femoral neck. Other common fracture sites include the proximal humerus, radius, vertebra, distal femur, pubic ramus, and rib. There is considerable overlap between type I and II osteoporosis, with type I often found in combination with type II in older women.[7,28–30]

Idiopathic osteoporosis refers to bone loss in young men and women without an identifiable underlying cause. It is an ill-defined disorder of increased bone turnover with a high level of resorption. The extent of loss is diagnosed more precisely by bone biopsy.

Secondary osteoporosis represents accelerated bone loss, as a result of another underlying disease process such as an endocrine, bone marrow, gastrointestinal, or connective tissue disorder. Immobilization, radiation therapy, and various medications (glucocorticoids, excessive thyroxine, and phenytoin) also contribute to bone loss.[30,32] Regardless of the type of osteoporosis, bone mass and integrity are compromised, with the incidence and prevalance of fractures increasing progressively as bone mass declines.

CLINICAL EXAMINATION

As noted, although postmenopausal osteoporosis is the most common form of the disease, there are other causes of decreased BMD. These processes may be acting alone or in combination with other mechanisms. Evaluation of patients should always begin with a thorough history and a review of systems, including risk factors, to determine the potential for developing osteoporosis and fractures. Knowledge of risk factors is important for identifying susceptible patients and allows physicians to develop a more appropriate osteoporosis treatment plan. Table 2 includes some factors that have been implicated as adversely affecting bone mass in the general population.[10–13,20,32–48]

When in doubt of the etiology, a comprehensive assessment would include a comparative measurement of height and weight with personal historical data, as well as the appropriate laboratory tests indicated by the history and physical examination findings. Although the workup should be individualized, the following tests should be considered to exclude secondary causes of osteoporosis: a complete blood cell count; serum chemistry group (calcium, phosphorus, and total alkaline phosphatase levels; liver enzymes, creatinine, electrolytes); and urinalysis including pH. If other causes of bone loss are suspected, additional laboratory tests may be warranted and may include erythrocyte sedimentation rate; either serum or urine protein electrophoresis; thyroid function tests; parathyroid hormone levels; serum cortisol levels; 25-hydroxyvitamin D levels; a 24-hour urinary calcium excretion; thyrotropin; and acid-base studies.[9,29,32,49] As these tests are usually normal in a patient with primary osteoporosis, they cannot be used as predictive measures of

Table 2. Risk factors associated with the development of osteoporosis

Genetic factors
   Female gender
   White or Asian
   Family history
   Low body mass
   Early menopause
Health status factors
   Oophorectomy
   Estrogen deficiency
   Intestinal malabsorption
   High gastric pH
   Vitamin D deficiency
   Amenorrhea
   Various metabolic disorders (hyperparathyroidism, hyperthyroidism, diabetes, Cushing's syndrome, metabolic acidosis)
   Various medications (prolonged corticosteroid therapy, aluminum antacids, anticonvulsants, lithium, loop diuretics, tetracycline, warfarin, prolonged use of high levels of thyroid hormone)
Nutritional factors
   Lifelong low calcium intake
   Very low or high protein intake
   High caffeine intake
   High phosphate intake
   High fiber intake
   High sodium intake
   Heavy alcohol consumption
Life activity choices
   Sedentary lifestyle
   Cigarette smoking
   Nulliparity
   Alcohol abuse
   Long-term intensive aerobic exercise

the disorder but instead are used to rule out secondary causes of osteoporosis. The most obvious benefit of obtaining these laboratory values is earlier and optimal intervention. However, a combination of some of these measures has been advocated when attempting to identify fast bone losers in perimenopausal women.[9]

Following the history, physical examination, and laboratory evaluation, an assessment of BMD is warranted. There are various methods for measuring or monitoring bone density including radiographic procedures, biochemical markers, and biopsy. The advantages of multiple diagnostic measures include diminished chance of error that is associated with tools that provide limited measures or are site-specific, such as certain types of imaging or biopsy, and more accessible monitoring.[12,27]

ADVANCED DIAGNOSTIC TESTING

There are a number of imaging techniques that may be used to evaluate bone integrity or determine the extent of bone loss: plain radiographs, radiogrammetry, single-photon absorptiometry (SPA), dual-photon absorptiometry (DPA), dual-energy X-ray absorptiometry (DEXA or DXA); quantitative computed tomography (QCT), quantitative ultrasound (QUS), and neutron activation analysis (NAA). Each of these procedures has inherent strengths and weaknesses. QUS, NAA, and vibrational tissue damping are still in the investigational stage. The four most widely utilized methods for evaluating bone mineral density are SPA, DPA, QCT, and DEXA. The choice of test is dictated by its availability.[32,50]

Conventional radiography

Conventional radiographic evaluation is still the primary clinical diagnostic tool for the assessment of fractures. Bone integrity changes such as accentuation of end-plate shadows or a change in vertebral body shape; diffuse demineralization with cortical thinning in long bones; fracture lines; and decreases in the trabecular pattern in the pelvis and proximal femur may be noted and are consistent with osteoporosis. This method is limited by the fact that detection of bone loss cannot be appreciated until a minimum of 30% to 50% of the bone material is depleted.[27,28,51] This fact is unfortunate for both patients and physicians as this procedure is the most readily available and is less expensive than advanced diagnostic methods.

SPA and DPA

Both the SPA and DPA methods use a radionuclide source to measure photon attenuation at the examination site. The attenuation is converted into bone mineral content in grams or to area bone mineral density in grams per square centimeter using a known standard.[51] SPA has a single photon beam and can be utilized only where soft tissue thickness is constant. Therefore, only measurements of the appendicular skeleton are practical, most often the distal radius and calcaneus. Another limitation is the inability to differentiate between cortical and trabecular bone.[9,21,27,32,51]

DPA applies the same principles as SPA but emits photons at two different energy levels. DPA has a better predictive value of future fractures as compared with SPA.[9,21,27,51] Another advantage is that DPA can be used to evaluate both the axial and appendicular skeleton. It can also measure both cortical and trabecular bone, although it cannot differentiate between the two. Limitations include the scan time and accuracy. The lengthy assessment time, 20 to 40 min, often makes it difficult for patients to remain still. Movement may result in less than optimal images, which can affect the density impression. Accuracy and reproducibility may be affected by vertebral compression fractures with callus formation, scoliotic and other spinal deformities, articular facet hypertrophy, sclerosis or marginal osteophytosis, and extraosseous calcification.[27,32]

DEXA

DEXA applies principles similar to DPA, utilizing a different energy source. DEXA replaces the radionuclide source with a more stable X-ray tube that reduces examination time and improves reproducibility of measurements. Unfortunately, it shares some of the same limitations as DPA. Performing both lateral and posterior imaging of the spine can address most of the accuracy problems, with the exception of a few levels where superimposition of the ribs or the iliac crest falsely increases the mineral content. DEXA has gained widespread acceptance in predicting future fractures and monitoring treatment response because of its high level of precision error of 0.5% to 2% and accuracy error of 2% to 5%.[21,29,32,51,52] Both DPA and DEXA assess the BMD and can typically provide the number of SDs above or below the mean SD, allowing an estimate of fracture risk.[32]

QCT

QCT can measure the vertebral body alone, separating the trabecular bone from the cortical bone, and measure the end plate.[21,50,51] It is also the only method that can give a true BMD estimate in milligrams per cubic centimeter. For the average adult between the ages of 20 and 40, BMD is approximately 175 mg/cm^3. This quantity decreases in both genders with aging. Levels less than 105 mg/cm^3 increase the risk for vertebral compression fractures. Therefore, QCT is an excellent device for predicting future fractures.[51]

Single energy, dual energy, and peripheral QCT measures are available. Unfortunately, QCT is not without limitations including questionable accuracy, high expense, and high doses of radiation. The accuracy is restricted by the amount of fat in the bone marrow, with demonstrable variations of 20% to 30%.[21,32] The addition of dual energy or biplanar QCT improves the chance of false readings from the fat and water variations; unfortunately it occurs at the expense of precision. QCT is most often used on the spine but peripheral scanners have recently been introduced. To date, the actual clinical utility of these peripheral scanners has not been determined.[21]

Other approaches

A number of other approaches to bone density assessment have been applied including combined calcium balance/calcium kinetic study, histomorphometry, and biochemical markers. The combined calcium balance/calcium kinetic study provides information about bone formation and resorption rates in the whole skeleton. However, it is very time-consuming, does not isolate areas, can be performed a limited number of times, and the results depend on mathematical models.[22,53]

Invasive procedures such a bone biopsies, although considered to be the most specific, should only be performed on patients whose low BMD has some unusual characteristic such as early onset, rapid progression, unusual severity, or an association with other systemic findings.[28] These histomorphologic studies provide excellent discernment of the architectural structure of the biopsied area, most often the iliac crests. The area evaluated, however, may not be representative of the rate of turnover for the body or specific areas, and the precision is poor.[53]

Assessing skin collagen levels obtained through tissue biopsy has also been researched. There appears to be a good correlation between bone mass and collagen levels in the skin, both decreasing with the loss of estrogen.[54,55] Another study[56] evaluated the same relationship using skin calipers instead of biopsy and compared the results with DEXA findings. This approach is not as invasive but does require skill. Again, a correlation was noted, but not as high as with biopsy.

Advances have been made over the past decade in the use of biochemical markers. They are gaining acceptance as a viable tool for the evaluation of bone density through assessment of the components of bone turnover. These serum or urinary markers may include enzymes associated with osteoblastic or osteoclastic activity, proteins synthesized by the bone forming cells, or components of the bone matrix that are released during resorption.[9,22,52,57] Notable bone formation markers include serum total and bone-specific alkaline phosphatase, osteocalcin (a bone Gla-protein), and procollagen I extension peptides.[57] Osteocalcin is a noncollagenous protein found in bone and dentin and can be measured in the serum by enzyme-linked immunosorbent assay (ELISA) or by radioimmunoassay. Although still in the research phase, serum osteocalcin has been demonstrated to be a sensitive and specific marker that accurately reflects increases in bone turnover.[52]

The bone resorption markers that are considered most efficient are urinary pyridinoline and deoxypyridinoline (collagen phosphate cross-links) and total and dialyzable hydroxyproline. Other potential, but perhaps less sensitive, markers include tartrate-resistant acid phosphatase, urinary hydroxylysine glycosides, and free gammacarboxy-glutamic acid, as well as a few other fragments of noncollagenous proteins.[57] With the discovery of polyclonal and monoclonal antibodies and measurement of the markers with ELISA, the sensitivity and specific index of bone resorption rate have increased considerably.[52,58,59]

The advantages of biochemical markers include noninvasiveness, ability to repeat measurements, and capability to show changes in the entire skeleton. However, with the questionable sensitivity of some markers, caution is advised.[53]

No matter which procedure is used to assess the BMD of patients, it is the physician's responsibility to stay current on the advantages and limitations of the method including the process, cost, risk-benefit, sensitivity and specificity, fracture predictive value, and availability. Although these techniques do have considerable overlap between persons with and without osteoporosis, they provide information as to the extent of bone loss that may allow for more informed decision making and compliance concerning the treatment regimen. For example, a study by Rubin and Cummings[60] demonstrated that a woman's decision to begin hormonal replacement therapy is significantly affected by her knowledge of her baseline BMD and the natural course of osteoporosis.

MANAGEMENT

In the study of osteoporosis, as with many other conditions, some erroneous and inappropriate assumptions have been made as a result of poor study design, which unfortunately may have an influence on clinical decision making. Heaney[11] performed an extensive review of the literature and noted many significant errors in study conclusions. Problems with study design, such as the population size of the study for both subjects and controls, have a significant impact on outcome findings. Too small a sample size may be inadequate to provide sufficient and accurate population level correlations. This problem seemed to be common in many studies, often resulting in inappropriate conclusions. Heaney also noted a recurrent compromise of outcome data due to utilization of weak or inaccurate tools for estimating BMD or tissue turnover. The inability to monitor subject compliance to the study parameters was also noted as a significant limitation. Last, subject group homogeneity was also compromised in many controlled studies. For example, many studies grouped all postmenopausal women into a single category. Due to the bone mass loss variances in early versus late menopause, the results did not reflect or provide a correct appraisal of the effects of an intervention. Therefore, therapeutic intervention provided by a physician should be based on repeatedly proven methods.

Preventive and treatment options for osteoporosis fall into two categories: those methods that attempt to prevent further bone loss and those that encourage bone remodeling. Each intervention attempts to influence bone mass and density. In chiropractic settings, prevention and education are essential, with therapy focusing on restoration and maintenance of joint biomechanics, exercise programs, nutritional supplementation, and patient education concerning treatment options. Treatments inhibiting bone turnover include the use of hormone (especially estrogen) replacement therapy (HRT), calcitonins, bisphosphonates, and calcium and vitamin D derivatives. The use of fluoride, anabolic steroids, parathyroid hormone and peptides, and intermittent calcitonin/phosphate therapy attempts to enhance bone formation.[61]

PREVENTIVE MEASURES

Prevention is the safest and most cost-effective treatment option. Such activities may fall into one of three levels: before bone loss has occurred through elimination of risk factors; after some evidence of bone loss, but in a reversible stage; and when therapy is applied to attempt to prevent further progression or to affect the associated disability.[13,17] Providing guidance and education to patients regarding the reduction of risk factors with an emphasis on diet and exercise could potentially decrease the severity of future changes associated with both type I and type II primary osteoporosis.

Exercise is an imperative component throughout life. It is well known that without mechanical loading of the musculoskeletal system, bone mass, muscle tone, and balance are diminished. Physical activity, especially early in life, promotes the development of high bone density. Continued activity can potentially create a reserve of bone mass.

This increase in BMD can help delay the clinical manifestations of osteoporosis.[31,50] In fact, positive lifetime effects on BMD have been noted with exercise alone or in combination with adequate levels of dietary calcium in young adults[62–64] and in older women and men.[65–70]

It is never too late to benefit from exercise. The course of exercise prescribed should be dependent on the patient's physical functioning capabilities.[65,66,71] Exercise that provides mechanical loading involves the pull of muscles on bone, for instance walking, jogging, or stair climbing. In older persons, flexion, high impact, and twisting exercises should be avoided because of excessive stress to osseous structures.[50,65,66,72]

The bone mass response will depend on the intensity and type of activity, hormonal level, and diet.[23,45,63,65,67,69] Fifty to 60 min of physical activity three times per week is necessary to be effective.[23,73]

After the onset of the disease, the aggressiveness of the treatment plan is dependent upon the level of bone density, general health status, and associated risk factors. The correlation between decreased incidence of hip fractures and the maintenance of some form of regular physical activity in older individuals has been repeatedly demonstrated.[48,71,74,75] It has been attributed to the improvement of coordination, balance, and muscle mass. Unfortunately, the benefits of exercise are dependent on the type of activity and continuation of that activity. Therefore, patients should be encouraged to continue their exercise regime, and physicians should counsel patients regarding the optimal form of exercise.

Regardless of the type of intervention for osteoporosis, appropriate diet and exercise should be a part of each program. The effect of calcium and vitamin D derivatives on osteoporosis has received the greatest amount of investigation. However, many other nutrients are essential for developing and maintaining a healthy skeleton. They include manganese, zinc, vitamin C, vitamin K, phosphorus, magnesium, and boron. The greatest influence of these substances occurs during the growth phase, with little definitive benefit of supplementation after maturity.[11] In addition, each of these nutrients must be in correct proportion to the others. Excess of one nutrient cannot substitute for deficiency of another.

CALCIUM

The skeleton is the storage site for 99% of the body's calcium. The remaining 1% is used for normal neural transmission, cardiac function, muscular contraction, and blood clotting. Total body calcium content cannot be diminished without affecting bone mass.[15,76] At birth, bones contain approximately 25 g of calcium. By maturity, this amount has increased to 1,000 to 1,200 g.[23,77] After peak bone mass is achieved, adequate calcium intake is essential to maintain the needs of metabolic demands. Diminished levels of calcium trigger the release of parathormone, which mediates bone loss through increased osteoclastic activity.[23]

Investigational studies of the effect of calcium supplementation on BMD are controversial. As noted earlier, appropriate study design, population size, type of intervention, and control of variables can significantly affect outcomes. Cummings[78] performed a meta-analysis of all studies through 1988 involving the effects of calcium intake on bone integrity and found a documented positive correlation between these two factors. The available data suggest that appropriate calcium intake has the greatest influence on bone density during the growth stage in children, during adulthood, and before and after the early phase of menopause in women. Unfortunately, as Heaney[11] noted, virtually all studies have shown little or no effect of dietary calcium during the 5-year period following the onset of menopause, the period of most extensive bone loss. This finding does not negate the benefit of sufficient calcium levels prior to this time, which has a significant impact on the integrity of the bone throughout life.

What is the adequate or threshold amount of calcium intake? Matkovic[79] analyzed the data from over 500 studies published since 1922 that investigated calcium balances in growing children. The results of his findings were alarming. The threshold amount of calcium intake necessary to maintain balance between bone growth and resorption was well above the recommended daily allowance. Matkovic[79] and Heaney[80] concluded that between the ages of 1 and 8, 1,000 mg/day is necessary; between the ages of 9 and 17, 1,600 mg/day is needed; and between the ages of 18 and 30 1,100 mg/day is required. Some of these levels are also higher than those suggested by the National Institutes of Health.[81]

Another variable is the amount of calcium absorbed into the system. Previously it was assumed that 50% of consumed calcium would be utilized by the body. In contrast, studies[82,83] have indicated that in growing children and adolescents only about 35% of ingested calcium is actually absorbed. Animal studies have shown that the size and shape of bones during the growth phase are not adversely influenced by low calcium intake levels, but the internal integrity is affected and is evidenced by increased porosity and a decrease in the cortical and trabecular thickness.[11] Obviously, this effect would potentially compromise and predispose someone to problems even before the physiologic process of bone mass loss is initiated.

For the osteoporotic population, the adequate or threshold amount of calcium is difficult to determine because of other complications of aging such as malabsorption. Approximately 75% of the older population demonstrate significant malabsorption of calcium.[84] Data indicate that the calcium intake requirement for women with intact hormone levels or women on estrogen replacement should be 1,000 mg/day and that of estrogen deficient women 1,500 mg/day.[77,80] These levels are consistent with those advocated by the 1994 NIH guidelines.[81] It has also been demonstrated that the mean calcium intake from food for the majority of middle-aged and older American women is only about 500 mg/day.[23,77] Therefore, calcium supplementation beyond what can be provided in the diet is essential and should be considered as a necessary component of a treatment plan.

Factors determining the bioavailability of calcium include the type of calcium consumed, both in foods and supplements; functional level of the gastrointestinal system to allow absorption; the availability of active vitamin D to facilitate absorption; and lifestyle factors. Dairy products provide the greatest usable amount of calcium by far.[15,29,76,85] However, many older individuals suffer from a lactose intolerance or other sensitivities prohibiting intake of some dairy products. Others are concerned about fat intake from dairy products. In these cases, lactose-reduced products are available such as Calcimilk®, which is also calcium fortified. Skim or 1% low-fat milk products are also available. Another source is juice fortified with calcium. Sardines (bone in), salmon cooked dry (bone in), tofu, and other soy products are very high in calcium. Green leafy vegetables such as collard greens and kale and fruits such as cooked rhubarb also provide calcium, but the amount available for absorption is less.[15,76,85]

When ingested food calcium levels are insufficient, supplements may be necessary. However, the ability of the supplement to dissolve in the stomach is an important consideration. Calcium carbonate, which is 40% elemental calcium, yields the highest amount of calcium per tablet at the least expense.[28,29,76] This form, however, may be of limited value for people with low acid secretion levels; therefore, it should be taken with meals.

Many references[23,49,73,85] advocate the use of the more soluble forms such as calcium citrate, citrate-malate, hydroxyapatite, or a combination with vitamin D. These forms of calcium are often better absorbed and tolerated, because nausea and constipation are also common side effects. Divided doses are also advised to decrease the chance of side effects.

Patients may also check the dissolvability of their calcium supplement by placing a tablet in a solution of water and vinegar (50-50). If it dissolves within 15 min it should readily dissolve in their stomach. Patients should also be advised to look for the USP (United States Pharmacopeia) symbol on the label. These voluntary standards for nutritional supplements ensure that the product will dissolve.

In general, calcium supplementation has its greatest effect on increasing or maintaining bone mass in cortical bone.[76] A study by Dawson-Hughes and associates[86] investigated the effect of calcium supplementation on BMD. They found that in women greater than 6 years postmenopausal, calcium carbonate supplementation maintained BMD at the femoral neck but not in the spine, while calcium citrate-malate prevented bone loss at all sites including the spine.

Last, various lifestyle components or habits such as inactivity, smoking, excessive alcohol ingestion, or high dietary fiber intake may either decrease calcium absorption or increase excretion.[15,76] When considering preventive measures, it has been demonstrated that BMD is much greater in those individuals who have had adequate lifelong calcium intake as compared with individuals who supplemented their diets at a single point in time. BMD is even higher when the lifelong calcium levels have been combined with lifelong physical activity.[28,62] It must be remembered that although calcium is a very necessary component, it is not the only determinant of bone integrity. Also, calcium is not a substitute for HRT, especially in the early postmenopausal phase.[5,74,77]

VITAMIN D

Vitamin D plays an important role in the regulation of bone formation and resorption. This process, although not completely understood, is associated with and somewhat dependent on vitamin D receptors (VDRs). These VDRs have been identified in the osteoblasts and osteoprogenitor cells in intact bone. It had been thought that the important and active metabolite 1,25-dihydroxyvitamin D was the only necessary vitamin D metabolite. However, VDRs have been identified in more than one of the vitamin D metabolites. This finding may suggest that multiple forms of vitamin D may be salient in maintaining skeletal homeostasis.[87]

Vitamin D also functions as a facilitator for stimulating calcium and phosphate absorption. In fact, it is considered the principal regulator of intestinal calcium absorption. Therefore, without sufficient levels of vitamin D, absorption of calcium and phosphate is impaired. Interestingly, 60% of patients with type I osteoporosis demonstrate low serum concentration levels of 1,25-dihydroxyvitamin D (calcitriol).[84] Conversely, many patients with postmenopausal osteoporosis and depleted calcium levels have no obvious serum deficiency of vitamin D. When a deficiency is found in this group, it is usually not appreciated before the age of 65.[87]

When present, depletion is attributed to the age-related decline in the ability to convert inactive vitamin D to the active forms D_2 and D_3 in the liver and kidney, as well as limited exposure to sunlight, which impairs vitamin D synthesis in the skin. Nevertheless, trabecular bone is most sensitive to decreased levels of vitamin D.[88] Some well-controlled studies[11,23,84,89–93] of populations deficient in vitamin D have demonstrated the benefit of supplementation of vitamin D alone or in combination with calcium supplementation for reducing the rate of cortical bone loss, increasing bone density, and reducing spinal or hip fractures.

Sunlight is a natural way to stimulate the body's production of vitamin D, with 15 min/day of exposure on the hands and face being sufficient to provide the amount needed for normal physiologic function. Cod liver oil is a good source of vitamin D, and milk and bread products are often fortified with vitamin D.[10,29] For supplementation, dosage is dependent on the form of vitamin D provided; however, 400 to 800 IU is considered a safe level.[5,29] Unlike the water-soluble vitamins, vitamin D is fat soluble and is not as readily excreted from the system. Accordingly, conflicting evidence regarding benefits, side effects, and risks of developing hypercalcemia or hypercalciuria is associated with this form of treatment for osteoporosis. A considerable amount of caution and monitoring should be applied when considering vitamin D supplementation.[7,10,13,92]

OTHER VITAMINS AND TRACE MINERALS

There are also other nutrients that are essential cofactors for enzymes involved in the synthesis of various bone matrix components. Vitamin K, for example, is important for the synthesis of osteocalcin, the principal noncollagenous bone protein. Osteocalcin is chemotactic for osteoclasts, which enhance the attachment of bone-resorbing cells. This feature affects bone remodeling and healing. Unless undergoing anticoagulant therapy, such as with coumadin, deficiency is relatively rare in adults and, although required during growth and development, the significance in osteoporotic bone remains unclear.[11,15,80,85,94]

Magnesium depletion may impair vitamin D metabolism.[95] It also regulates active calcium transport.[85,96] Vitamin C deficiency can affect the integrity of the collagen molecule, which constitutes more than 90% of the organic material of bone matrix.[15,97] Zinc, copper, and manganese are all elements for organic bone matrix synthesis.[85] Phosphorus makes up roughly one half of the bone mineral weight. However, most Americans obtain more than adequate amounts in their diets, and caution should be exercised to avoid excess due to the potential harm. Increased phosphorus amounts lead to transient imbalance of calcium remodeling and resorption. Older individuals with declining renal function comprise the population most at risk for phosphorus deficiency.[11]

CALCITONIN

Receptors for calcitonin have been identified on osteoclasts and renal cell membranes. These receptors inhibit osteoclast function and increase renal tubular reabsorption of various ions, including sodium and calcium.[7] Calcitonin appears to be most effective in conditions causing high rates of bone resorption and of limited value in states of low resorption.[98]

Salmon calcitonin is considered to be a safe drug and a preferred choice for the treatment of osteoporosis for patients with contraindications to the use of HRT.[29,99,100] Calcitonin has also demonstrated some analgesic effect in vertebral compression fractures.[20] Side effects have been reported in 10% to 50% of patients. Reactions include skin flushing, nausea, vomiting, and diarrhea. Nausea may be reduced by lowering the dosage.[20,22,101]

The initial mode of administration was subcutaneous injection, which was associated with poor compliance. Development of rectal suppositories and nasal spray has led to better tolerance and compliance. More research is necessary to determine the long-term effects of calcitonin.[92]

ESTROGEN

Numerous studies have evaluated the effect of HRT, especially estrogen, on bone mass in postmenopausal women. A vast amount of evidence indicates that HRT can prevent or slow bone loss, even that occurring during the accelerated phase in early postmenopause. Estrogen increases the amount of both vitamin D and intestinal calcium absorption, reduces the rate of remodeling, and improves the balance between formation and resorption in all skeletal sites prone to easy fracture. Prospective and retrospective studies of HRT have demonstrated a significant reduction in the incidence of fracture occurrence with as much as a 70% to 80% reduction of vertebral fractures and an overall fracture incidence decrease of 50%.[7,10,20,25,102–104]

HRT should be considered a therapeutic approach for women under the age of 50 who have had an oophorectomy. Also, patients who have a personal or strong family history of low bone mass fall into a high-risk category, as well as older women who have been diagnosed with low bone mass or osteoporotic-related fractures.

The recommended dosage of estrogen is 0.625 mg/day, optimally started in early menopause with a minimum of 7 years of HRT necessary after menopause for any long-term protection to be appreciated.[7,20,29,99,105] However, rapid bone loss, approaching a level equal to that of natural menopause, occurs with discontinued use. Therefore, many advocate HRT indefinitely to prevent this rebound effect.[7,104,106]

Controversy exists on the beneficial effect of HRT in women 75 years of age or older.[10,25,104,105,107] However, the benefits derived from delayed onset of bone loss that HRT does provide supercede these concerns. Other positive benefits associated with HRT include protection from cardiovascular disease through alteration of lipid metabolism,[7,29,103,105,108] relief of menopausal symptoms,[85] and healthier genital tissue, which diminishes the occurrence of chronic recurrent urinary tract infections.[29,103,105]

Patients should be made aware of possible side effects associated with the use of HRT such as vaginal bleeding, nausea, vomiting, diarrhea, fluid retention, breast tenderness, hypertension, and thromboembolic disease.[85,90,109] For these reasons compliance level is often adversely affected. An increased incidence of breast and endometrial cancer in women treated with HRT has also been reported. Epidemiologic studies[105,108,110] suggest that long-term use (greater than 10 years) increases the risk of neoplastic development, perhaps as much as 30% for breast cancer. However, mortality rates are significantly lower in women who take HRT.[105,108] It may be attributed to more frequent required evaluations for and earlier detection of cancer. In women with an intact uterus, the addition of progestin for 10 to 12 days each month eliminates the risk of endometrial cancer.[20,29,105]

HRT is highly contraindicated in women who have a personal history of breast or endometrial cancer, a strong family history of breast cancer, or unexplained vaginal bleeding.[29,99,105] Smoking may also eliminate the protective effect of HRT.[37,104] Continued monitoring of BMD is warranted as not all women respond to estrogen replacement therapy.[85]

BISPHOSPHATES

Bisphosphates, previously called diphosphates, are a class of carbon-substituted compounds similar to pyrophosphate. There are over 300 compounds in this category, but the most commonly used are alendronate, etidronate, tiludronate, and pamidronate. They bind to the hydroxyapatite in bone and prevent bone resorption by exerting an inhibitory effect on osteoclastic activity resulting in increases in bone density.[6,11,73] The gain is permanent as long as the reduced level of remodeling activation persists.[111] First generation bisphosphates appear to be effective in preventing bone loss associated with BMD deficiency from glucocorticoid therapy and prolonged mobilization, by partially reversing the bone loss. Excessive side effects have been noted such as diarrhea, nausea, gastrointestinal problems, acute renal failure, hypocalcemia, and toxic skin reactions.[112,113] Although the use of etidronate (Didronel) was reported to decrease risk for fractures,[112] it was denied approval by the Food and Drug Administration (FDA) because it also inhibits bone formation.[101]

Conversely, alendronate (Fosamax) appears to have great promise for the prevention of fractures. FDA recently approved Fosamax for the treatment of osteoporosis with a daily dose of 10 mg. In two concurrent 3-year clinical trials conducted by Liberman and coworkers,[114] alendronate therapy was compared with a placebo in 994 postmenopausal osteoporotic women. In both groups, 500 mg of calcium was administered daily. In the alendronate group BMD increased by 8.8% in the spine and 5.9% in the femoral neck. The incidence of vertebral fractures was reduced by 48%. The most common side effects of Fosamax are gastrointestinal symptoms such as abdominal pain, nausea, constipation, and diarrhea. Long-term effects of the antiresorptive drugs have not been determined, indicating a need for more research.[92]

FLUORIDE

The use of sodium fluoride for the treatment of osteoporosis has been studied extensively with controversial outcomes. Fluoride therapy is reported to halt bone mass loss and increase BMD, especially cortical bone. Treatment effects include an increase in BMD in a range of 3% to 6% in the spine and an associated decrease in vertebral fracture rate.[7,115,116] However, the effect on cortical bone is not as favorable. Some evidence suggests an increased rate of hip fracture.[7,9,117] Also, therapeutic doses have a high incidence of side effects such as gastric irritation and lower extremity pain.[13,99,117] Response to treatment is also unpredictable with up to 40% of patients receiving no benefit.[7,117] Due to these erratic consequences of fluoride use, it is not usually considered a first-line therapy for osteoporosis.[73]

ANABOLIC THERAPY

Androgens, derivatives, and analogues of testosterone have produced an increase in bone mass, although study results are controversial.[118] Many consider it a treatment option for men suffering from the effects of osteoporosis.[16] However, the use of androgens for the treatment of osteoporosis in women has caused some unfavorable side effects in 25% to 50% of the patients such as virilization, voice changes, edema, and liver damage. Therefore, the use of these compounds must be considered experimental.[7,92]

FRACTURE TREATMENT

Osteoporotic fractures have three distinctive features. First, incidence rates are greater for women (39.7%) than men (13.1%). Second, fracture rate increases with age. Last, there is a predilection for skeletal sites containing a predominant proportion of trabecular bone.[4,12]

Patients with vertebral compression fractures may experience severe pain and muscle spasm. A short period of bedrest to diminish compressive forces is often beneficial, but should be kept to a minimum to avoid increased bone loss and muscle weakness. Mechanical bracing may also be appropriate for the first few weeks after a fracture, but should be discontinued as soon as the pain decreases to avoid muscle weakness and promote postural changes.[28] Symptomatic relief may also be obtained with the initial use of ice to decrease inflammation, progressing to the use of moist heat as the inflammation dissipates. Soft tissue massage may be utilized to decrease muscle spasm. Analgesics or nonsteroidal anti-inflammatory agents are often utilized.[28] Calcitonin has demonstrated moderate analgesic effect for vertebral fractures.[20]

When the acute phase subsides, the patient should be encouraged to resume normal daily activities. Mechanical changes in the spine are inevitable after sustaining a vertebral fracture, which may result in more stress to the adjacent structures. Thus, appropriate extension exercises must be initiated, beginning with less stressful exercises and low repetitions, progressing in intensity to patient tolerance. A routine exercise program that is performed at least three times per week should be the goal. Dietary habits including calcium and vitamin D supplementation should be considered as well as modification of detrimental lifestyle habits and environmental factors. In women identified as being in a high-risk category for fracture, hormone replacement therapy is considered the most consistent treatment because of patient compliance. In patients with contraindications or poor tolerance of HRT, other options such as alendronate or calcitonin are available.[5,13,28,62]

Treatment of unstable vertebral fractures has consisted of surgical fusion. Various types of prostheses have been developed for fractures of the femoral neck, head, or shaft through stabilizing or replacement procedures. Although still in the experimental state, a less invasive treatment has been developed for extremity fractures. This process involves an in situ formation of a bone mineral stabilizer. A combination of monocalcium phosphate, monohydrate, alpha-tricalcium phosphate, and calcium carbonate is mixed with a sodium phosphate solution. This paste compound is surgically implanted by injection and dries within 10 min. It is accepted by and crystallizes with the existing bone carbonate apatite, called dahllite, becoming morphologically similar to the bony material.[119,120] This technique may eventually be of benefit to patients with osteoporotic fractures.

It is imperative for physicians to perform annual follow-up assessments of all high-risk patients or any patient on an osteoporosis prevention or treatment plan. The evaluation should consist of an interim history; physical examination including stature measurement, breast examination, and pelvic examination; assessment of compliance and activity level; and reinforcement of the therapeutic program. BMD measurements should also be obtained periodically to monitor changes in bone mass. A change of 5% in BMD in less than 2 years with DEXA technique is considered clinically significant.

The following guidelines are recommended by the American Association of Clinical Endocrinologists for performing DEXA BMD measurements.[121] For patients with a normal baseline BMD (T score >1.5), follow-up measurements should be obtained every 2 to 3 years. For patients in an osteoporosis treatment program, a BMD evaluation should be performed every 1 to 2 years until bone mass stabilizes. Then it should be performed every 2 to 3 years. For patients who have accelerated bone loss due to medications or secondary conditions, BMD assessment should be performed yearly.

SUMMARY

Osteoporosis is a very common disorder affecting the quality of life through pain, fracture, and disability. Genetics plays the major role in bone mass integrity. However, lifestyle factors are extremely important in the development of osteoporosis. The development of fractures is multifactorial and dependent on skeletal fragility and risk of trauma. There is an inverse relationship between bone mass and fracture risk. As bone mass decreases, fracture rate increases significantly. The areas most commonly affected are the spine, femur, and wrist. Vertebral fractures occur most often when spinal compressive forces exceed the strength of the compromised skeleton. These forces are often not greater than those of daily living; therefore bending, lifting, sneezing, and coughing are frequent initiating factors. A fracture of the wrist or hip, on the other hand, is most often associated with a fall.

A thorough evaluation is warranted for those at risk for developing osteoporosis. The evaluation should consist of a history, general appearance and measure of stature, appropriate laboratory work, and the assessment of bone density. Algorithm 1 offers insight on osteoporosis prevention strategies.

There are many treatment options available. The treatment selected should be dictated by the specific needs of each patient, although intervention through prevention can be introduced to patients at any age. Appropriate lifestyle changes, which include diet, physical activity, and social activities, should be considered in all patients. Exercise, especially weight-bearing exercises, should also be considered as an intervention that may prevent bone loss and enhance bone formation. An exercise program should be started in early adulthood, and it should be a definite part of a treatment plan for perimenopausal women and postmenopausal women.

Minimizing risk for falls in older persons is also an important consideration. Although exercise may help with muscle strength and balance, other recommendations may be necessary such as use of non-skid rugs or mats, removal of clutter or wires from walk areas, installation of handrails in bathrooms, use of proper shoes, and maintenance of appropriate lighting. A well-balanced diet is essential for the prevention and treatment of osteoporosis. It has been demonstrated that many people do not receive the necessary amount of nutrients, especially calcium, which indicates the need for supplementation. Available forms, dosage, and ability to tolerate the supplement are important features that the patient and physician must consider. More aggressive therapy may be necessary for patients who demonstrate an excessive loss or accelerated loss of BMD. Nutritional and hormonal replacement therapy, either alone or in combination, appear to provide prophylactic benefit. The use of synthetic compounds, such as the bisphosphonates, may also be considered. To date, Fosamax (alendronate) has shown the most promise. However, the efficacy and safety beyond 3 years have not been established, and more research is necessary. As with any treatment plan, monitoring and follow-up assessments are imperative.

In the treatment of osteoporosis, prevention of fractures is considered a successful outcome. As Stevenson[14] noted, by delaying bone loss and therefore fracture for even 5 years, the incidence of fracture could be reduced by 50%. If bone loss could be delayed 7 to 8 years, a reduced fracture incidence of 75% could be expected. In chiropractic health care, maintenance of normal joint mechanics and reduction of stress to the various systems including musculoskeletal is a principal goal of treatment. Conservative care always includes education related to disease prevention and therapies to enhance a patient's quality of life. Truly, the treatment of choice for osteoporosis should be prevention throughout life.

REFERENCES

1. Consensus development conference: prophylaxis and treatment of osteoporosis. *Osteoporos Int.* 1991;1:114–117.
2. Melton L, Chrischilles E, Cooper C, et al. How many women have osteoporosis? *J Bone Miner Res.* 1992;7:1005–1010.
3. Peck W, Riggs B, Bell N, et al. Research directions in osteoporosis. *Am J Med.* 1988;84:275–282.
4. Cooper C, Melton LJ. Magnitude and impact of osteoporosis and fractures. In: Marcus R, Feldman D, Kelsey J, eds. *Osteoporosis.* San Diego, Calif.: Academic Press; 1996.
5. Riggs BL, Melton LJ. The prevention and treatment of osteoporosis. *N Engl J Med.* 1992;327:620–627.
6. Silver JJ, Einhorn TA. Osteoporosis and aging. *Clin Orthop.* 1995;316:10–20.
7. Weinerman SA, Bockman RS. Medical therapy of osteoporosis. *Orthop Clin North Am.* 1990;21(1):109–124.
8. Hunder GG, Kaye RL, Williams RC. Osteoarthritis, osteoporosis, fibromyalgia: advances in understanding and management. *J Musculoskel Med.* 1993;10(9):16–34.
9. Baran DT. Osteoporosis: monitoring techniques and alternative therapies. *Obstet Gynecol Clin North Am.* 1994;21(2):321–335.
10. Nevitt MC. Epidemiology of osteoporosis. *Rheum Dis Clin North Am.* 1994;20:535–559.
11. Heaney RP. Nutritional factors in osteoporosis. *Annu Rev Nutr.* 1993;13:287–316.
12. Ross PD. Risk factors for fracture. *Spine: State of the Art Reviews.* 1994;8(1):91–110.
13. O'Neill TW, Silman AJ. Prevention of vertebral osteoporosis. *Spine: State of the Art Reviews.* 1994;8(1):171–187.
14. Stevenson JC. Pathogenesis, prevention, and treatment of osteoporosis. *Obstet Gynecol.* 1990;75(4):36s–41s.
15. Einhorn TA, Levine B, Michel P. Nutrition and bone. *Orthop Clin North Am.* 1990;21(1):43–50.
16. Niewoehner CB. Osteoporosis in men, is it more common than we think? *Postgrad Med.* 1993;93(8):59–70.
17. Lindsay R. Prevention of osteoporosis. *Prev Med.* 1994;23:722–726.
18. Cooper C. Epidemiology of vertebral fractures in western populations. *Spine: State of the Art Reviews.* 1994;8(1):1–12.
19. Jenkins EA, Cooper C. The epidemiology of osteoporosis: who is at risk? *J Musculoskel Med.* 1993;10(3):18–33.
20. Lindsay R. Osteoporosis: a clinical overview of diagnosis and therapy. *J Musculoskel Med.* 1993;10(8):31–41.
21. Hagiwara S, Yang SO, Giver CC. Noninvasive bone mineral density measurement in the evaluation of osteoporosis. *Rheum Dis Clin North Am.* 1994;20(3):651–669.
22. Eriksen EF, Langdahl B, Kassem M. The cellular basis of osteoporosis. *Spine: State of the Art Reviews.* 1994;8(1):23–62.
23. Breslau NA. Calcium, estrogen, and progestin in the treatment of osteoporosis. *Rheum Dis Clin North Am.* 1994;20(3):691–716.
24. Johnston CC, Miller JZ, Slemenda CW, et al. Calcium supplementation and increases in bone mineral density in children. *N Engl J Med.* 1992;327:82–87.
25. Sobel NB. Progestins in preventive hormone therapy. *Obstet Gynecol Clin North Am.* 1994;21(2):311–312.
26. Parfitt AM. Bone remodeling: relationship to the amount and structure of bone, and the pathogenesis and prevention of fractures. In: Riggs BL, Melton LJI, eds. *Osteoporosis: Etiology, Diagnosis, and Management.* New York: Raven Press; 1988.
27. Dequeker J, Geusens P. Measurements of bone mass. *Spine: State of the Art Reviews.* 1994;8(1):133–154.
28. Lukert BP. Osteoporosis: prevention and treatment. *Compr Ther.* 1990;16(4):36–42.
29. Babbitt AM. Review: osteoporosis. *Orthopedics.* 1994;17(10):935–941.
30. Riggs BL, Melton LJ. Evidence for two distinct syndromes of involutional osteoporosis. *Am J Med.* 1983;75:899–901.
31. Mosekilde L. Vertebral bone quality and strength. *Spine: State of the Art Reviews.* 1994;8(1):63–81.
32. Gamble CL. Osteoporosis: making the diagnosis in patients at risk for fracture. *Geriatrics.* 1995;50:24–33.

33. Metz JA, Anderson JJB, Gallagher PN. Intakes of calcium, phosphorus, and protein, and physical activity are related to radial bone mass in young adult women. *Am J Clin Nutr.* 1993;58:537–542.
34. Wahlqvist M, Strauss B. Clinical nutrition in primary health care. Part 2: assessment, diagnosis, presentation and management. *Aust Fam Physician.* 1992;21:1633–1640.
35. Sambrook P, Birmingham J, Kelly P. Prevention of corticosteroid osteoporosis: a comparison of calcium, calcitriol, and calcitonin. *N Engl J Med.* 1993;328:1747–1752.
36. Hollenbach KA, Barrett-Connor E, Edelstein S. Cigarette smoking and bone mineral density in older men and women. *Am J Public Health.* 1993;83:1265–1270.
37. Kiel DP, Baron JA, Anderson JJ. Smoking eliminates the protective effect of oral estrogens on the risk of hip fracture among women. *Ann Intern Med.* 1992;116:716–721.
38. Harris SS, Dawson-Hughes B. Caffeine and bone loss in healthy postmenopausal women. *Am J Clin Nutr.* 1994;60:573–578.
39. Hernandez-Avila M, Colkitz GA, et al. Caffeine, moderate alcohol intake, and risk of fractures of the hip and forearm in middle-aged women. *Am J Clin Nutr.* 1991;54:157–163.
40. Gavaler JS. Alcohol and nutrition in postmenopausal women. *J Am Coll Nutr.* 1993;12(4):349–356.
41. Lukert BP, Raisz LG. Glucocorticoid-induced osteoporosis. *Rheum Dis Clin North Am.* 1994;20(3):629–650.
42. Massey LK, Whiting SJ. Caffeine, urinary calcium, calcium metabolism and bone. *J Nutr.* 1993;123:1611–1614.
43. Weaver CM, Plawecki KL. Dietary calcium: adequacy of a vegetarian diet. *Am J Clin Nutr.* 1994;59(suppl):1238s–1241s.
44. Greendale GA, Barrett-Connor E, Edelstein S. Dietary sodium and bone mineral density: results of a 16-year follow-up study. *J Am Geriatr Soc.* 1994;42:1050–1055.
45. Knox TA, Kassarjian Z, Dawson-Hughes B, et al. Calcium absorption in elderly subjects on high and low fiber diets: effect of gastric acidity. *Am J Clin Nutr.* 1991;53:1480–1486.
46. Hirota T, Nara M, Ohguri M. Effect of diet and lifestyle on bone mass in Asian young women. *Am J Clin Nutr.* 1992;55:1168–1173.
47. Wolman RL. Osteoporosis and exercise. *Br Med J.* 1994;309:400–403.
48. Farmer ME, Harris T, Madans JH, et al. Anthropometric indicators and hip fracture: the NHANES I epidemiologic follow-up study. *J Am Geriatr Soc.* 1989;37:9–16.
49. Murray C, O'Brien K. Osteoporosis workup: evaluating bone loss and risk of fractures. *Geriatrics.* 1995;50:41–53.
50. Pomerantz EM. Osteoporosis and the female patient. *Orthop Phys Ther Clin North Am.* 1996;5:71–84.
51. Van Kuijk C, Hagiwara S, Genant HK. Radiologic assessment of osteoporosis. *J Musculoskel Med.* 1994;11(4):25–32.
52. Arnaud CD. Osteoporosis: using bone markers for diagnosis and monitoring. *Geriatrics.* 1996;51(4):24–30.
53. Eastell R. Biochemical markers. *Spine: State of the Art Reviews.* 1994;8(1):155–170.
54. Castelo-Branco C, Pons F, Gratacos E, et al. Relationship between skin collagen and bone changes during aging. *Maturitas.* 1994;18:199–206.
55. Castelo-Branco C, Duran M, Gonzalez-Merlo J. Skin collagen changes related to age and hormone replacement therapy. *Maturitas.* 1992;15:113–119.
56. Chappard D, Alexandre CH, Robert JM, Riffat G. Relationship between bone and skin atrophies during aging. *Acta Anat.* (Basel) 1991;141:239–244.
57. Delmas PD. Biochemical markers of bone turnover: methodology and clinical use in osteoporosis. *Am J Med.* 1991;91(suppl 5B):59S–63S.
58. Garnero P, Gineyts E, Riou JP, Delmas PD. Assessment of bone resorption with a new marker of collagen degradation in patients with metabolic bone disease. *J Clin Endocrinol Metab.* 1994;79(3):780–785.
59. Gertz BJ, Shao P, Hanson DA. Monitoring bone resorption in early postmenopausal women by an immunoassay for cross-linked collagen peptides in urine. *J Bone Miner Res.* 1994;9(2):135–142.
60. Rubin SM, Cummings SR. Results of bone densitometry affect women's decisions about taking measures to prevent fractures. *Ann Intern Med.* 1992;116(12):990–995.
61. Kanis JA. The restoration of skeletal mass: a theoretic overview. *Am J Med.* 1991;91(suppl 5B):29S–36S.
62. Anderson JJB, Metz JA. Contributions of dietary calcium and physical activity to primary prevention of osteoporosis in females. *J Am Coll Nutr.* 1993;12:378–383.
63. Fehily AM, Coles RJ, Evans WD. Factors affecting bone density in young adults. *Am J Clin Nutr.* 1992;56:579–586.
64. Alekel L, Clasey JL, Fehling PC, et al. Contributions of exercise, body composition, and age to bone mineral density in premenopausal women. *Med Sci Sports Exerc.* 1995;27:1477–1485.
65. Vargo MM. Osteoporosis: strategies for prevention and treatment. *J Musculoskel Med.* 1995;12:19–30.
66. Dalsky GP. The role of exercise in the prevention of osteoporosis. *Compr Ther.* 1989;15:30–37.
67. Eisman JA, Sambrook PN, Kelly PJ. Exercise and its interaction with genetic influences in the determination of bone mineral density. *Am J Med.* 1991;91(suppl 5B):5S–9S.
68. Nelson ME, Fisher EC, Dilmanlan FA. A 1-year walking program and increased dietary calcium in postmenopausal women: effects on bone. *Am J Clin Nutr.* 1991;53:1304–1311.
69. Krall EA, Dawson-Hughes B. Walking is related to bone density and rates of bone loss. *Am J Med.* 1994;96:20–26.
70. Dalsky GP, Stocke KS, Ehsani AA, et al. Weightbearing exercise training and lumbar bone mineral content in postmenopausal women. *Ann Intern Med.* 1988;108:824–829.
71. Barry HC, Rich BSE, Carlson RT. How exercise can benefit older patients. *Physician Sportsmed.* 1993;21(2):124–140.
72. Adachi JD. Current treatment options for osteoporosis. *J Rheumatol.* 1996;23(suppl 45):11–14.
73. Bellantoni MF. Osteoporosis prevention and treatment. *Am Fam Physician.* 1996;54(3):986–992.
74. American College on Sportsmedicine. American College on Sportsmedicine: position stand on osteoporosis and exercise. *Med Sci Sports Exerc.* 1995;27(4):i–vii.
75. Wickham CAC, Walsh K, Cooper C, et al. Dietary calcium, physical activity, and risk of hip fracture: a prospective study. *Br Med J.* 1989;299:889–892.
76. Harward MP. Nutritive therapies for osteoporosis. *Med Clin North Am.* 1993;77(4):889–898.
77. Heaney RP. Effect of calcium on skeletal development, bone loss and risk of fractures. *Am J Med.* 1991;91(suppl 5B):23S–28S.
78. Cumming RG. Calcium intake and bone mass: a quantitative review of the evidence. *Calcif Tissue Int.* 1990;47:194–201.
79. Matkovic V. Calcium metabolism and calcium requirements during skeletal modeling and consolidation of bone mass. *Am J Clin Nutr.* 1991;54:245s–260s.
80. Heaney RP. Bone mass, nutrition and other lifestyle factors. *Am J Med.* 1993;95(suppl 5A):29S–33S.

81. Proceedings from the National Institutes of Health: consensus development conference statement—optimal calcium intake. *JAMA.* 1994;272(24):1942–1948.
82. Miller JZ, Smith DL, Flora L, et al. Calcium absorption in children estimated from single and double stable calcium isotope techniques. *Clin Chem Acta.* 1989;183:107–113.
83. Miller JZ, Smith DL, Flora L, et al. Calcium absorption from calcium carbonate and a new form of calcium (CCM) in healthy male and female adolescents. *Am J Clin Nutr.* 1988;48:1291–1294.
84. Gallagher JC. The role of vitamin D in the pathogenesis and treatment of osteoporosis. *J Rheumatol.* 1996;23(suppl 45):15–18.
85. Cook A. Osteoporosis: review and commentary. *J Neuromuskoskel Syst.* 1994;2(1):9–18.
86. Dawson-Hughes B, Dallal GE, Krall EA, et al. A controlled trial of the effect of calcium supplementation on bone density in postmenopausal women. *N Engl J Med.* 1990;323:878–883.
87. Bikle DD. Role of vitamin D, its metabolites, and analogs in the management of osteoporosis. *Rheum Dis Clin North Am.* 1994;20(3):757–775.
88. Dawson-Hughes B, Dallal GE, Krall EA. Effect of vitamin D supplementation on wintertime and overall bone loss in healthy postmenopausal women. *Ann Intern Med.* 1991;115:505–512.
89. Nordin BEC, Baker MR. A prospective trial of the effect of vitamin D supplementation on metacarpal bone loss in elderly women. *Am J Clin Nutr.* 1985;42:470–474.
90. Gallagher JC, Goldgar D. Treatment of postmenopausal osteoporosis with high doses of synthetic calcitriol. *Ann Intern Med.* 1990;113:649–655.
91. Tilyard MW, Spears GFS, Thomson J. Treatment of postmenopausal osteoporosis with calcitriol or calcium. *N Engl J Med.* 1992;326:357–362.
92. Gallagher JC. Antiresorptive therapy in osteoporosis. *Spine: State of the Art Reviews.* 1994;8(1):199–223.
93. Chapuy MC, Arlot ME, Duboeuf F. Vitamin D_3 and calcium to prevent hip fractures in elderly women. *New Engl J Med.* 1992;327:1637–1642.
94. Rosen HN, Maitland LA, Suttle JW. Vitamin K and maintenance of skeletal integrity in adults. *Am J Med.* 1993;94:62–68.
95. Rude RK, Adams JS, Ryzen E. Low serum concentrations of 1,25-dihydroxyvitamin D in human magnesium deficiency. *J Clin Endocrinol Metab.* 1985;61:933–940.
96. Sojka JE, Weaver CM. Magnesium supplementation and osteoporosis. *Nutr Rev.* 1995;53(3):71–80.
97. Robey PG, Fisher LW, Young MF, Termine JD. The biochemistry of bone. In: Riggs BL, Melton LJ, eds. *Osteoporosis: Etiology, Diagnosis, and Management.* New York: Raven Press; 1988.
98. Civitelli R, Gonnelli S, Zacchei F, et al. Bone turnover in postmenopausal osteoporosis: effect of calcitonin. *J Clin Invest.* 1988;82:1268–1274.
99. El-Choufi L, Nelson J, Kleerekoper M. Therapeutic options in osteoporosis. *J Musculoskel Med.* 1994;11(10):15–21.
100. Reginster JY. Effect of calcitonin on bone mass and fracture rates. *Am J Med.* 1991;91(suppl 5B):19s–22s.
101. Gamble CL. Osteoporosis: drug and nondrug therapies for the patient at risk. *Geriatrics.* 1995;50(8):39–43.
102. Ettinger B, Genant HK, Cann CE, et al. Postmenopausal bone loss is prevented by treatment with low-dosage estrogen with calcium. *Ann Intern Med.* 1987;106:40–45.
103. Griffing GT, Allen SH. Estrogen replacement therapy at menopause. *Postgrad Med.* 1994;96:131–140.
104. Felson DT, Zhang Y, et al. The effect of postmenopausal estrogen therapy on bone density in elderly women. *N Engl J Med.* 1993;329:1141–1146.
105. Prestwood KM, Raisz LG. Using estrogen to prevent and treat osteoporosis. *J Musculoskel Med.* 1994;11(5):17–27.
106. Heaney RP. Estrogen-calcium interactions in the postmenopause: a quantitative description. *Bone Miner.* 1990;11:67–84.
107. Lindsay R. Estrogens, bone mass, and osteoporotic fracture. *Am J Med.* 1991;91(suppl 5B):10S–13S.
108. Cummings SR. Evaluating the benefits and risks of postmenopausal hormone therapy. *Am J Med.* 1991;91(suppl 5B):14S–18S.
109. Barlow DH. Estrogen treatment of established osteoporosis. *Spine: State of the Art Reviews.* 1994;8(1):189–197.
110. Colditz GA, Hankinson SE, Hunter MB, et al. The use of estrogens and progestins and the risk of breast cancer in postmenopausal women. *N Engl J Med.* 1995;322:1589–1593.
111. Parfitt AM. Use of bisphosphonates in the prevention of bone loss and fracture. *Am J Med.* 1991;91(suppl 5B):42S–46S.
112. Watts NB. Treatment of osteoporosis with bisphosphonates. *Rheum Dis Clin North Am.* 1994;20(3):717–734.
113. Riggs BL. Treatment of osteoporosis with sodium fluoride of parathyroid. *Am J Med.* 1991;91(suppl 5B):37S–41S.
114. Liberman UA, Weiss SR, Broll J, et al. Effect of oral alendronate on bone mineral density and the incidence of fractures in postmenopausal osteoporosis. The alendronate phase III osteoporosis treatment study group. *N Engl J Med.* 1995;333:1437–1443.
115. Pak CYC, Sakhaee K, Zerwekh JE, et al. Safe and effective treatment of osteoporosis with intermittent slow release sodium fluoride: augmentation of vertebral bone mass and inhibition of fractures. *J Clin Endocrinol Metab.* 1989;68(1):150–159.
116. Riggs BL, Seeman E, Hodgson SF, et al. Effect of the fluoride/calcium regimen on vertebral fracture occurrence in postmenopausal osteoporosis. *N Engl J Med.* 1982;306:446–450.
117. Boivin G, Meunier PJ, Reeve J. Treatments that are anabolic for osteoblasts: fluoride and parathyroid peptides. *Spine: State of the Art Reviews.* 1994;8:225–250.
118. Ebeling P. Male osteoporosis. *Aust Fam Physician.* 1994;23:1967–1969.
119. Pool R. Coral chemistry leads to human bone repair. *Science.* 1995;267:1772.
120. Constantz BR, Ison IC, Fulmer MT. Skeletal repair by in situ forma-tion of the mineral phase of bone. *Science.* 1995;267:1796–1798.
121. Hodgson SF, Johnston CC. *AACE Clinical Practice Guidelines for the Prevention and Treatment of Postmenopausal Osteoporosis.* Brandamore, Pa: American Association of Clinical Endocrinology; 1996.

Algorithm 1

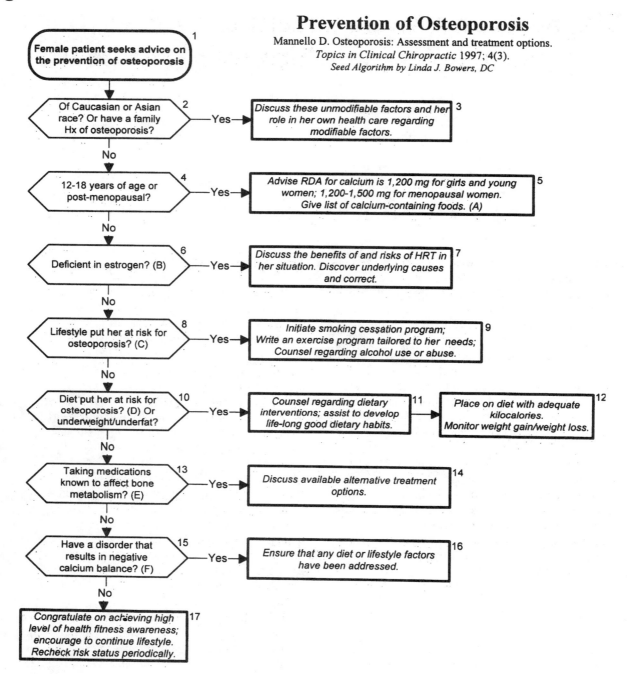

Prevention of Osteoporosis
Mannello D. Osteoporosis: Assessment and treatment options.
Topics in Clinical Chiropractic 1997; 4(3).
Seed Algorithm by Linda J. Bowers, DC

Annotations:
(A) e.g., yogurt, milk, cheese, calcium-fortified orange juice, broccoli, kale, spinach, sardines/salmon with the bones.
(B) post-menopausal, early menopause, early oophorectomy, hypogonadism due to excessive exercise.
(C) e.g., sedentary, cigarette smoking, alcohol abuse, long term intensive aerobic exercise.
(D) e.g., excessive caffeine, fiber, sodium, phosphorus, and protein intake; inadequate calcium, vitamin D or protein intake; excessive alcohol use.
(E) e.g., exogenous thyroid, steroids, aluminum-containing antacids, tetracycline, anticonvulsants.
(F) e.g., hyperparathyroidism, hyperthyroidism, diabetes mellitus, Cushing's, metabolic acidosis, chronic renal failure, chonic diarrhea or malabsorption, chronic obstructive lung disease, subtotal gastrectomy, hemiplegia.

11

Diagnosis and Management of Premenstrual Syndrome in the Chiropractic Office

Tolu A. Oyelowo

Premenstrual syndrome (PMS) was first characterized in 1931 by a gynecologist named T. Frank.[1] It is a catch-all term used to describe a wide array of often debilitating symptoms experienced by women during the luteal phase of the menstrual cycle. The general criteria for a diagnosis of PMS are symptoms that commonly begin shortly after ovulation, peak prior to menstruation, and stop or subside within a day or two after the onset of menstrual bleeding. These symptoms must be documented over several menstrual cycles, they must not be caused by any other physiologic or psychologic disorder, and they must be severe enough to disrupt the patient's lifestyle.[2,3] Common symptoms of PMS are listed in Table 1.

The American Psychiatric Association has further proposed that women with severe PMS actually have a psychologic disorder termed premenstrual dysphoric disorder (PDD). The criteria for a diagnosis of PDD require that 5 of 11 listed symptoms must be severe premenstrually and resolve postmenstrually and that the five symptoms must include at least one dysphoric symptom such as depression. These criteria are listed in Table 2.[4]

PREVALENCE

Estimates of the prevalence of PMS range from 10% to 90%. This large discrepancy is due to the differing modes of assessment. Approximately 40% of women of reproductive age suffer from true PMS, and about 9% suffer from PDD using the previously described criteria.

THE MENSTRUAL CYCLE

The bleeding phase of the menstrual cycle (days 1 through 5) is characterized by very low levels of estrogen and progesterone. These levels are insufficient to support uterine endometrial tissue, which then breaks down. This tissue, blood, and other secretions are released from the cervix and vagina. The low levels of estrogen and progesterone stimulate the hypothalamus to secrete releasing factors that affect the anterior pituitary, causing the release of follicle stimulating hormone (FSH) and luteinizing hormone (LH). FSH stimulates the primordial cells of the ovary, and although several primordial follicles are stimulated, usually only one follicle is recruited. This dominant follicle progresses in maturation and function and begins to secrete estrogen, causing proliferation of the uterine lining of the endometrium and the glandular and ductal tissue of the breast (days 6 through 13).

The rising levels of estrogen have a negative effect on pituitary production of FSH and a positive effect on pituitary production of LH. This action results in a surge of LH, which causes the dominant (graafian) follicle to release an egg. Ovulation occurs on or around the 14th day in a woman who has a 28-day menstrual cycle.

Within the ruptured graafian follicle, the corpus luteum develops and secretes progesterone (days 15 through 28). Progesterone is a thermogenic hormone that thickens the endometrial lining by inducing the secretory abilities of the endometrial cells. Rising levels of progesterone have an inhibitory effect on the continued secretion of LH by the pituitary gland. The low levels of LH cause the corpus luteum to regress, resulting in a

---

Adapted from *Top Clin Chiro* 1997; 4(3): 60–67
© 1997 Aspen Publishers, Inc.

The author thanks Dr. Linda Bowers for her professional expertise.

Table 1. Common symptoms of PMS

- Headaches
- Migraines
- Food cravings
- Allergic rhinitis
- Depression
- Irritability
- Confusion
- Violent behavior
- Breast tenderness
- Bloating/water retention
- Back pain

Sources: Cohen K. *Clinical Management of Women in the Childbearing Years.* Extension Press; 1991. Lark, SM. *Dr. Susan Lark's Premenstrual Syndrome Self-Help Book. A Woman's Guide to Feeling Good All Month.* Los Angeles: Forman Publishing; 1984. Walter DS. *Applied Kinesiology.* Pueblo, Colo: Systems DC; 1981.

decline in progesterone production and leading once again to the breakdown of the endometrial lining.[5,6]

ETIOLOGY

Hippocrates blamed premenstrual tension on the "agitated blood of a woman seeking a way of escape from the womb."[1(p30)] It suffices to say that establishing a cause for PMS has "agitated" countless minds over the years. The following text is an overview of proposed etiologies.

Decreased serotonergic activity

Serotonin is formed from tryptophan and is released from mast cells and blood platelets. It is a precursor of melatonin, as well as a central neurotransmitter. Studies[7,8] of women with PMS reveal decreased serotonin levels in platelets and whole blood. Decreased serotonergic activity has been shown to cause depression, a common PMS symptom.

Estrogen excess or progesterone deficiency

Symptoms of PMS intensify late in the luteal phase as progesterone levels decline. Declining progesterone gives rise to a relative estrogen excess. This excess may cause fluid retention, hyperplasia of breast tissue, and abnormal carbohydrate metabolism. Elevated levels of estrogen may also cause symptoms of nervous tension and anxiety, irritability, and insomnia. In addition, elevated levels of estrogen stimulate the renin angiotensin system resulting in increased aldosterone production. Increased levels of aldosterone promote sodium and water retention, manifested by symptoms of bloating, weight gain, swelling of the extremities, and breast tenderness.[2,7,9–11]

Altered thyroid function

Normal thyroid function is essential for normal functioning of the menstrual cycle. Thyroid stimulating hormone is secreted by the anterior pituitary gland via stimulation by thyroid releasing hormone, which also controls the anterior

Table 2. Criteria for Premenstrual Dysphoric Disorder

A. In most menstrual cycles during the past year, five (or more) of the following symptoms were present for most of the time during the last week of the luteal phase, began to remit within a few days after the onset of the follicular phase, and were absent in the week postmenses, with at least one of the symptoms being either (1), (2), (3), or (4):
  1. markedly depressed mood, feelings of hopelessness, or self-deprecating thoughts
  2. marked anxiety, tension, feelings of being "keyed up" or "on edge"
  3. marked affective lability (eg, feeling suddenly sad or tearful or increased sensitivity to rejection)
  4. persistent and marked anger or irritability or increased interpersonal conflicts
  5. decreased interest in usual activities (eg, work, school, friends, hobbies)
  6. subjective sense of difficulty in concentrating
  7. lethargy, easy fatigability, or marked lack of energy
  8. marked change in appetite, overeating, or specific food cravings
  9. hypersomnia or insomnia
  10. a subjective sense of being overwhelmed or out of control
  11. other physical symptoms, such as breast tenderness or swelling, headaches, joint or muscle pain, a sensation of "bloating" or weight gain
B. The disturbance markedly interferes with work or school or with usual social activities and relationships with others (eg, avoidance of social activities, decreased productivity and efficiency at work or school).
C. The disturbance is not merely an exacerbation of the symptoms of another disorder, such as major depressive disorder, panic disorder, dysthymic disorder, or a personality disorder (although it may be superimposed on any of these disorders).
D. Criteria A, B, and C must be confirmed by prospective daily ratings during at least two consecutive symptomatic cycles. (The diagnosis may be made provisionally prior to the confirmation.)

Sources: Cohen K. *Clinical Management of Women in the Childbearing Years.* Extension Press; 1991. Lark, SM. *Dr. Susan Lark's Premenstrual Syndrome Self-Help Book. A Woman's Guide to Feeling Good All Month.* Los Angeles: Forman Publishing; 1984. Walter DS. *Applied Kinesiology.* Pueblo, Colo: Systems DC; 1981. American Psychiatric Association. *Diagnostic and Statistical Manual of Mental Disorders.* 4th ed. Washington, DC: American Psychiatric Association; 1994.

pituitary's release of prolactin. Elevated levels of thyroid releasing hormone, as occurs with hypothyroidism, may induce hyperprolactinemia. Although the evidence linking premenstrual syndrome with hyperprolactinemia is inconclusive, prolactin levels do increase mid cycle, and suppression of prolactin secretion in women with premenstrual syndrome has been shown to relieve breast symptoms. Furthermore, the general effect of thyroid hormone on tissue metabolism is important to proper functioning of the neurohormonal axis. Thyroid hormone is also important in the cellular metabolism of the ovary. Abnormal thyroid function may therefore result in PMS symptomatology.[5,12–15]

Deficient cofactors

Dopamine is a decarboxylated form of dopa found in the adrenal glands. The production of dopamine relies on vitamin B_6 and magnesium as cofactors. Therefore, suboptimal levels of vitamin B_6 result in suboptimal production of dopamine. As dopamine functions as an aldosterone antagonist, low levels of dopamine may result in higher than normal levels of aldosterone.[5,16] Increased levels of aldosterone promote sodium and water retention.

Estrogen is excreted through the elimination of estrogen conjugates, which are produced in the liver. This reaction requires the presence of glucuronide and vitamins such as B_6 to function as coenzymes. Suboptimal levels of vitamin B_6 could therefore lower the hepatic rate of estrogen clearance.

Vitamin B_6 acts as a coenzyme (pyridoxal phosphate) in the synthesis of serotonin. Therefore, suboptimal levels of vitamin B_6 could result in a deficiency of serotonin. As previously stated, a deficiency of serotonin may cause depression. Calcium and magnesium are cofactors in the synthesis of many neurotransmitters. For example, the conversion of tryptophan to serotonin requires calcium and magnesium. Suboptimal levels of these minerals could result in low serotonin levels. Magnesium is required for the phosphorylation of B vitamins, whereby they become active coenzymes. A magnesium deficiency may cause a relative B vitamin deficiency.[16]

Altered blood sugar levels

Blood glucose levels in the healthy individual remain within a range of about 30 mg/dL. When food is ingested, the blood glucose level rises and then gradually drops as insulin is released from the pancreas. This process is repeated continuously throughout the day. If food is not ingested, the blood glucose level will continue to fall until it reaches a baseline level. It is prevented from going beneath the baseline by the body's built-in homeostatic mechanisms. Once the blood sugar level reaches the baseline, in the absence of ingested food, adrenalin (epinephrine) is released, which mobilizes stored carbohydrate. As adrenalin is the hormone responsible for the body's "fright and flight" response, symptoms of fear, anxiety, and heart pounding may be experienced by some women with PMS. During the premenstruum, changes in hormonal levels alter the blood glucose level, raising the lower level of the baseline and producing an increased appetite and craving for sweets.[10]

Prostaglandins

Increased production of certain prostaglandins causes bone resorption and dysmenorrhea and influences glucose metabolism. In addition, there are elevated prostaglandin concentrations in the central nervous system. Prostaglandins influence the excitability of neurons,[5] and they may account for PMS symptoms such as heart palpitations, panic attacks, headaches, migraines, feelings of dizziness, mood swings, and fainting spells.

Psychologic factors

For decades, physicians who were unable to account for the wide array of PMS symptoms told women that it was "all in their heads." Unfortunately, these women suffered tremendously due to this ignorance. However, there is a strong indication of a psychologic component to PMS, as women frequently relate the onset or worsening of symptoms following stressful situations, emotional trauma, rape, or other physical abuse.

Psychoneuroendocrine mechanisms

A recent theory regarding the cause of PMS states that normal ovarian function rather than hormone imbalance is the cyclical trigger for biochemical events within the central nervous system and other target tissues. A psychoneuroendocrine mechanism triggered by the normal endocrine events of the ovarian cycle is now considered to be a plausible explanation for PMS.[7,8,11]

DIAGNOSTIC CRITERIA

To diagnose PMS, a clear pattern of symptoms that begin prior to menses (during the luteal phase) and improve or disappear once menses begins needs to be documented. These symptoms should be severe enough to cause a disruption in the patient's lifestyle (ie, have a subjective impact on the woman's relationships with others or her ability to function at home or work) and be recurrent (ie, occur over several menstrual cycles). The symptoms can be physical (eg, fatigue, abdominal distention, headaches, and migraines) or psychologic (eg, mood swings, anxiety, depression, loss of control, and tension).[3,17]

Although it is always important for the physician and patient to work together, it is even more so for a woman with PMS because she must keep careful records of her symptoms and signs. The patient should be advised to keep a daily diary of pertinent signs and symptoms of PMS for 2 to 3 months. This approach allows evaluation of the timing, characteristics, and severity of symptoms. The diary should include dates of menstrual blood loss, dates of ovulation, and character and severity of symptoms. The patient can use her own diary or may wish to utilize other daily assessment measures. These measures may include the Patient Daily Self-Assessment Form, the Visual Analogue Scale, and the modifications of the Moos Menstrual Distress Questionnaire (Figure 1).[18]

The physician should perform a complete physical examination, including pelvic, abdominal, and rectovaginal examinations. Although there is no pathognomonic symptom, sign, lab test, or finding to diagnosis PMS, a Pap smear, blood chemistries, routine urinalysis, and thyroid function tests should be ordered or performed. Several studies report abnormally low thyroid function in many women with PMS.

The chiropractic physician should perform a complete neuromusculoskeletal examination. Particular attention should be given to the region from T-11 through S-3, as this region is the one from which sympathetic and parasympathetic innervation to the reproductive organs originate. Stude[19] reports a case of improved premenstrual syndrome symptomatology following spinal manipulation. Browning[20–22] demonstrated a link between pelvic pain and organic dysfunction as a result of sacral nerve compromise.

Particular attention should be paid in the evaluation of the range of motion of the femur at the hip. The function of the adductor and psoas major muscles, which are innervated by nerve roots L2–4, is to adduct and medially rotate the femur at the hip. It is this author's clinical observation that these muscles are frequently hypertonic in patients with menstrual disorders, causing restricted movement in abduction and lateral rotation of the femur at the hip.

The use of hormone assays of estrogen and progesterone levels taken at 7-day intervals during the course of one menstrual cycle has been advocated. However, physicians may choose an initial trial of conservative therapy including diet modification, exercise, and nutritional supplementation prior to ordering these blood tests due to their high costs.

Another author[7] suggested the use of the drug goserelin as a diagnostic measure. It is a gonadotrophin releasing hormone (GnRH) analogue that is given for 3 months to eliminate cyclical ovarian function. Complete elimination of symptoms after 3 months of use implies that the symptoms are solely dependent on ovarian activity and supports the diagnosis of PMS.[7]

Referral for psychologic evaluation may be necessary if a diagnosis of PMS is unclear or if the patient's symptoms are severe and/or uncharacteristic.

MANAGEMENT

For several years, it was believed that the cause of PMS was low levels of progesterone. Progesterone replacement thus became the treatment of choice for patients with PMS. It has become apparent, however, that while progesterone therapy is beneficial for some patients, it is not the cure for all patients with PMS. The only clear conclusion that can be drawn from a review of the literature on treatment modalities for PMS is that no clear conclusions can be made and that further research is needed. The following text presents an overview of management approaches that have been reported to have beneficial effects. It is understood that correction of any existing thyroid abnormalities would be undertaken in addition to these therapeutic interventions. Algorithm 1 reviews management options.

Lifestyle modifications and psychosocial interventions

Education and reassurance are central and critical to the management of patients with PMS.[5] The patient should be informed that the disorder is common in women in their reproductive years. The physician should briefly explain PMS and assure the patient that her symptoms are real and that she is not crazy. She should be taught the basics of the menstrual cycle. She should be assisted in determining stressors in her life, and recommendations should be made for stress reduction techniques such as yoga, biofeedback, and the "relaxation response" (Table 3).[23] These stress reduction techniques have been demonstrated to decrease the severity of physical and emotional premenstrual symptoms.[23] The physician should encourage her to get adequate rest so that she can function at an optimal level when symptoms occur.

Table 3. The Relaxation Response

1. Sit quietly in a comfortable position.
2. Deeply relax all muscles, beginning with the face and progressing down to the feet.
3. Breathe through the nose. Become aware of your breath. As you breathe out, say the word "One."
4. Maintain a passive attitude and permit relaxation to occur at its own pace. Do not worry about being successful in achieving a deep level of relaxation. When a distracting thought comes to mind, simply say "Oh well" and go back to the word "One."
5. Practice the technique 15 to 20 min twice each day.

Sources: Cohen K. *Clinical Management of Women in the Childbearing Years.* Extension Press; 1991. Lark, SM. *Dr. Susan Lark's Premenstrual Syndrome Self-Help Book. A Woman's Guide to Feeling Good All Month.* Los Angeles: Forman Publishing; 1984. Walter DS. *Applied Kinesiology.* Pueblo, Colo: Systems DC; 1981. Goodagle II, Domar AD, Benson H. Alleviation of premenstrual syndrome symptoms with the relaxation response. *Obstet Gynecol.* 1990;75:649–655.

PATIENT DAILY SELF-ASSESSMENT FORM

Name: _____ Cycle number: _____

Date: _____ Day number: _____

Please rate the way you feel in terms of the dimension below. Regard the lines as representing the full range of each dimension. Rate your feelings as they are at the moment. Mark clearly and perpendicularly across each line. Please complete at the same time each day.

Alert _____	Drowsy
Calm _____	Excited
Strong _____	Feeble
Fuzzy _____	Clear-headed
Well-coordinated _____	Clumsy
Lethargic _____	Energetic
Contented _____	Discontented
Troubled _____	Tranquil
Mentally slow _____	Quick witted
Tense _____	Relaxed
Attentive _____	Dreamy
Incompetent _____	Proficient
Happy _____	Sad
Antagonistic _____	Friendly
Interested _____	Bored
Withdrawn _____	Sociable
Depressed _____	Elated
Self-centered _____	Outward going
Bloated _____	Thin
Irritable _____	Calm

Fig 1. Daily PMS assessment measures. *Source:* Reprinted with permission from B. Faratian, A. Gaspar, and P.M. O'Brien, Premenstrual syndrome, *American Journal of Obstetrics and Gynecology,* Vol. 150, No. 2, pp. 200–204, © 1984.

Coping mechanisms

The patient should be taught to schedule activities with PMS in mind (ie, not to overschedule when symptoms are apt to be at their worst). Self-education should also be encouraged. Books such as *Dr. Susan Lark's Premenstrual Syndrome Self-Help Book*[24] and *How To Cope with Menstrual Problems*[25] give helpful insights for managing premenstrual syndrome. Encourage the patient to carry small, low-calorie snacks in her purse for times when symptoms such as fatigue, difficulty concentrating, and irritability occur.[6,25] If she smokes, cessation should be encouraged.[26]

Exercise

There is no evidence that one specific type of exercise (eg, weight-bearing or non-weight-bearing) is better for the management of PMS. There is evidence that exercise influences levels of estradiol.[27] Patients who exercise regularly obtain systemic benefits that may temper the symptoms of PMS. General recommendations include a daily, light aerobic workout, such as a brisk walk. This exercise encourages the release of endorphins and the stimulation of the immune system. Sporadic exercise during or before the premenstruum could strain muscles, resulting in a perceived increase of symptomatology.[28–30]

Diet

Nine recommendations relative to diet are offered:

1. Encourage the patient to eat small, regular meals that include whole grains, green leafy vegetables, and fruit. Small, frequent meals during the luteal phase can be helpful in reducing the postprandial rebound hypoglycemia.[1,5,28] Carbohydrate consumption without protein has been shown to increase serotonin synthesis and release by increasing brain uptake of the serotonin precursor, tryptophan.[8]
2. Limit red meats, dairy items, and fried foods. They are sources of arachidonic acid, a precursor in the synthesis of prostaglandins E and Falpha, which have been implicated in primary dysmenorrhea. A preliminary double-blind, placebo-controlled study showed some alleviation of the symptoms of PMS with the administration of a prostaglandin synthetase inhibitor.[1,5,26,28]
3. Limit or eliminate caffeine, as it can intensify anxiety and has been linked to PMS.[1,5,31] Patients should be educated as to common sources of caffeine in their diets such as coffee, tea, cola, and certain over-the-counter medications.
4. Limit or eliminate foods with a high sugar content. Rossignol and Bonnlander[32] demonstrated that foods and beverages that are high in sugar may be associated with an increased prevalence of premenstrual symptoms in women between the ages of 18 and 22.
5. Screen the diet for excessive yeast intake or possible food allergies. Researchers studying the yeast Candida found an estrogen binding protein in *Candida albicans*.[33,34]
6. Avoid or limit salt, especially during the luteal phase, to reduce the risk of perceived or actual water retention.
7. Dietary fiber intake should be increased, as this increase may aid in the clearance and fecal excretion of estrogen.[35]
8. Increase water intake to six to eight glasses per day to achieve a natural diuresis.
9. Decrease or eliminate alcohol consumption, as data suggest an association between alcohol use and PMS.[36]

Nutritional supplementation

The clinician should tailor any nutritional supplementation advice given to a woman with PMS. He or she should consider the patient's present diet and symptoms of PMS when prescribing nutritional supplements and advise her that supplements cannot offset poor dietary habits. Supplementation should be used in addition to other conservative measures and never as a shotgun measure.

Some useful recommendations concerning supplementation follow:

1. Primrose oil: 1,000 to 2,000 mg daily as a source of omega six fatty acids; precursors in the synthesis of prostaglandin E1.[1,26,28,37]
2. Flaxseed and borage oil: as a source of the omega three fatty acids, also precursors in the synthesis of anti-inflammatory prostaglandins.[1] Although there are some contradictory studies,[38,39] there is evidence that supplementation with omega-six and omega-three fatty acids reduces premenstrual breast tenderness, mood swings, and irritability.[1,28,37,40]
3. Magnesium: 400 to 1,000 mg daily for reasons previously given.[28,37,41,42]
4. Vitamin B$_6$: 50 to 500 mg daily for reasons previously given.[28,37,43,44] *Note:* At doses over 600 mg, vitamin B$_6$ (pyridoxine) has been associated with peripheral neuropathy.[45] Patients should therefore be cautioned about excessive dosages.
5. St. John's wort: an herb that has been shown to be effective in the treatment of depression.[46] It may be useful for women suffering from mild depression.
6. Zinc: evaluate levels. Chuong and Dawson[47] demonstrated a zinc deficiency and copper excess in a small group of patients with PMS.

Spinal manipulation

There is a little information in the chiropractic practice literature regarding PMS and manipulation or chiropractic care of women with PMS. The few reports available indicate favorable response with manipulation. Particular attention should be given to areas of innervation to the breasts and pelvic organs.

Browning[21] reports improvement in symptoms relating to the pelvis following distractive decompressive manipulation in patients with lower sacral nerve root compression. Liebl and Butler[48] report improved symptoms of dysmenorrhea following manipulation of primarily L-1, L-2, L-5, and the sacroiliac joints. Stude[19] reports a case of improved premenstrual syndrome symptomatology following manipulation of the lumbar and lumbosacral spine.

Furthermore, it is this author's observation that the sacral base angle is frequently increased in women with menstrual cycle–related disorders. Adjustive procedures designed to reduce the sacral base angle appear to be beneficial. In cases where anxiety and irritability are presenting complaints, low force techniques such as Logan Basic and Spinal Touch may be utilized.[16,49]

Neurolymphatic stimulation

This approach may be instituted. Points that correlate to the areas of complaint should be used[16,24,50] (see Table 4).

Reflexology

Ear, hand, and foot reflexology may be recommended. Oleson and Flocco[51] report a significantly greater decrease in premenstrual symptoms for women given reflexology treatment than for women in a placebo group.

Pharmacologic agents

There is as yet no scientifically rational, validated, and proven drug treatment for PMS.[5] However, there are three classes of pharmacologic agents that are widely used in the treatment of PMS: (1) serotonin reuptake inhibitors (eg, fluoxetine and nefazodone); (2) hormones (eg, Lupron and oral contraceptives), and (3) benzodiazepines (eg, alprazolam). It is prudent to keep the number of medications prescribed to a minimum (preferably one).[5]

Serotonin reuptake inhibitors such as fluoxetine help to increase the pool of available serotonin. There is increasing evidence that abnormal synthesis or release of serotonin is involved in the pathogenesis of PDD, a severe form of PMS. There is also evidence that platelet serotonin uptake and blood serotonin concentrations are depressed during the luteal phase of the cycle in women with PDD.[24] The efficacy of fluoxetine as it pertains to depression has been demonstrated to be superior to that of tricyclic antidepressants. It does, however, have several reported side effects including agitation, insomnia, headaches, and gastrointestinal disturbances. Fluoxetine has also been reported to cause birth defects in animals when given in large doses.[45]

Another class of drugs that alters the normal menstrual cycle is hormones. Lupron, a GnRH agonist, is proposed to work by causing pituitary desensitization to GnRH. The production of LH and FSH is substantially reduced, as is ovarian production of estrogen and progesterone, resulting in a menopausal state. The patient therefore experiences few PMS symptoms but may experience symptoms of menopause such as vaginal dryness, hot flushes, and insomnia.[45]

Danazol is a testosterone derivative that suppresses the mid cycle surge of FSH and LH, which in effect eliminates menstrual cyclicity. It has been shown to be beneficial in treating PMS-associated migraines. Side effects include acne, weight gain, decreased breast size, and, on occasion, overt masculinizing effects such as a deepening voice. In addition, there have been reports of hepatotoxicity. Based on the risk-benefit ratio, Danazol is a poor choice for most women with PMS.[45]

Studies[7,45] of oral contraceptive use in the treatment of PMS are inconclusive. Some women report relief, but for

---

Table 4. Neurolymphatic treatment points for symptoms of PMS

Breast tenderness, anxiety, mood swings
  Anterior—Between the fifth and sixth intercostal spaces. Just lateral to the sternum.
  Posterior—Between the transverse processes of the fifth, sixth, and seventh thoracic vertebrae.
Fluid retention
  Anterior—One inch superior and 1 inch lateral to the umbilicus.
  Posterior—On the lamina of the twelfth thoracic and the first lumbar vertebrae.
Pelvic pain
  Anterior—Over the pubic ramus.
  Posterior—On the lamina of the second, third, and fourth lumbar vertebrae.

Points should be stimulated for 5 to 10 seconds with about as much pressure as can be tolerated on the eyeball. Movement should be in a circular pattern.

Sources: Cohen K. *Clinical Management of Women in the Childbearing Years.* Extension Press; 1991. Lark, SM. *Dr. Susan Lark's Premenstrual Syndrome Self-Help Book. A Woman's Guide to Feeling Good All Month.* Los Angeles: Forman Publishing; 1984. Walter DS. *Applied Kinesiology.* Pueblo, Colo: Systems DC; 1981.

others the adverse effects of oral contraceptives (ie, mood swings, appetite changes, and bloating) are precisely those from which they are trying to obtain relief. In general, oral contraceptives are not an effective treatment for PMS.

Progesterone increases monoamine oxidase (MAO) levels in the plasma during the luteal phase. One theory relates MAO levels to depression as a result of deficiency in catecholamines. If the progesterone feedback pathway in the synthesis of MAO were faulty, then, in theory, adding progesterone might help.[2,7,9,23,33]

During the luteal phase of the menstrual cycle, endorphins are elevated and inhibit catecholamines. A decreased level of catecholamines is associated with depression, and an increased level causes irritability. Progesterone therapy can maintain a level of endorphins that does not overly inhibit catecholamines, but prevents a rise to a magnitude that leads to irritability and tension.

Synthetic progestins do not have the same molecular structure as natural progesterone. They do, however, allow the treating physician to better regulate the quantity of progesterone being taken by the patient. Natural progesterone found in placentas and plants such as wild yams is most similar to that normally produced by the female. It can be given sublingually, orally, vaginally, rectally, or intramuscularly.[1-3,7,23,25,33,52,53]

Patients have reported improvement in symptoms when antianxiety medications are taken during the luteal phase. There is, however, a risk of adverse effects such as lethargy, fatigue, drowsiness, and drug dependence. There have also been cases of withdrawal symptoms similar to those seen in barbiturate withdrawal such as nausea, tremors, and muscle cramps.[2,45]

Diuretics such as spironolactone are used to treat the water retention symptoms of PMS. Side effects include hypokalemia.[2,45]

Nonsteroidal anti-inflammatory drugs are primarily used to treat dysmenorrhea. They are not very helpful with PMS symptoms.[2,45]

Surgical intervention

There is evidence that symptoms of PMS diminish following hysterectomy.[52] Of note is the contradictory evidence that PMS symptoms do not diminish following hysterectomy without bilateral ovariectomy.[54] If we are to accept the latter, then the result is a low estrogen state that predisposes the patient to increased bone loss and other menopausal symptoms. Surgical therapy for the PMS patient should only be a last resort[9] and may be a technique that can be reserved for older, severely symptomatic women if less invasive methods have failed.[2] If it remains a consideration, the risks should be weighed, and the benefits and disadvantages should be clear to the patient.[2,45]

CONCLUSION

Additional research on chiropractic and other conservative treatment approaches for PMS is needed. PMS is a serious and complex condition that appears to be amenable to conservative care. As more invasive treatment approaches have not consistently shown greater efficacy, conservative care should be encouraged as an initial trial of therapy. Treatment options, although broad, can and should be tailored to the patient's needs, and the patient should be encouraged to actively participate in her recovery.

REFERENCES

1. Norris R, Sullivan C. *PMS/Premenstrual Syndrome*. New York: Berkeley Printing; 1985.
2. Moline ML. Pharmacologic strategies for managing premenstrual syndrome. *Clin Pharm*. 1993;12(3):181–196.
3. Parker PD. Premenstrual syndrome. *Am Fam Physician*. 1994;50(6):1309–1317.
4. American Psychiatric Association. *Diagnostic and Statistical Manual of Mental Disorders*. 4th ed. Washington, DC: American Psychiatric Association; 1994.
5. Clarke-Pearson DL, Dawood Y. *Green's Gynecology: Essentials of Clinical Practice*. 4th ed. Boston: Little, Brown; 1990.
6. Youngkin E, Davis M. *Women's Health*. Norwalk, Conn: Appleton & Lange; 1994.
7. O'Brien PM. Helping women with premenstrual syndrome. *Br Med J*. 1993;307:1471–1475.
8. van Leusden HAIM. Serotonin and premenstrual dysphoric disorder. *Lancet*. 1996;347:470–471.
9. Barnhart KT, Freeman EW, Sondheimer SJ. A clinicians' guide to the premenstrual syndrome. *Med Clin North Am*. 1995;79:1457–1472.
10. Dalton K. *Once a Month*. Claremont, Cal.: Hunter House Inc; 1983.
11. van Leusden HAIM. Premenstrual syndrome no progesterone; premenstrual dysphoric disorder no serotonin deficiency. *Lancet*. 1995;346(8988):1443–1444.
12. Leibenluft E, Fiero PL, Rubinow DR. Effects of the menstrual cycle on dependent variables in mood disorder research. *Arch Gen Psychiatry*. 1994;51:761–781.
13. Mortola J. Assessment and management of premenstrual syndrome. *Curr Opin Obstet Gynecol*. 1992;4(6):877–885.
14. Brayshaw N. Thyroid hypofunction in premenstrual syndrome. *N Engl J Med*. 1986;315(23):1486–1487.
15. Schmidt PJ, Grover GN, Roy-Byrne PP. Thyroid function in women with premenstrual syndrome. *J Clin Endocrinol Metab*. 1993;76:671–674.
16. Cohen K. *Clinical Management of Women in the Childbearing Years*. Santa Cruz, Cal.: Extension Press; 1991.
17. Rubinow DR. The premenstrual syndrome. New news. *JAMA*. 1992;268:1908–1912.
18. O'Brien PMS. *Premenstrual Syndrome*. Boston: Blackwell Scientific Publications; 1987.

19. Stude DE. The management of symptoms associated with premenstrual syndrome. *J Manipulative Physiol Ther.* 1991;14:209–215.
20. Browning JE. Chiropractic Distractive Decompression in the treatment of pelvic pain and organic dysfunction in patients with evidence of lower sacral nerve root compression. *J Manipulative Physiol Ther.* 1988;11:426–432.
21. Browning JE. Pelvic pain and organic dysfunction in a patient with low back pain: response to distractive manipulation: a case presentation. *J Manipulative Physiol Ther.* 1987;10:116–121.
22. Browning JE. The recognition of mechanically induced pelvic pain and organic dysfunction in the low back pain patient. *J Manipulative Physiol Ther.* 1989;12:369–373.
23. Goodagle Il, Domar AD, Benson H. Alleviation of premenstrual syndrome symptoms with the relaxation response. *Obstet Gynecol.* 1990;75:649–655.
24. Lark SM. *Dr. Susan Lark's Premenstrual Syndrome Self-Help Book. A Woman's Guide to Feeling Good All Month.* Los Angeles: Forman Publishing; 1984.
25. Goldbeck N. *How To Cope with Menstrual Problems: A Holistic Approach.* New Canaan, Conn: Keats Publishing; 1983.
26. Wilson JR, Carrington ER. *Obstetrics and Gynecology.* 8th ed. St. Louis, Mo: Mosby; 1987.
27. Reis E, Frick U, Schmidtbleicher D. Frequency variations of strength training sessions triggered by the phases of the menstrual cycle. *Int J Sports Med.* 1995;16:545–550.
28. Havens CS, Sullivan ND, Tilton P. *Manual of Outpatient Gynecology.* 2nd ed. Boston: Little, Brown; 1991.
29. Choi PY, Salmon P. Symptom changes across the menstrual cycle in competitive sportswomen, exercisers, and sedentary women. *Br J Clin Psychol.* 1995;34(Pt 3):447–460.
30. Steege JF, Blumenthal JA. The effects of aerobic exercise on premenstrual symptoms in middle-aged women: a preliminary study. *J Psychosom Res.* 1993;37:127–133.
31. Rossignol AM, Bonnlander H. Caffeine containing beverages, total fluid consumption and premenstrual syndrome. *Am J Public Health.* 1990;80:1106–1110.
32. Rossignol AM, Bonnlander H. Prevalence and severity of the premenstrual syndrome. Effects of foods and beverages that are sweet or high in sugar content. *J Reprod Med.* 1991;36:131–136.
33. Frederickson HL, Wilkins-Haug L. *Ob/Gyn Secrets.* Philadelphia: Hanley & Belfus; 1991.
34. Skowronski R, Feldman D. Characterization of an estrogen-binding protein in the yeast *Candida albicans. Endocrinology.* 1989;124:1965–1972.
35. Goldin BR, Adlercreutz H, Gorbach SL. Oestrogen excretion patterns and plasma levels in vegetarian and omnivorous women. *N Engl J Med.* 1982;307:1542–1547.
36. Chuong CJ, Durgos DM. Medical history in women with premenstrual syndrome. *J Psychosom Obstet Gynaecol.* 1995;16(1):21–27.
37. Gerber JM. *Handbook of Preventive and Therapeutic Nutrition.* Gaithersburg, Md: Aspen Publishers; 1993.
38. Cerin A. Hormonal and biochemical profiles of premenstrual syndrome. Treatment with essential fatty acids. *Acta Obstet Gynecol Scand.* 1993;72:337.
39. Collins A. Essential fatty acids in the treatment of premenstrual syndrome. *Obstet Gynecol.* 1993;81:93.
40. McFayden IJ, Forrest AP, Chetty U, Raab G. Cyclical breast pain—some observations and the difficulties in treatment. *Br J Clin Pract.* 1992;46(3):161–164.
41. Rosenstein DL, Ryschon TW, Neimela JE. Skeletal muscle intracellular ionized magnesium measured by 31-P-NMR spectroscopy across the menstrual cycle. *J Am Coll Nutr.* 1995;14:486–490.
42. Seelig MS. Interrelationship of magnesium and estrogen in cardiovascular and bone disorders, eclampsia, migraine and premenstrual syndrome. *J Am Coll Nutr.* 1993;12:442–458.
43. Brush MG, Perry M. Pyridoxine and the premenstrual syndrome. *Lancet.* 1985;1:1339.
44. Klein TA. Office gynecology for the primary care physician, Part II. Pelvic pain, vulvar disease, disorders of menstruation, premenstrual syndrome and breast disease. *Med Clin North Am.* 1996;80:321–336.
45. Mortola JF. A risk-benefit appraisal of drugs used in the management of premenstrual syndrome. *Drug Saf.* 1994;10:160–169.
46. Linde K, Ramirez G, Mulrow CD. St John's wort for depression—an overview and meta-analysis of randomized clinical trials. *Br Med J.* 1996;313(7052):253–258.
47. Chuong CJ, Dawson EB. Zinc and copper levels in premenstrual syndrome. *Fertility and Sterility.* 1994;62(2):313–320.
48. Liebl NA, Butler LM. A chiropractic approach to the treatment of dysmenorrhea. *J Manipulative Physiol Ther.* 1990;13:101–106.
49. Rosquist LW. *Encyclopedia of Spinal Touch.* Salt Lake City: German Therapology; 1975.
50. Walter DS. *Applied Kinesiology.* Pueblo, Colo: Systems DC; 1981.
51. Oleson T, Flocco W. Randomized controlled study of premenstrual symptoms treated with ear, hand, and foot reflexology. *Obstet Gynecol.* 1993;82(6):906–911.
52. Braiden V, Metcalf G. Premenstrual tension among hysterectomized women. *J Psychosom Obstet Gynaecol.* 1995;16:145–151.
53. Dalton K. *The Premenstrual Syndrome and Progesterone Therapy.* Chicago, Ill.: Year Book Medical Publishers; 1984.
54. Backstrom T, Boyle H, Baird DT. Persistence of symptoms of premenstrual tension in hysterectomized women. *Br J Obstet Gynaecol.* 1981;88:530–536.

Algorithm 1

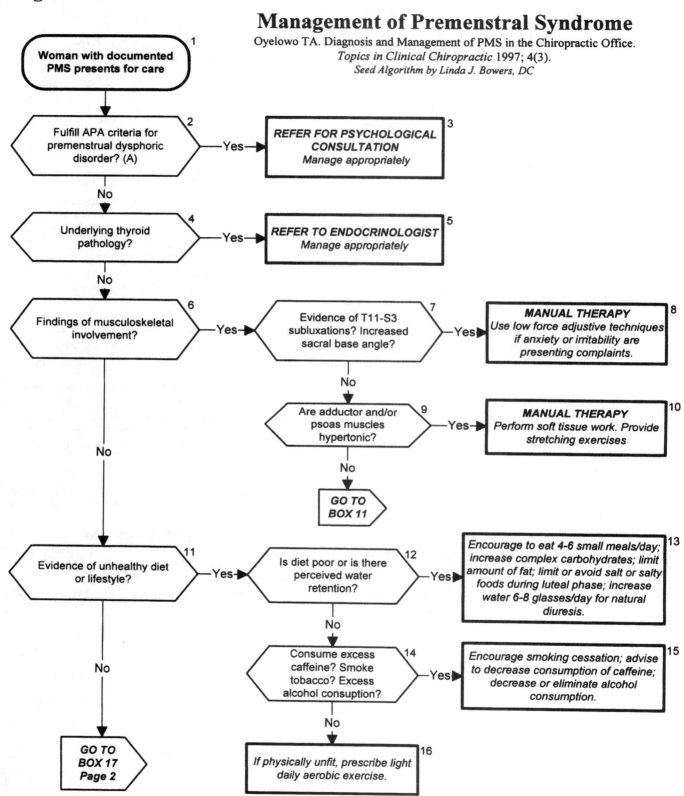

Management of Premenstral Syndrome
Oyelowo TA. Diagnosis and Management of PMS in the Chiropractic Office.
Topics in Clinical Chiropractic 1997; 4(3).
Seed Algorithm by Linda J. Bowers, DC

Algorithm 1, continued

Management of Premenstral Syndrome - Page 2

Oyelowo TA. Diagnosis and Management of PMS in the Chiropractic Office.
Topics in Clinical Chiropractic 1997; 4(3).
Seed Algorithm by Linda J. Bowers, DC

Annotations:
(A) American Psychiatric Association. Diagnostic and Statistical Manual of Mental Disorders 4th Ed. 5/11 symptoms, at least one of the symptoms being either 1, 2, 3 or 4.
(B) Primrose oil (1,000-2,000 mg/day), flaxseed or borage oil, magnesium (400-1,000 mg/day), vitamin B6 (50 mg/day).

12

Breast Cancer: A Current Summary

Leona Berestiansky Sembrat

Breast cancer continues to be the most commonly diagnosed cancer among Canadian and American women.[1,2] As portal-of-entry physicians, it is crucial that chiropractors have a working knowledge of the risks, developments, and treatments of this disease and be aware of preventive tools to use in patient education. It also is paramount to understand the nature and appearance of recurrence and metastasis. This understanding enables the clinician to respond confidently and accurately to patient inquiries and concerns and, most important, allows timely referral to the appropriate health care professional.

Breast tissue is mainly composed of milk glands and ducts. Because it changes in response to alterations in hormone production at various stages in a woman's life cycle, many women develop breast lumps. Fortunately, most are benign. In premenopausal women, lumps or breast changes are common prior to menstruation. Postmenstruation, any lump that has not entirely disappeared requires further investigation. For postmenopausal women, a change in an existing lump, or discovery of a new lump, warrants investigation. For those lumps that are malignant, early detection is key. With improved screening, including mammography, the survival rate for breast cancer is now greater than 60%.[3]

It is critical that the chiropractor be aware that one of every nine women will develop breast cancer[1] and that breast cancer risk increases with age.[1] In fact, women over 50 years of age account for 70% of all cases. Though it is unlikely that the initial diagnosis of breast cancer will take place in the chiropractic office, it is not an impossible scenario. One of the most simple and effective tools for identifying the patient with breast cancer is a good history.[4] A thorough history will illuminate risk factors, including family history, and can identify those patients who have had breast cancer in the past. This knowledge is especially useful because relapse can occur at any time. Though most recurrences develop within the first 2 to 6 years following the initial diagnosis and treatment,[1] they can occur 15 to 30 years after treatment.[1,3] In fact, 50% of breast cancer survivors will develop metastasis.[1] This statistic is valuable knowledge for the chiropractor, as 40% to 60% of metastasis appears in bone and 7% to 15% appears in soft tissue.[1]

BREAST CANCER EPIDEMIOLOGY

Over the past 10 years, the incidence of breast cancer has consistently risen.[1,3] Breast cancer rates in Canada are amid the highest globally, after those in the United States. According to the Canadian Cancer Society, it is mainly due to increased awareness and education, and a larger number of early stage breast cancers being detected by a higher number of screening mammograms.[1] In addition, age at first live birth, at menarche, and at menopause, a growing population of women over 50 years of age, environmental factors, hormone use, lifestyles, and improved statistical reporting all contribute to the higher incidence.[1] Breast cancer incidence is lowest among African and Asian women. However, as these women move to regions where the incidence is higher, breast cancer among their descendants will increase until it matches that of the new region.[1,5,6]

In 1997, the number of new breast cancer cases was expected to be double the estimated cases of lung and colorectal cancer.[1] Breast cancer is second only to lung cancer as the number one cause of cancer death for Canadian[1] and most American[7] women. Breast cancer is second to gallbladder cancer among the American Indians of New Mexico, and it is the leading cause of death for those American women of Filipino background.[7] Of women who develop

Adapted from *Top Clin Chiro* 1999; 6(1): 9–17
© 1999 Aspen Publishers, Inc.

breast cancer, one third will die from it.[2] While it is debatable whether the death rate due to cancer of the breast has decreased slightly,[1] or remained unchanged,[3] the survival rate has risen.[3] The median survival is greater than 5 years.[3] Thus, breast cancer is one of the most treatable cancers, and puts it in the group of cancers where the prognosis is very good.[1,3]

In most cases, for a tumor to be large enough to be detected, it must grow for several years.[3] This timing gives it ample opportunity to spread, either by direct extension or microscopically via lymph and blood channels.[1,3] Half of all tumors arise in the milk ducts, and a third arise in the lobules.[3] Possibly because it is larger, more tumors develop in the left breast than in the right.[1] Tumors most frequently occur in the upper, outer quadrant.[1]

With statistics such as these, it becomes obvious that, though they do not treat breast cancer directly, chiropractors do treat patients who have, will have, or have had breast cancer.

RISK FACTORS

Many factors influence a woman's individual susceptibility to breast cancer. Some are more strongly linked than others. Risk factors serve mainly to aid in identifying those women who require close monitoring and screening.[1]

Factors strongly associated with breast cancer

The most obvious and unavoidable risk factor is gender. Of all cases of breast cancer, 99% occur in women.[1] In 60% of cases, the only identifiable risk factor is female gender.[1] As mentioned previously, the chance of developing breast cancer increases with age.[1,2] Incidence increases steeply until menopause, after which rates continue to rise, but not as sharply.[1]

Family history, or having a relative who has a history of breast cancer, is mistakenly thought by many to be the most important risk factor. Though it is a strong risk factor, only an average of 5% of women develop breast cancer as a direct result of family history.[1] This risk rarely exceeds 30%.[2] When assessing risk due to family history, the degree of relation is pertinent.[1,2] If the family member is a first-degree relative, such as a mother, sister, or daughter, the risk is greater than if the family member is a second-degree relative, such as a grandmother, aunt, or cousin.[1] A positive history in paternal female relatives also seems to increase the risk, though the extent to which it does is unknown.[1] The number of first-degree relatives with breast cancer augments risk[1,2] as well as whether the cancer was diagnosed premenopausally[1] and in both breasts.[1] A family history of cancer such as cervical, uterine, colorectal, or ovarian cancer also appears to increase breast cancer risk.[1]

Personal history of breast cancer is another major risk factor. If the previous diagnosis involved breast lobules, lobular carcinoma in situ (LCIS), or if the cancer was diagnosed before menopause, risk of another primary breast tumor is three to four times greater.[1,2] Chances are even higher if the woman also has a positive family history.[1] The opposite breast or remaining tissue in the original breast can be a site of a second primary breast cancer.[1]

Duration of menstrual life also can elevate risk.[1,2] Early onset of menarche, defined as before age 12 years, or late onset of menopause, defined as after age 55 years, lengthens the time that breast cells are exposed to estrogen.[1,2] The longer the duration of exposure, the greater the likelihood of breast cancer.[1] This is not because estrogen causes cell mutation, but rather because it may promote the growth of established cancer cells.[1] Those women who reach menopause before the age of 45 have half the incidence of breast cancer when compared with those who enter menopause after the age of 55.[1,2] Early menstrual regularity also may affect risk. The risk is three times greater for women who establish regular periods during their first year of menstruation, than for women who do not.[1] The role of other female hormones, such as estradiol, prolactin, and progesterone, is still under investigation.[1] In the laboratory, prolactin has been shown to play a role in the development of breast cancer cells.[1]

Pregnancy causes a decrease in the levels of circulating prolactin, imparting a protective effect. This protection seems to be heightened with each subsequent pregnancy, and it may be lifelong, regardless of age in pregnancy.[1] However, pregnancy in later life is associated strongly with elevated breast cancer incidence,[1,8] as is nulliparity.[1,2] This is due mainly to the effect that a steady exposure of circulating estrogen has on breast tissue.[1] Pregnancy interrupts this otherwise constant exposure, but the protective effect is only seen before age 30.[1] The risk for a woman whose first live birth is after age 30 is double that of a woman who gives birth before age 20.[2] A woman who has never been pregnant has one and a half times the risk of a woman who has had a full-term pregnancy between the ages of 20 and 30.[1] A first full-term pregnancy between ages 30 and 34 carries a risk similar to nulliparity,[1,2] but giving birth after age 35 carries a fivefold risk of breast cancer.[1] All of this is thought to be the result of the uninterrupted exposure to estrogen prior to pregnancy, combined with other age-related risk factors.[1]

The genetics of hereditary breast cancer syndromes also plays a strong role in the development of breast cancer. Mutations to the gene BRCA1, located on chromosome 17, increase a carrier's lifetime risk by up to 85%.[1,2] In these women, the chance of acquiring a second primary breast tumor is 65%. They also have a 40% to 60% chance of developing ovarian cancer.[1] Early onset, bilateral breast involvement, evidence in third-degree relatives, and tendencies to develop cancers in sites such as the colon, ovary, and uterus, all characterize hereditary breast cancer.[1] Men can carry this mutated gene and pass it, and the associated risks, on to their daughters. In another syndrome, the tumor suppressor gene p53, also located on chromosome 17, is inactivated, rendering it unable to control the growth of cancer cells.[1,2] This genetic mutation is associated with the Li-Fraumeni syndrome, a familial syndrome of early-onset breast cancer with associated tumors, such as soft tissue sarcomas.[1] The alteration of a third gene, BRCA2, located on chromosome 13, may increase the risk of breast cancer in both men and women.[1,2] Other hereditary syndromes that elevate breast cancer risk include Cowden's syndrome, Muir syndrome, and Louis-Bar syndrome, or ataxia telangiectasia.[1]

Other major risk factors include a previous abnormal breast biopsy, especially if the lesion was proliferative[1,2]; previous exposure to large amounts of radiation, especially as a child, when breast tissue is most sensitive to radiation effects; and being the female descendant of a European Jew.[1] Table 1 provides a comprehensive list of the major risk factors.

Factors associated with breast cancer whose role is unclear

Women who do not breast feed elevate their risk of breast cancer slightly. The exact mechanism is unknown, and further investigation is required.[1] Heavy intake of alcohol, defined as more than two drinks per day, before age 30 is a potential risk factor.[1,8] The thought behind this factor is that breast cells in the younger woman are more susceptible to the potentially harmful effect of alcohol.[1] Factors such as socioeconomic status and lifestyle play a role, however, further research is necessary.[1]

Other dietary factors also seem to come into play. While some still support the theory that a diet high in total fat increases the incidence of breast cancer,[5] recent data have challenged this theory.[1,6] It has been suggested that increased dietary fat may increase body fat mass, which may augment breast cancer risk by elevating available estrogen concentration.[5] Again, more research is needed to clarify the role of a high percentage of dietary fat energy.[1]

Researchers now are investigating the role individual fatty acids play in the incidence of breast cancer. It is known that a high-fat diet that is also high in linoleic acid promotes the growth and the metastasis of human breast cancer cells.[9] A high, unbalanced, dietary ratio of linoleic acid to linolenic acid may also be detrimental.[5,6,10,11] A protective effect is seen when the diet contains higher amounts of linolenic acid,[5,9,10] oleic acid,[5,6,9] and conjugated linoleic acid.[10] Researchers are also trying to determine how a low fat diet may decrease breast cancer risk, by decreasing breast tissue density.[1] In any event, even if total fat consumption does not have a strong influence in breast cancer development, there are other important reasons, such as protection from other cancers and heart disease, to recommend diets with a low percentage of energy from fat.[11]

As mentioned earlier, higher amounts of circulating estrogen are related to increased breast cancer risk.[5] For postmenopausal women, estrogen contribution from the ovaries is no longer a factor, as estrogen levels are dependent on how much adipose tissue there is.[12] Adipose tissue contains an enzyme capable of converting estrone and estradiol into estrogen. Thus, the more adipose a woman has, the higher the levels of estrogen.[1] Obese women also have lower amounts of a protein, sex hormone binding globulin (SHBG), which binds to estradiol, impeding its conversion to estrogen.[1] Without the control of SHBG, cancer cells requiring estrogen to grow have an unlimited hormonal nutrient supply.[1] Consequently, obesity in menopausal women seems to increase the risk of breast cancer.[1,12] In addition, weight gain in adulthood,[8,12] modest or large, and central adiposity "have been consistently and independently found to confer an increased risk for postmenopausal breast cancer."[12(p439S)] Unfortunately, adult weight loss has not been shown to decrease the risk.[12]

Conversely, at higher risk than postmenopausal obese women are lean premenopausal women.[1] The tumors they tend to develop, however, are usually small and nonmetastatic.[1] Heavier premenopausal women seem to have a lower incidence of premenopausal breast cancer,[12] but if a tumor is diagnosed, they have lower survival rates and a shortened period to recurrence.[12] The entire area of body weight, and its effects on breast cancer incidence, requires more investigation.[1]

Oral contraceptive use is still considered a questionable risk.[1,8] Data in this area are contradictory and inconclusive. Some studies claim there is no risk, while others cite factors such as age, length of use, prolonged use prior to first pregnancy, and length of time since discontinuation. Further research is needed to clarify this risk.[1]

Table 1. Major risk factors

Female gender
Increasing age
Family history
Personal history
Onset of menarche before age 12 years
Onset of menopause after age 55 years
First live birth after age 35 years
Alterations to the genes BRCA1, BRCA2, and p53
Cowden's syndrome
Muir syndrome
Louis-Bar syndrome
Previous abnormal breast biopsy
Previous exposure to large amounts of radiation, especially as a child
Being a female descendant of a European Jew

Similarly, hormone replacement therapy (HRT) is thought to increase risk.[1,8] Again, data on the effects of unopposed estrogen replacement therapy (ERT) and combined estrogen-progesterone therapy are contradictory.[1] HRT for more than 9 years, higher hormone dose, and the combination of estrogen and progesterone are all thought to increase risk.[1] However, some research[1] indicates that breast cancer rates after 15 years of ERT are only slightly increased. Nevertheless, the most consistent factors known to increase breast cancer risk are all hormonally related.[5] Research in this area is ongoing. Table 2 provides a complete list of those factors weakly associated with breast cancer.

Factors not associated with breast cancer

The following factors, independent of other factors, have not shown any conclusive association with breast cancer: caffeine intake, cerumen, coffee intake, exposure to dichlorodiphenyltrichloroethane (DDT), exposure to electromagnetic fields, exposure to polychlorinated biphenyl (PCB), fibrocystic breasts, hair dyes, induced abortion, multiple pregnancies, personality type, smoking, and stress.[1,2] However, Sharpe[8] suggests that tobacco use during adolescence may increase breast cancer risk among some women. In addition, while some studies[6,10] claim that breast cancer risk is unrelated to the presence of the transconfiguration of polyunsaturated fatty acids, others[5,11] state that it cannot be ruled out.

Although there are many theories regarding risk factors for developing breast cancer, it should be emphasized that the fundamental cause of breast cancer remains a mystery. As a result, women should not be cavalier regarding their personal risk because the more commonly identified risk factors (such as family history) may not apply. Vigilance in performing monthly self-examination and regular mammograms, as appropriate, should be exercised even in the absence of common risk factors.

CAUSATION THEORIES

There is no one specific factor known to cause breast cancer. Thus far, researchers have only identified risk factors, which in combination, seem to have a definite effect.[1] Two out of three breast cancer cases will have no identifiable cause.[1] With this statistic in mind, there are some theories discussed in the literature. Most have taken a strong risk factor, worked back to discover the mechanisms of action, and come up with hypotheses to support a theory.

The importance of a high-fat diet, and its role in the circulating concentrations of estrogen, is the key issue in a number of theories.[5,9,11] Specifically, dietary fat influences body fat, which makes the amount of available estrogen higher and the likelihood of breast cancer stronger.[5,9,11] Estrogen, itself, is not thought to be the main factor in cell alteration, but it is considered to cause proliferation of established cancer cells.[1] Thus other hypotheses state that there are key periods, such as puberty or menopause, when estrogen has its strongest effect.[8,12]

Other hypotheses also center around key periods of sensitivity. All cancers are caused by an alteration in gene expression, such as the activation of oncogenes or inactivation of tumor suppressor genes.[8] A combination of negative risk factors, such as early menarche brought on by a high-fat diet and lack of exercise, radiation exposure during multiple chest radiographs for chronic bronchitis, and an inherited or acquired genetic alteration of a tumor suppressor gene, may occur throughout a woman's early life. A developing breast is more vulnerable to various carcinogens because a genetic hit in one cell could be passed on to its daughter cells during breast growth.[8] Thus the pathogenesis of breast cancer could be lifelong, and preventive efforts should begin in childhood.[8,12]

Other theories discuss the effects of individual fatty acids, specifically linoleic and linolenic polyunsaturated fatty acids.[5,9] Very simply put, we are what we eat. Fatty acids can affect both breast cancer cell proliferation, and the expression of metastatic phenotype.[9] Ingesting higher amounts of linoleic acid may alter phospholipids in tumor cell membranes, influencing growth.[5,9] Conversely, linolenic acid interferes with cell growth through the formation of oxidation products.[5] Research[13] has shown the effectiveness of a diet containing linolenic acid—and its derivatives docosahexaenoic acid (DHA) and eicosapentaenoic acid (EPA)—in suppressing tumor growth, arresting tumor progression, and inhibiting the formation of metastasis.[5,9] Linoleic acid is found in commonly used vegetable oils. Linolenic acid is most concentrated in flax seeds. Flax seeds, bottled flax seed oil, and

---

Table 2. Weak risk factors

Never having breast fed
Heavy alcohol intake, more than two drinks per day, before age 30 years
High dietary fat
Diet high in linoleic acid, especially when linolenic acid intake is low
Obesity in menopause
Adult weight gain
Being lean and premenopausal
Oral contraceptive use
Hormone replacement therapy

Source: Canadian Cancer Encyclopedia—CCE. Rev. ed: Cancer Information Service, Canadian Cancer Society; 1998.

nutritional flax supplements are now available. DHA and EPA are available in supplement form, and they occur naturally in deep, cold-water fish.[13]

PREVENTION

Factors that may lower breast cancer risk

Though it is a small list, some circumstances are known to lower the incidence of breast cancer. One factor is natural or surgically induced menopause, prior to 45 years of age, in the absence of hormone replacement therapy.[1,2] This factor is thought to reduce breast cancer incidence by up to 50%.[1]

First full-term pregnancy before the age of 20 is another modifying factor.[1,8] A woman who gives birth before age 20 has half the breast cancer risk of a nulliparous woman.[1] Breast cells at this age are still developing, and the interruption of the constant estrogen supply at this time provides a protective effect.[1] It also is known that breast tissue fully differentiates, or matures, with pregnancy, which seems to be protective.[1,8] In addition, the earlier this maturation occurs, the greater the degree of protection.[1]

Last, Japanese women living in Japan have the lowest incidence of breast cancer in the world.[1,9] As these women move to areas of higher incidence, however, the incidence in their offspring rises.[1,5,6] The exact reason for this rise is unknown, but current theories include factors such as a change in exercise habits,[1] alcohol and drug use,[1] hormone therapy use,[1] and a lack of soy products.[5,14]

Primary prevention

The best way to fight breast cancer is to prevent it from occurring in the first place. Although risk factors such as age and gender cannot be changed, modifying other risk factors may decrease overall incidence.

The easiest items to change are the ones over which women have the most control. Lifestyle changes, like increasing exercise, reducing stress, and eating a balanced diet, seem prudent.[1] A body mass index (BMI) of greater than or equal to 27.3 is the point at which the risk of postmenopausal breast cancer increases.[12] Exercise can, among myriad other benefits, help prevent adult weight gain, which is a risk factor in itself.[12] Exercise also can reduce body fat,[1,12] thereby decreasing postmenopausal estrogen concentrations. Though not an independent risk factor, stress can negatively affect the function of the immune system, possibly increasing susceptibility to various diseases.[1]

A balanced diet can provide antioxidants, such as vitamins A, C, and E and carotenoids. These vitamins have been suggested to be protective against breast cancer.[1,15] Also in terms of diet, it appears that less fat and more fiber can significantly reduce estrogen concentrations.[5] Though there is conflicting evidence,[6] it seems wise to increase daily intake of linolenic acid, EPA, and DHA to achieve the protective effect of a more balanced ratio of linolenic to linoleic acid.[5,6,10,11] Though better than saturated fat, high amounts of the polyunsaturated linoleic acid in adipose tissue have been associated with a higher individual risk of breast cancer, as well as recurrence.[5] High concentrations of linoleic acid may facilitate metastasis by enhancing angiogenesis and invasion negotiated by tumor cells.[9] Current data on the protective effect of monounsaturated oleic acid, found in olive oil, as an independent factor are not convincing.[10,11] However, in olive oil–consuming countries, some dietary studies[5,6,9] have shown an inhibitory effect. It may be due to the resultant decrease in linoleic acid intake,[10] or to other components,[5] such as phenolic compounds.[11] In any event, there is no harm in using olive oil more often.

Another primary preventive tool is decreased use of oral contraceptives and HRT.[1] Much debate surrounds this issue, and each woman must weigh her individual risk-benefit ratio with her health care professional.[1]

The nonsteroidal antiestrogen, tamoxifen, used as primary chemoprevention, has received a lot of media coverage. The newest research is promising,[1,16] but it may only be useful for a certain, high-risk segment of women.[16] As with most drug therapies, tamoxifen has complicating factors and negative side effects, specifically endometrial carcinoma.[17] Tamoxifen-like drugs, such as raloxifene and toremifene, are currently under investigation.[18]

Prophylactic mastectomy is an infrequent form of primary prevention.[1,2] It is usually reserved for high-risk women, for example, those carrying the altered BRCA1 or BRCA2 genes.[1] There are two types: subcutaneous mastectomy and simple, or total, mastectomy.[2] Neither procedure removes all of the breast tissue, thus neither provides absolute protection against tumor development.[1,2] Total mastectomy is the preferable choice, as it removes the highest percentage of breast tissue.[2] Breast cancer can occur in even the smallest amount of remaining tissue.[1,2]

Choosing prophylactic mastectomy is never an emergency, as there are no absolute indications. It should only be performed following a second opinion.[2] The patient should clearly understand that the decision to operate is based on the risk of developing breast cancer, not the risk of dying from breast cancer.[2] As many as 33% of women have moderate to severe sexual dysfunction following mastectomy.[2] In addition, when breast cancer is detected, it is usually advanced.[2] This is typically because the woman feels a false sense of security that all risk has been eliminated.[2] The alternative, for these high-risk women, is monthly breast self-examination (BSE), annual mammograms, and clinical breast examinations at 4- and 6-month intervals.[2]

Secondary prevention

Any measure that prevents cancer from developing too far is defined as secondary prevention. BSE, clinical breast examination by a physician, and mammography are all screening procedures aimed at preventing morbidity and mortality.[1]

Screening is important for all women. Women age 20 and older should perform a monthly BSE 1 week after menstruation, a period sufficient to allow the tissue to return to normal. Repetition is the key to detection of breast changes. It is only with practice that a woman will know what is normal when palpating her breast tissue. To ensure that the woman is performing the BSE accurately, proper instruction should be given by a trained professional.[1]

Clinical breast examinations should be performed as part of a woman's annual physical by her physician. For women age 39 and younger, a clinical breast examination should be done at least every 3 years. For women 40 years of age and older, examinations should be annual.[1]

Mammography is the most effective screening method.[1] Forty percent of all breast cancers are found by mammography.[3] However, 10% to 15% of tumors will be missed on a mammogram, but detected by physically examining the breast.[1,3] Thus, to provide complete protection, all three methods of screening must be used.[1]

The standard screening mammogram procedure includes two views, one at 90° to the other, of each breast.[1] The X-ray dose is very low, typically 0.15 radiation absorbed dose (rad) per breast.[1,3] Combined with the fact that the breast tissue of a woman age 40 or older is less sensitive to radiation effects, the risk from screening mammography is almost nil. Current data from the Canadian National Breast Screening Study suggest that to improve accuracy in premenopausal women, screening mammograms should be performed in the first 2 weeks of the menstrual cycle.[1] This is recommended because hormonal changes in the latter 2 weeks can cause breast tenderness, preventing adequate compression of breast tissue. It may result in inferior quality mammograms and a higher false negative rate.[1]

There are conflicting views on the frequency required for screening mammograms and the appropriate age to begin screening. Prior to age 30, mammography is unreliable, due to the density of breast tissue.[3] The Canadian Cancer Society (CCS) recommends that women between the ages of 50 and 69 years have a screening mammogram biennially.[1] Women whose risk is high should be treated individually; they may need mammography more frequently and before the age of 50.[1] This guideline is supported by data showing that half of a woman's risk of developing breast cancer occurs after the age of 65 years.[2] The CCS also cites the findings of a consensus panel commissioned by the National Institutes of Health (NIH). The panel was unable to reach a consensus on the data, as there was no difference in the number of breast cancer deaths between women screened in their forties and those screened in their fifties.[1] The NIH statement was, therefore, that the decision to undergo mammography must be made individually by each woman.[1]

On March 21, 1997, the American Cancer Society (ACS) changed its guidelines on screening mammography, when it came to light that a considerable proportion of the premature deaths from breast cancer were in women who were diagnosed in their forties.[19] The new recommendations state that annual screening mammograms should begin at age 40, with no upper age limit specified, and that clinical breast examinations be conducted around the time of the mammogram.[19] Supporting data for this change were provided by two trials in Sweden, the Gothenburg trial and the Malmo trial.[19] Combined, the trials showed a reduction in mortality for women between the ages of 40 and 49 years who underwent screening mammography. Thus, the ACS finds that "data for this age group now meet the same criteria of benefit that has been the basis for concluding that mammography was beneficial for women aged 50 years or older."[19(p151)] The ACS also states that in younger women there is a higher proportion of tumors that grow faster. Thus, in order to reduce premature mortality, women, both older than and younger than 50 years of age, should be screened annually.[19]

Tertiary prevention

Limiting complications, enhancing rehabilitation for women diagnosed with breast cancer, and preventing advanced recurrence is the aim of tertiary prevention. Examples include postoperative care, follow-up visits, and patient education.[1] As a health care professional current on the realities of breast cancer, the chiropractor can play an important role in increasing patient awareness and education.

CLASSIFICATION AND STAGING

Classification

Breast tumors are classified by the region from which they arise and by the degree of invasiveness. Noninvasive breast tumors are thought to be signs of early stage cancer, or even precancerous.[1] Noninvasive cancer arising from the milk ducts is referred to as ductal carcinoma in situ (DCIS).[1] Similarly, cancer arising in the lobules is known as LCIS.[1] Noninvasive tumors account for slightly more than 10% of all breast cancer cases.[1]

DCIS develops in both pre- and postmenopausal women. On mammogram, DCIS is seen as clusters of microcalcification, making it appear multicentric, when in fact it is not. Nipple discharge may be the only sign of DCIS, but it normally forms a palpable mass. It most commonly localizes to one quadrant, and axillary lymph node involvement is rare. Without treatment, most cases of DCIS will become invasive. Even following total excision, 40% will develop into invasive cancer.[1]

DCIS has two subtypes: comedo and non-comedo. Comedo types are generally more invasive that non-comedo types, and they carry an increased risk of local recurrence within the first 10 years. Non-comedo types grow more slowly, over a longer period of time.[1]

LCIS is most common in premenopausal women.[1] A diagnosis of LCIS is considered to be more of a risk factor than an actual precursor to breast cancer.[1,2] Though LCIS has no specific mammographic characteristics, it is multicentric and, in 30% of cases, found bilaterally.[1] It is unusual for LCIS to present with a palpable mass.[1] Most cases of LCIS are discovered by a pathologist, after examining tissue that was removed during a routine procedure for a benign breast condition. Even 40 years after treatment, 25% to 35% will develop into a more invasive form.[1]

The most common type of invasive breast cancer is ductal carcinoma. It comprises 80% of all cases of breast cancer.[1] The main types of invasive ductal cancer are adenocarcinoma, tubular carcinoma, mucinous or colloid carcinoma, and medullary carcinoma.[1] Prognosis varies depending on the type, stage, and grade of the tumor.[1]

Accounting for the last 10% of breast cancer cases is invasive lobular carcinoma.[1] It is usually detected by women in their early fifties as a thickening of the breast, rather than as a lump.[1] Invasive lobular carcinoma is often multicentric, and it most commonly consists of adenocarcinomas.[1]

Staging

To provide information on recurrence risk, and to guide the choice of treatment, breast tumors are divided into stages. There are two main types of staging.[1] Tumor, lymph node, metastasis (TNM) staging is used primarily for research purposes.[1,3] The type of staging used more in clinical situations divides tumors into four groups.[1] A rating of zero (0) is reserved for those lesions found in situ that are noninvasive.[1] Stage one (I) includes early breast cancer, where the lesion is smaller than 2 cm and has no lymph node involvement.[1] A stage two (II) designation is used for either tumors less than 2 cm with lymph node involvement, lesions 2 to 5 cm with or without lymph node involvement, or lesions greater than 5 cm without lymph node involvement.[1] Stage three (III) lesions are more advanced, are larger than 5 cm with lymph node involvement, and may initially be inoperable.[1] Stage four (IV) is assigned when metastasis is present.[1]

SIGNS AND SYMPTOMS

The signs and symptoms associated with breast cancer are not exclusive to breast cancer. Any abnormality should be investigated by a physician who examines and treats breast conditions on a regular basis.[4]

Usually, the first sign is detection of an abnormal lump during a monthly BSE.[1] The lump may be hard and irregular, and it may feel as if it is attached to the skin.[1,4] The lump is not usually painful, but it may be tender.[1,4] Any other change in breast tissue size or shape also may be a warning sign.[1,4] Other signs include spontaneous and/or bloody discharge from the nipple, or surface changes such as crusting, ulceration, or eczema.[1,4] Neither non-bloody discharge nor discharge that occurs bilaterally is thought to be a sign of malignancy.[4] Distended veins forming an irregular pattern; "peau d'orange" or an orange peel appearance; and any redness, increased warmth, or edema may indicate breast cancer.[1]

It is worth noting that deep-seated, boring bone pain is often a symptom of metastasis to the bone, which is a very common occurrence.[1] It is likely that over a lifetime of practice a chiropractor will see this in his or her office. As stated by the Canadian Cancer Society, it is imperative that a woman with diagnosed breast cancer who is experiencing back pain have "a chest X-ray before having any chiropractic or massage treatments."[1] This precaution will help to avoid the potential complications of manipulating an area weakened by bony metastasis.[1]

LABORATORY MARKERS

There are a number of genetic markers and histologic factors that signify an increased risk of breast cancer or an increased risk of recurrence or that affect the prognosis once a diagnosis has been made. Hereditary genetic abnormalities include BRCA1, BRCA2, and the altered tumor suppressor gene, p53.[1,2] Other markers are the oncogenes HER2/neu and cyclin D1.[1] The higher the level of oncogenes expressed, the greater the risk of tumor recurrence.[1] Comedo subtypes of DCIS express large amounts of these oncogenes.[1] Comedo subtypes also lack the tumor suppressor gene, p53, and the gene bcl-2, which promotes the proliferation and survival of normal cells.[1] In addition, comedocarcinoma cells are aneuploid, meaning their amount of deoxyribonucleic acid (DNA) is abnormal.[1] The higher the degree of aneuploid, the more aggressive the tumor.[1]

Normal breast tissue has receptors for hormones such as progesterone and estrogen.[3] Hormone receptor status, therefore, is a measure of how similar to normal tissue the tumor cells are.[1,3] Breast tumors that are positive for estrogen receptors are more differentiated and thus less aggressive.[3] If the tumor is highly positive, especially for both estrogen and progesterone, it will likely respond well to hormonal therapy.[1,3] LCIS is a tumor that is commonly estrogen-receptor positive.[1]

Another relevant laboratory finding is the presence of cancer cells in the lymph nodes or blood vessels surrounding the primary tumor. If microscopic vascular invasion is present, the lesion is more aggressive and likely to metastasize.[3]

Tumor grade pertains to how abnormal the cancer cells are. The lower the grade, the more differentiated, or closer to normal, the cells appear. Thus a high-grade tumor is an aggressive tumor, and it will likely metastasize.[3]

The TRUQUANT BR RIA test is a blood test that detects serum levels of the antigen CA27.29. This antigen is a tumor marker that is shed by cancer cells as they metastasize. The test is most effective for women who were treated for stage II or stage III cancer. High serum levels indicate that the cancer has recurred.[1]

Blood counts and chemistry panels provide information on the function of organs and organ systems. High levels of serum calcium point to more serious disease. However, only 10% of women with advanced breast disease have hypercalcemia.[1]

DIAGNOSIS AND TREATMENT

Diagnosis

Diagnosis of breast cancer usually begins by investigation of a breast lump or other change found by the woman or her physician.[3,4] An irregularity detected by mammography is investigated differently than a suspicious lump detected by a physical examination.[4,20] A flow chart detailing diagnostic protocols and treatment procedures can be found in Algorithm 1.

Any suspicious change found by a woman should be examined by her physician.[4] The physician typically will begin with a thorough history and physical examination including palpation of the breast tissue and lymph nodes to detect axillary and supraclavicular lymphadenopathy.[3,4] Then the woman is sent for either a diagnostic mammogram,[3,4] depending on her age, or for fine-needle aspiration (FNA).[4] Ultrasonography is sometimes used instead of FNA, particularly to distinguish between a cyst and a solid tumor.[3,4] Scintimammography is occasionally used if the mammographic image is difficult to read.[1] If it is still questionable whether the lesion is benign or malignant, a biopsy is performed.[4] A core biopsy can be used to exclude or establish malignancy by allowing histologic diagnosis such as the determination of hormone receptor status and degree of invasiveness.[4] Should a surgical biopsy be performed, the intent is to remove the entire lesion along with some normal tissue surrounding it.[4] If metastasis is suspected, the woman may undergo chest radiographs, a bone scan, and a liver scan.[1,3] Positron emission tomography (PET) is a new technique useful in the detection of axillary lymph node involvement.[1] Thermography and light scanning are not endorsed as diagnostic procedures.[4] The value of magnetic resonance imaging is currently under investigation.[1,4] Algorithm 2 summarizes diagnosis and treatment protocols.

Traditional therapies

Generally, cancerous breast tumors require surgery or surgery plus radiation treatment.[3] Most women diagnosed with stage I or stage II breast cancer are candidates for breast conserving surgery (BCS), or lumpectomy, and radiotherapy in place of radical mastectomy.[3,21] Mastectomy should be considered if the risk of local recurrence is high, if the use of radiotherapy is not possible or contraindicated, if the tumor is very large, or if the patient clearly prefers it.[21] Data from clinical trials conclusively show that BCS and radiation offer the same survival rates as mastectomy.[3] Adjuvant therapy is used as preventive treatment.[3] It includes chemotherapy, hormonal therapy, or both, depending on the type, the grade, and the stage of the cancer.[3]

Unconventional therapies

This year, the Canadian Breast Cancer Research Initiative set up a task force to review the literature on six unconventional therapies used in the treatment of cancer.[22] The task force found that, when used appropriately, some positive effects can be seen with the following: vitamins A, C, and E used in combination; Essiac; green tea; Iscador; hydrazine sulfate; and 714-X.[15,22–26] These results are encouraging, but more research is needed.

SUMMARY

Breast cancer is a vast and complex disease. Although chiropractors rarely serve in primary diagnosis and care roles for the disease, an understanding of the epidemiology and risk factors is necessary to answer questions posed by patients. In addition, the chiropractor emphasizing wellness and prevention may provide a forum for breast cancer education and awareness.

Menopause prior to age 45 and full-term pregnancy prior to age 20 reduce breast cancer risk. More controllable factors that may enhance prevention include increasing exercise, reducing stress, and eating a balanced diet. However, the extent and certainty of these factors require more research. Genetic and ethnic factors also may contribute to risk.

Diagnosis is usually based on self- or provider-performed examination that identifies a lump in the breast. Mammogram or fine-needle aspiration is usually used for confirmation. Principal conventional treatments include mastectomy, breast conserving surgery, and radiation therapy. In terms of secondary prevention, chemotherapy and hormonal replacement therapy may be used. A handful of unconventional interventions have been studied (vitamins A, C, and E used in combination; Essiac; green tea; Iscador; hydrazine sulfate; and 714-X) with some encouraging preliminary results. However, these interventions need to undergo further research before definitive recommendations can be offered.

REFERENCES

1. *Canadian Cancer Encyclopedia—CCE™*. Rev. ed.: Cancer Information Service, Canadian Cancer Society; 1998.
2. Bilimoria M, Morrow M. The woman at increased risk for breast cancer: evaluation and management strategies. *CA Cancer J Clin.* 1995;45(5):263–278.
3. Breast cancer and you. *Curr Opin Oncol.* 1996;3(3, suppl):S1–S32.
4. The palpable breast lump: information and recommendations to assist decision-making when a breast lump is detected. *Can Med Assoc J.* 1998;158(3, suppl):S3–S8.
5. Kohlmeier L. Biomarkers of fatty acid exposure and breast cancer risk. *Am J Clin Nutr.* 1997;66(suppl):1548S–1556S.
6. Willett W. Specific fatty acids and risks of breast and prostate cancer: dietary intake. *Am J Clin Nutr.* 1997;66(suppl):1557S–1563S.
7. Parker S, Davis K, Wingo P, Ries L, Heath C. Cancer statistics by race and ethnicity. *CA Cancer J Clin.* 1998;48:31–48.
8. Sharpe C. A developmental hypothesis to explain the multicentricity of breast cancer. *Can Med Assoc J.* 1998;159(1):55–59.
9. Rose D. Dietary fatty acids and cancer. *Am J Clin Nutr.* 1997;66(suppl):1581S–1586S.
10. Ip C. Review of the effects of trans fatty acids, oleic acid, n-3 polyunsaturated fatty acids, and conjugated linoleic acid on mammary carcinogenesis in animals. *Am J Clin Nutr.* 1997;66(suppl):1523S–1529S.
11. Dwyer J. Human studies on the effects of fatty acids on cancer: summary, gaps, and future research. *Am J Clin Nutr.* 1997;66(suppl):1581S–1586S.
12. Ballard-Barbash R, Swanson C. Body weight: estimation of risk for breast and endometrial cancers. *Am J Clin Nutr.* 1996;63(suppl):437S–441S.
13. Mahan L, Arlin M. *Krause's Food, Nutrition, and Diet Therapy.* Philadelphia: WB Saunders Co; 1992.
14. Negata C, Kabuto M, Kurisu Y, Shimizu H. Decreased serum estradiol concentration associated with high dietary intake of soy products in premenopausal Japanese females. *Nutr Cancer.* 1997;29(3):228–233.
15. Kaegi E. Unconventional therapies for cancer: 5 A, C and E. *Can Med Assoc J.* 1998;158(11):1483–1488.
16. Robert N. Clinical efficacy of tamoxifen. *Oncology.* 1997;11(2, suppl 1):15–20.
17. Carcangui M. Uterine pathology in tamoxifen treated patients with breast cancer. *Anat Pathol.* 1997;2:53–70.
18. Powles T. Status of antiestrogen breast cancer prevention trials. *Oncology.* 1998;12(3, suppl 5):28–31.
19. Leitch A, Dodd G, Costanza M, et al. American Cancer Society guidelines for the early detection of breast cancer: update 1997. *CA Cancer J Clin.* 1997;47(3):150–153.
20. Investigation of lesions detected by mammography. *Can Med Assoc J.* 1998;158(3, suppl):S9–S14.
21. Mastectomy or lumpectomy? The choice of operation for clinical stages I and II breast cancer. *Can Med Assoc J.* 1998;158(3, suppl):S15–S21.
22. Kaegi E. Unconventional therapies for cancer: 1. Essiac. *Can Med Assoc J.* 1998;158(7):897–901.
23. Kaegi E. Unconventional therapies for cancer: 2. Green Tea. *Can Med Assoc J.* 1998;158(8):1033–1035.
24. Kaegi E. Unconventional therapies for cancer: 3. Iscador. *Can Med Assoc J.* 1998;158(9):1157–1159.
25. Kaegi E. Unconventional therapies for cancer: 4. Hydrazine sulfate. *Can Med Assoc J.* 1998;158(10):1327–1330.
26. Kaegi E. Unconventional therapies for cancer: 6. 714-X. *Can Med Assoc J.* 1998;158(12):1621–1624.

Algorithm 1

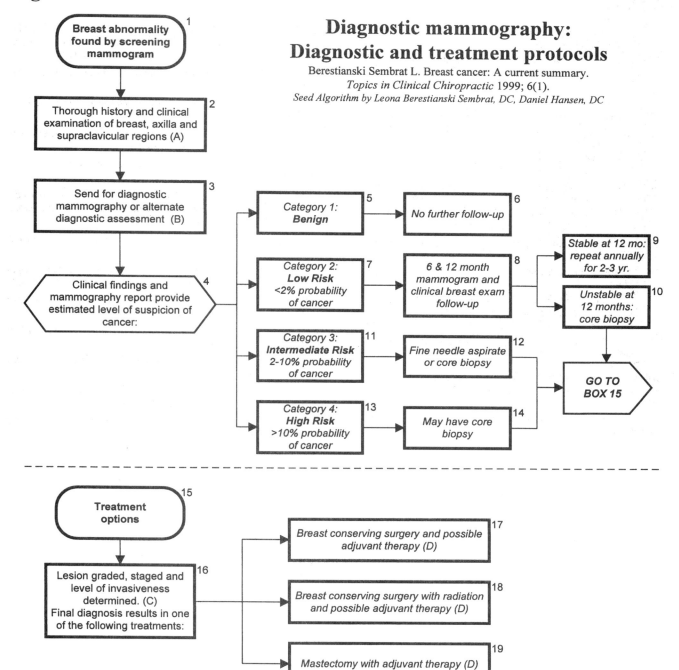

Annotations:
(A) Including palpation of the breast tissue and lymph nodes, to detect axillary and supraclavicular lymphadenopathy
(B) Consider ultrasonography or fine needle aspiration procedures, depending on patient's age, nature of lump, local availability, reliability of technology and/or physician preference
(C) May or may not include axillary dissection
(D) Includes chemotherapy, hormonal therapy, or both depending on the type, the grade and stage of cancer. Is used as preventative treatment.

Algorithm 2

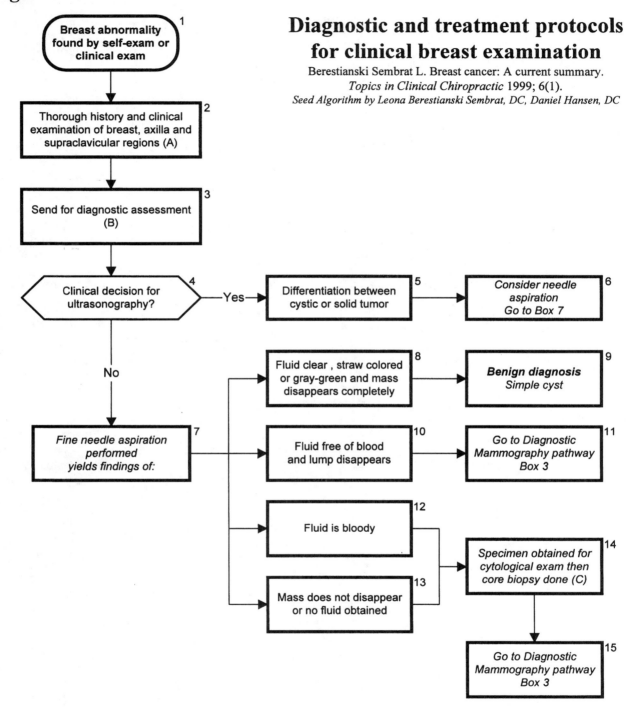

Diagnostic and treatment protocols for clinical breast examination

Berestianski Sembrat L. Breast cancer: A current summary.
Topics in Clinical Chiropractic 1999; 6(1).
Seed Algorithm by Leona Berestianski Sembrat, DC, Daniel Hansen, DC

Annotations:
(A) Including palpation of the breast tissue and lymph nodes, to detect axillary and supraclavicular lymphadenopathy
(B) Consider ultrasonography or fine needle aspiration procedures, depending on patient's age, nature of lump, local availability, reliability of technology and/or physician preference
(C) Core biopsy used to exclude or establish malignancy through histological diagnosis

13

Considerations in Adjusting Women

Kevin M. Bartol

According to chiropractors' self-reports, female patients comprise approximately 59% of patients seeking chiropractic care.[1] A 1987 epidemiologic survey compared the incidence of musculoskeletal problems among patients in Finland, Norway, and Sweden. The results revealed that women have a higher incidence of musculoskeletal problems than men, particularly pain or discomfort in the neck or shoulder region.[2] It is therefore reasonable to suspect that a higher incidence of musculoskeletal conditions exists within the female population in any industrialized, free-world country.

There are many reasons for this phenomenon. As more women enter the work force, the diseases and discomforts associated with job-related stress are affecting them. This factor, when superimposed on biomechanical attributes unique to female skeletal structure and other stresses that may ensue from pregnancy, leisure activities, and physical demands of daily activities, can pose particular challenges for practitioners of manual methods.

Anatomic differences, such as an increased Q angle at the knee and an increased sacral base angle, may contribute to the higher prevalence of musculoskeletal conditions in women. According to McPoil and coworkers,[3] 97% of all women over the age of 18 have a pronated foot. Unilateral pronation may lead to a physiologic short leg on the affected side. Rothbart and Estabrook[4] report that 97% of the time a low iliac crest will be found on the same side as the pronated foot. A pronated foot causes a shift in the center of gravity, as well as asymmetry of motion leading to altered forces on tissues. Such stresses and strains may contribute to a number of compensatory conditions (Table 1).[5-29]

Several factors may predispose women to development of a pronated foot. High heels cause an anterior shift in weight bearing that can lead to pronation. An increased Q angle, genu valgus, genu recurvatum, leg length inequality, and a wide pelvis also contribute to pronation, which may be unilateral or bilateral depending on the structural fault.

During the third trimester of pregnancy, hormonal factors can also increase pronation. The hormone relaxin is released, which increases the elasticity of connective tissue. This increase allows the plantar ligamentous fibers, plantar capsular fibers, and the plantar fascia to soften and elongate, leading to dropped arches of the foot. As a result, pronated feet are more likely to occur during pregnancy along with an increase of weight distribution on the feet and the anterior shift of the weight-bearing line.[30-34]

Given the high percentage of female patients seeking chiropractic care, along with the high prevalence of women suffering from various musculoskeletal conditions, consideration of the uniqueness of female patients is important for all chiropractors.

CHIROPRACTIC CLINICAL CONSIDERATIONS IN WOMEN'S CARE

Table 2 provides a glossary of terms related to manipulative and adjustive procedures.[35-39] The definitions are based in part on formal consensus exercises undertaken by the chiropractic profession. Some key concepts associated with the provision of chiropractic care for women follow.

Reprinted from *Top Clin Chiro* 1997; 4(3): 1–10
© 1997 Aspen Publishers, Inc.

The author thanks the model for her assistance. Illustrating set-ups on a pregnant individual greatly enhances the usefulness of the manuscript, and her willingness and patience were greatly appreciated.

Table 1. Symptoms or conditions that may be associated with a leg length inequality

Pelvic tilt	Patella tendinitis
Scoliosis	Patellofemoral syndrome
Asymmetric facet joint angle	Plantar fascitis
Facet arthrosis	Medial tibial stress syndrome
Lumbar end plate concavity	
L-5 wedging	Metatarsalgia
Traction spurs	Iliotibial band syndrome
Lateral disc compression	Trochanteric bursitis
Disc bulge	Sacroiliac pain
Paraspinal muscle imbalance	Knee pain
	Achilles tendinitis
Hip arthrosis	Sciatica
Knee arthrosis	

INITIAL EVALUATION

As always, an initial patient visit includes the patient's history and a thorough physical examination. The resultant data are assessed to establish a clinical impression and care plan prior to implementing specific treatment. Strategies for monitoring progress and assessing outcome also should be developed and agreed to prior to treatment. Ideally, the chiropractic examination provides a conceptual biomechanical and/or physiologic model of the patient's "structural status," which tissues are affected, and how they are affected. Once a conceptual model of the causative factors has been developed, an optimal treatment that focuses on the intended outcomes can be tailored to the patient's individual needs.[38]

Three unique considerations may attenuate the choice of thrusting procedures in the care of women: flexibility, osteoporosis, and pregnancy. In designing an optimal treatment program, the following questions must be answered:

- What conditions are responsible for the dysfunction?
- Are these conditions reversible?
- What forms of intervention will affect the reversible pathology?
- What can be done to optimize residual function if the condition is irreversible?
- What can be done to prevent recurrences, secondary problems, and progression of the existing disorders?[36]

FLEXIBILITY

Differences in flexibility between the genders are multifactorial. A person's degree of flexibility may be acquired, such as a pronated foot or performing back walkovers; may

Table 2. Terminology related to manipulation and adjustment

Term	Definition
Adjustment	"Any chiropractic therapeutic procedure that utilizes controlled force, leverage, direction, amplitude, and velocity which is directed at specific joints or anatomical regions. Chiropractors commonly use such procedures to influence joint and neurophysiological function."[35(p308)]
Manipulation	"A manual procedure that involves a directed thrust to move a joint past the physiological range of motion, without exceeding the anatomical limits."[35(p308)]
Open pack (Loose pack)	The position of the articulating surfaces where the joint is not maximally congruent, the capsular and ligamentous fibers are maximally lax so the joint surfaces can distract, and one half of the motion segment can be freely pushed in relation to the other half. The open-pack position of a joint is the position in which joint play is evaluated.[36]
Closed pack	The position of the articulating surfaces where the joint is maximally congruent, the capsular and ligamentous fibers are pulled taut so the articulating surfaces are as close together as possible, and the joint is locked so no further movement is possible in that direction is called the closed-pack position.[36]
Articular lock up Lock up, Removal of slack	A doctor-induced closed-pack position. The joint is moved in such a manner that the capsular and/or ligamentous fibers to be affected are pulled tight, removing any slack in them but not so much that the joint cavitates. If cavitation occurs, then, by definition, a manipulation has been performed.
Long lever arm procedures	Procedures where the force is created distal to the axis of rotation.[37]
Short lever arm procedures	Procedures where the force is created proximal to the axis of rotation.[37]
Force	Force is a function of velocity and amplitude.

be developmental, such as genu valgus or genu recurvatum; may be genetic; or may be affected by biochemical and hormonal variations. *Flexibility* is the resistance to stress imparted by the capsular and ligamentous fibers (ie, the degree of mobility). In general, women tend to have greater flexibility than men. For example, genu recurvatum of up to 15° is common in women.[40] It indicates that the posterior knee capsular fibers, as well as the posterior one half of the medial collateral ligament, the anterior cruciate, the posterior cruciate, the arcuate, and the oblique popliteal ligaments, are elongated.

Normal lumbar spine extension measures about 10° more in normal, healthy women than in men.[41] This finding is due to an elongated anterior longitudinal ligament that allows the lumbar vertebrae to separate anteriorly. The anterior aspects of the zygapophyseal joint capsular and ligamentous fibers are also stretched during extension. Gymnasts, especially female gymnasts, can display an acquired increase in lumbar extension.

Normal hip abduction measures 30° to 50°.[40] Athletic training may stretch the connective tissues that normally restrict hip abduction allowing the hip to abduct more than 90°. Hip abduction, hip flexion, lumbar extension, and anterior pelvic tilting are required to achieve 90° of hip abduction.[42] The ability to perform front splits is common in gymnasts, ballerinas, figure skaters, and persons involved in martial arts.

Testing joint play assesses the integrity of the capsular fibers. The joint is placed in the open-pack position, and the examiner pushes one half of the motion segment in a translatory direction. Generally, the amount of joint play is freer in female patients compared with male patients. Although no documentation exists regarding this phenomenon, it may be due to the length, thickness, or ratio of elastic to plastic qualities of the capsular fibers. It may lead to a softer (more give with less force) and a greater amount of motion in a woman's joint play.

End-play or *end-feel* is the springiness felt at the end of the passive range of motion. Depending on the motion segment, end-play tests the integrity of muscles, ligaments, capsular fibers, or a combination of the three. Stress tests, such as the valgus stress test at the knee, the anterior Drawer sign at the ankle, or Ludington's test for the shoulder, assess the integrity of the ligamentous fibers. When performing the ligamentous stress tests, or checking the end-play in women, the quality will be looser and softer than in men.

It is important to reiterate that these are generalizations regarding flexibility. There are male patients with hypermobile joints and female patients with hypomobile joints. Yet overall the average female is more hypermobile than the average male.[43] Age-related differences in the amount of resistance to stress provided by the capsular and ligamentous fibers also exist. Under the age of 14 years, males and females have about the same degree of mobility or quality of resistance to stress in the joints. However, mobility decreases during puberty in males, and it continues to decrease with aging depending on physical activities and trauma.

Females usually maintain a high degree of mobility as evidenced by lax, softer, more elastic capsular and ligamentous fibers in their joints until the age of menopause. Mobility may vary depending on physical activities and trauma. Research regarding age-related factors of flexibility has demonstrated that as women get older, the ligaments, tendons, and capsular fibers shorten and become stiffer.[44,45] It has been found that osteoporosis is associated with decreased mobility of the thoracic spine and ribs causing predictable respiratory impairment.[46] During pregnancy, especially the latter part, the hormones relaxin, pregnanediol, and estriol are released, causing the connective tissues (eg, ligaments, tendons, capsular fibers, plantar fasciae) to lose some of their viscous qualities and become more elastic.[33,47,48]

When a joint is cavitated with an adjustive or manipulative thrust, the capsular or ligamentous fibers absorb the force of the thrust, causing them to be maximally stretched. If a person has lax capsular or ligamentous fibers, the intent of the thrusting procedure should not be to stretch them even further. Therefore, it is important to select thrust procedures that minimize force beyond the anatomic end range. The integrity of the capsular and ligamentous fibers must be assessed. If these structures are found to be normal or lax, then the most appropriate thrusting procedure should be performed in the open-pack (loose-pack) position, employing a very short lever arm, a high velocity, and a very low amplitude thrust.

There are numerous hypothesized causes of joint restriction of motion such as decreased elasticity of the capsular or ligamentous fibers, mistracking of the articular surfaces, meniscoids, capsular entrapments, and loose bodies. Restriction of motion is often detected in a motion segment even though the capsular and ligamentous fibers may range from normal to lax. In this case, the chiropractor should choose a corrective procedure that keeps the capsular or ligamentous fibers from stretching further. Although this principle is important in the care of all patients, it is even more important in the female population because of the status of the capsular and ligamentous fibers (ie, their relative laxity or softness).

OSTEOPOROSIS

Bone is a dynamic tissue that is constantly being remodeled. If bone production is in balance with bone resorption, osteoporosis does not occur. Typically, the ability to produce new bone decreases with age and an overall loss of bone ensues. Many factors influence this balance. With age, an individual's skin may be less able to produce vitamin D from exposure to ultraviolet radiation in sunlight. In addition, many older individuals may not get out as much and therefore suffer from a decrease in ultraviolet exposure.

As individuals age, their diets tend to change. This transition can be due to changes in personal taste for various foods, loss of taste sensation, cooking for convenience rather than nutrition, inability to prepare certain foods, lack of interest or motivation to eat properly, or mental confusion. Aging may also bring about decreased production of digestive enzymes as well as decreased intestinal motility.[49,50] These changes result in an inability to digest foods and absorb and utilize the necessary nutrients.

Individuals also tend to become more sedentary as they age. New bone formation is stimulated when stress is placed on the bones. Many older patients suffer from chronic pain, arthritis, tendinitis, and muscle pain syndromes and, as a direct response, decrease their level of physical activity. Patients with heart conditions, arteriosclerosis, and hypertension will also restrict their activities proportional to the severity of their condition. As the level of physical activity decreases, the degree of osteoporosis increases. Osteoporosis may cause chronic pain, further decreasing activity levels. As the level of physical activity decreases, these original contributors will also worsen, resulting in a steady decrease in the overall health status of the patient.

Estrogen stimulates osteoblasts to form new bone. The onset of menopause causes the level of estrogen to decrease, resulting in a more rapid loss of bone. Menopausal women or women with a deficiency of estrogen for other reasons are at risk of developing osteoporosis.

One third of women over the age of 65 will suffer from spinal fractures due to osteoporosis.[51] Fifteen percent of women will suffer from hip fractures, which is three times the incidence in males.[51] Hip fractures due to osteoporosis cost the health care system an estimated $6 billion annually.[51] Unfortunately, 12% to 20% of all hip fractures result in death.[51] Manipulation does not appear to increase the risk of fractures;[52] however, as the most common site of fractures related to osteoporosis is the spine, chiropractors should always consider osteoporosis in their management of patients, especially in older persons. Under the age of 75 the incidence of osteoporosis is much greater in women than in men. This fact poses unique clinical considerations in care.

Chiropractic adjustments or manipulations are not contraindicated in patients with osteoporosis; in fact, they should be part of the management protocol. Chiropractic adjustments or manipulations are thought to relieve somatic dysfunction and associated pain and stiffness in older persons.[53] Pain causes inactivity, and inactivity promotes osteoporosis. If pain and stiffness are reduced, it may be easier for an individual to become more active, thus slowing the progression of osteoporosis.

Due to the shortening and stiffening of capsular fibers, restriction of movement in motion segments is almost always associated with osteoporosis. It is hypothesized that the shortening and stiffening are due to an increase in the number of cross-links between the adjacent collagen molecules.[44]

A management goal for osteoporotic patients is to restore the capsular and ligamentous fibers to a more elastic state.

Three modifications to thrusting procedures to be considered in treating patients with osteoporosis are: (1) the use of broader and less specific contacts, (2) slow mobilizing procedures, and (3) light force adjustments.[54] Mobilizing procedures can be employed to facilitate a plastic deformation of the restricting structures. Mobilizing procedures should begin with long axis distraction. After long axis distraction is applied to the motion segment, distraction should be maintained while the motion segment is moved through its gross ranges of motion. All procedures should be performed to the patient's tolerance. Although light force adjustments are suggested, the force should be of high velocity and low amplitude. The total amount of force utilized should reflect the mechanical aberrancies identified as well as the patient's condition and tolerance to the prestress. It is recommended that the thrust be performed using long axis distraction and removing articular slack to protect any degenerating articular cartilage. The goal of the high velocity, low amplitude thrusts is to restore elasticity by breaking cross links in the restricting connective tissues.

It should always be remembered that losses of elasticity develop over a long period of time. It is unrealistic to believe that they will be reversed overnight. Patience and moderation are therefore essential. Attempting to get too much correction too quickly is a common mistake. This approach can aggravate the condition and result in greater temporary discomfort for the patient.

PREGNANCY

Understanding changes associated with pregnancy is of paramount importance in determining why, when, and how to adjust a pregnant patient. Mechanical stress variations; the effects of relaxin, pregnanediol, and estriol; patient comfort; and applicable boundary issues are important factors for caring for pregnant patients. This discussion raises a number of common issues, but it is not intended to be comprehensive for all situations that may occur during different pregnancies.

Biomechanical changes affecting posture during pregnancy result from the increase in weight, an anterior weight distribution, and expansion of the uterus, which crowds the internal organs. These changes are progressive throughout pregnancy, most of them becoming demonstrable by the second trimester.

The gravitational weight line normally lies just anterior to the second sacral tubercle. As the fetus develops, the uterus (which lies anterior to the gravity line) pulls the sacral base anterior, causing an anterior tilting of the pelvis and flexion at the hips. To compensate, the shoulder region is drawn posterior, causing an accentuation of the lumbar lordosis and thoracic kyphosis. To compensate for the thoracic kyphosis, there is an anterior translation of the cervical spine and an extension of the occiput on the atlas, causing possible suboccipital muscle spasm or suboccipital headache.

Progressive thoracic kyphosis, anterior translation of the cervical spine, and increased weight of the breasts may cause the patient to develop cervical-thoracic syndromes such as pain in the cervical-thoracic region, thoracic outlet syndromes, or myofascial pain syndromes. The anterior displacement of the gravity line and the flexion of the hips place hyperextension stress on the knees, causing a slow stretch of the posterior capsular and ligamentous fibers of the knee. Eventually these fibers undergo elongation due to plastic deformation, and genu recurvatum may result.[31]

Normally 50% of the body's weight is borne by the calcaneus.[34] As the center of gravity migrates anterior, less of the body's weight is placed on the calcaneus. Therefore, more weight is placed on the metatarsal arches. Also, as the fetus grows and develops, the woman will usually increase in weight. This weight is transmitted to the arches of the feet, the plantar fasciae, long and short plantar ligaments, and plantar capsular fibers. These tissues begin to undergo plastic deformation, allowing the arches of the feet to drop. As the arches of the feet drop, the talus internally rotates and adducts in relation to the calcaneus. If the talus internally rotates, the tibia will also internally rotate, as long as the anterior and posterior tibiofibular ligaments are intact.

As the pelvis tilts anteriorly and the lumbar lordosis increases, increased activity in the psoas muscle and the multifidi muscle occurs. This activity may result in a sacroiliac syndrome, lumbosacral or lumbar facet syndrome, or sciatica.

As the fetus develops and the uterus expands, the abdominal muscles and their investing fasciae become stretched. By the seventh month the fetus has developed enough to put pressure on the diaphragm, causing diaphragmatic muscle spasms, and approximately a 4-cm decrease in the vertical height of the rib cage.[31,32] Inferior to superior compression of the rib cage results in intercostal myalgia, neuralgia, and costovertebral pain.

The cephalad expansion of the gravid uterus changes the position of the heart. As the uterus continues to expand, it places pressure on other internal organs. The iliac veins may compromise venous return, causing possible edema or varicose veins. Pressure on the lymphatic channels can also cause edema. Pressure on the intestines may cause constipation.

The entire spine may experience problems due to the postural changes associated with pregnancy. Adjusting or manipulating the spine during pregnancy is effective for numerous neuromusculoskeletal conditions such as leg, groin, and back pains; sciatica; and headaches.[55] Furthermore, no evidence exists of any side effects related to spinal thrusting procedures on adjusting pregnant females.[55,56]

Low back pain is very common in pregnancy. Fast and coworkers[57] report that 56% of pregnant women suffer from low back pain. Melzack and Schaffelberg[58] report back labor in 74% of women. Chiropractic adjustments or manipulations relieve low back pain in 84% of women suffering from pregnancy-related low back pain as well as significantly decrease the incidence of back labor.[56] An important consideration during the ninth month of pregnancy is to ensure the mobility of the sacroiliac joints in preparing for labor and delivery.[31]

Pelvic and lumbar adjusting procedures should be limited to light force adjustments. When performing pelvic or lumbar thrust procedures, the patient should experience no abdominal pressure. Modifications to side-lying lumbar or pelvic adjustments/manipulations/mobilizations include flexing the hip less than usual, positioning the patient further away from the doctor, and placing a small pillow or folded towel between the abdomen and the table to support the weight of the fetus (Fig 1).[31,59] The first two modifications place the doctor at a mechanical disadvantage, but the hormonally related increase in tissue elasticity seems to compensate for this disadvantage by necessitating less effort to apply the corrective force. These modifications are also recommended when applying a posterior to anterior thrust to the lower ribs or applying a rotatory thrust to the lower thoracic vertebrae in a side-lying posture. The thrusts for these side-lying techniques can be a single, high velocity, low amplitude thrust in the open-pack position, or six to eight repetitive mobilizations utilizing a low velocity and low amplitude type of force. If the patient is uncomfortable in the side-lying position, the procedure can be performed in the sitting position.

An alternative method of mobilizing the sacroiliac joints is to have the patient in a side-lying position with a pillow placed under the abdomen to help support the fetus. The doctor stands behind the patient and contacts the second sacral

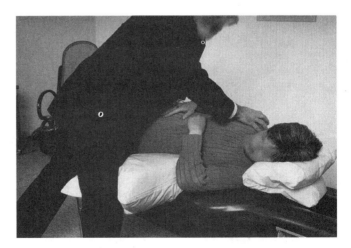

Fig 1. Modification of side-lying adjusting posture—Note placement of pillows.

tubercle with his or her cephalad hand stabilizing the sacrum. The caudal hand grasps the patient's top knee. The doctor flexes the patient's thigh until the knee is opposite the second sacral tubercle. The patient's thigh is internally and externally rotated until the thigh is in the neutral position as it relates to internal and external rotation. As the patient inhales, the doctor slowly circumducts the hip in the following direction: abduction, extension, adduction, flexion. The circumduction is performed to the point of the physiologic barrier of the hip (end play). As the doctor is circumducting the hip, a palpable or audible pop in the sacroiliac joint may occur. This procedure is repeated on the opposite side (Fig 2).

The following text describes an alternative procedure for correcting an anterolisthesis or a rotated fifth lumbar vertebra. The patient lies supine. The doctor stands on either side of the patient at the level of the patient's hips, facing cephalad. The patient's legs are flexed. The doctor places his or her inside hand under the sacrum with fingers pointing toward the head of the table; the middle and index fingers straddle the spine of the sacrum, and the finger tips are at the lumbosacral junction. The patient is asked to flex and abduct her thighs fully, causing the plantar surface of her feet to touch. The patient inhales deeply. When full inspiration is reached the doctor tractions the sacrum in a superior to inferior direction, moving the apex of the sacrum anterior. Maintaining traction on the sacrum, the patient is asked to extend her hips rapidly, keeping the plantar surfaces of her feet together. This procedure is thought to move the base of the sacrum posteriorly and caudally, allowing the fifth lumbar vertebra to drop posteriorly (Fig 3).

A modification of the previous technique can be used to correct restriction of motion or a rotatory misalignment of the lower thoracic and lumbar vertebrae. The patient is

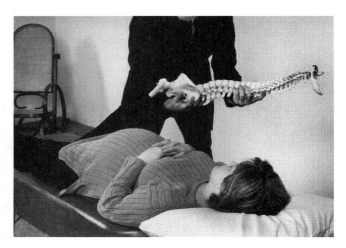

Fig 3. Alternate technique to adjust an anterolisthesis of L5.

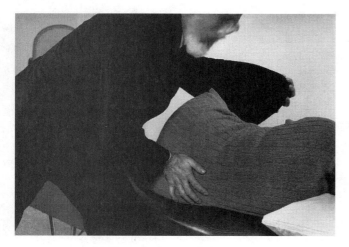

Fig 2. Alternate sacroiliac adjustment.

placed in the same position. The doctor's hand is placed under the patient's back, fingers pointing cephalad and contacting the lower half of the motion segment. The middle finger is placed on the spinous process of the vertebra, and the second and fourth fingers on the mamillary processes. The doctor tractions the lower half of the motion segment caudally. If rotation, or a rotational distortion exists, the doctor may augment the procedure by creating a torque to the lower segment. The patient inhales deeply, and at full inspiration the patient rapidly extends her hips, keeping the plantar surface of her feet together.

Osteitis pubis is a very common condition that occurs during the last trimester of pregnancy. It is due to the anterior shift in weight bearing, the increased weight gain, and the release of relaxin, pregnanediol, and estriol. The hormones cause the connective tissues holding the pubic bones together to soften and become more elastic. Trauma to the pubic symphysis is also very common during vaginal childbirth. Osteitis pubis is usually very painful. It is much easier to correct a pubic misalignment while the connective tissue is still soft and elastic. To correct for a pubic misalignment, the practitioner has the patient lie supine with her knees flexed 90° to 100° and feet flat on the table. The doctor stands at the side of the table, at the level of the patient's knees, facing cephalad. The doctor places his or her right hand on the medial aspect of the patient's right knee and his or her left hand on the medial aspect of the patient's left knee. The patient adducts her thighs against resistance. After the patient's adductors are contracted, the doctor gives a quick short thrust to abduct the patient's thighs (Fig 4).

The last four techniques are progressively more effective in treating joint dysfunction from the 12th week of pregnancy onward, due to the release of relaxin, pregnanediol, and estriol. They also place the patient in a compromising

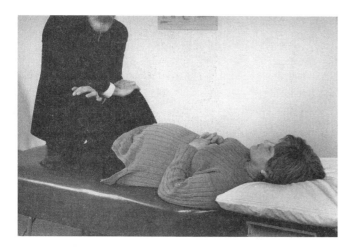

Fig 4. Pubic misalignment adjustment.

position. Every attempt should be made to protect the patient's level of comfort through appropriate gowning or use of towels and informing the patient as to why the procedure is necessary. The clinician should explain any procedures prior to performing them.

After the fifth month of pregnancy many patients will not be comfortable lying prone. Patient comfort is a vital consideration in all examination and treatment procedures. If it is necessary to have the patient prone during an examination or treatment procedure, the doctor should make every attempt to take pressure off of the abdominal region. This goal can be accomplished by placing pillows under the patient's pelvic and chest regions (Fig 5). If the doctor has an adjusting table with an adjustable abdominal section, it may suffice to just lower the abdominal section. If the abdominal section is spring loaded, the tension should be reduced to lessen pressure on the abdomen. To further enhance patient comfort, the knees should be flexed to relieve pressure on the hamstrings and gastrocnemius muscle groups. It can be accomplished by raising the footrest, if possible, or by placing another pillow under the ankles. Whenever the patient is lying supine, her head and shoulders should be elevated and her knees should be flexed. The practitioner should place a pillow under the patient's head and shoulder region (do not just rely on elevating the headrest) and another pillow under the patient's knees, supporting them in a flexed position (Fig 6).

Pregnancy will usually cause the breasts to enlarge and become more sensitive to pressure. Lying prone may cause discomfort for the patient. Commercially made breast pillows can be used to allow the patient to lie prone with less discomfort. The pillows may allow the patient to relax more, making the adjustments more effective with less force.

Many women may develop somatic dysfunction in the thoracic region due to the postural changes during pregnancy as well as the fetus compromising the thoracic region. This condition may be manifested as intercostal neuralgia and myalgia, costovertebral pain, intervertebral pain, or pulmonary distress. Correcting the static misalignments and maintaining motion in the thoracic spine and the costovertebral joints may prevent or eliminate these symptoms. The patient lies in the supine position. The doctor stands at the side of the table at the level of the patient's low back, facing cephalad, in a broad fencer stance. The patient's arms are crossed tightly over her chest with the arm furthest from the doctor on top. The doctor demonstrates the amount of pressure the

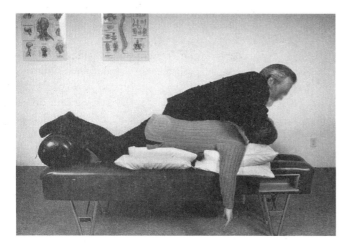

Fig 5. Modification of prone adjusting posture—Note placement of pillows.

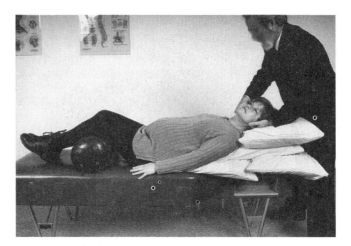

Fig 6. Modification of supine adjusting posture—Note placement of pillows.

patient will experience with this adjustment by pressing the patient's elbows toward her chest. The doctor places his or her cephalad hand (indifferent hand) behind the patient's cervicothoracic region and pulls the patient into a sitting position (Fig 7). The patient should remain relaxed throughout the procedure and not attempt to assist by sitting up. A common mistake is for the doctor to contact behind the patient's head and create too much stress on the patient's cervical spine. The doctor should reach behind the patient with his or her other hand (contact hand) contacting the thoracic spine just below the segment to be adjusted. The doctor may use an open-hand contact with the patient's spine placed along the distal palmar crease, or the doctor may fully flex the distal interphalangeal joint and proximal interphalangeal joint, placing the patient's spine along the distal palmar crease. The doctor contacts the patient's elbows just below the doctor's coracoid process (contact hand side). The patient is held in a tight flexed position by the doctor's indifferent hand for the entire procedure, and the doctor firmly grasps the patient between the contact hand and the coracoid process. The patient is slowly rolled backward toward the table until the doctor's hand touches the table.

Usually the vertebra will adjust at this point. If not, the doctor should lean into the patient's elbows with the coracoid process slightly in a posterior and superior direction. To augment the adjustment, the contact hand should traction the spine slightly caudally. Although this position allows for a high degree of control and finesse, it places the doctor and the patient in a compromising posture. A modification that sacrifices control yet is not as compromising is to have the patient clasp her hands behind her lower neck, bringing her elbows together (Fig 8). This modification is also very useful for female patients with large or painful breasts. If clasping the hands behind the neck sacrifices too much control, the doctor should place a roll of toweling along the sternum (Fig 9). The practitioner should have the patient cross her arms over the toweling. This modification will not only protect from compression of pain-sensitive breasts but also may help to lessen the compromising nature of the procedure.

The preceding procedure can be modified for the correction of thoracic rotational restriction or malpositions by rolling the patient backward with slightly more pressure on the right or left side of the spine and torquing in a corrective

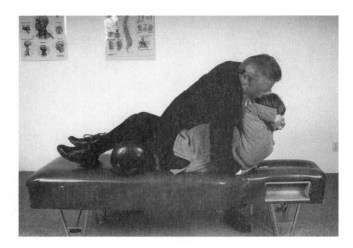

Fig 8. Hands behind the head thoracic anteriority adjustment for extended and/or rotated thoracic segments.

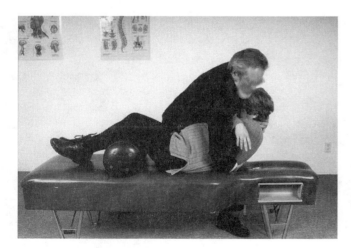

Fig 7. Crossed-arm thoracic anteriority adjustment for extended and/or rotated thoracic segments.

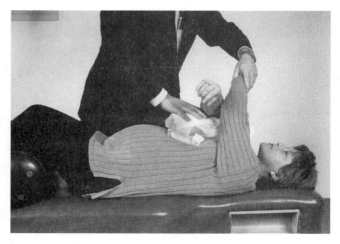

Fig 9. Pillow placement to optimize patient comfort in performing crossed-armed thoracic anteriority adjustment.

rotatory fashion with his or her contact hand. The doctor should move the contact point on the patient a little more lateral to adjust for a posterior rib.

Prone adjustments can also be attempted. However, much of the posterior to anterior thrust will be absorbed by the pillow located under the patient's chest. If the prone adjustments increase the pressure on the patient's abdomen and cause discomfort, they should be avoided. The upper thoracic spine and lower cervical spine can also be adjusted in the sitting or side-lying positions, and the lower thoracic spine can be adjusted using the knee-chest position. There are numerous prone, sitting, and side-lying techniques. For a more detailed description of these procedures, the author recommends the text *Chiropractic Technique*.[39]

Most patients are more comfortable with the supine and sitting positions than with the prone position for cervical and occipital adjusting procedures. However, any of the three positions may be used. When adjusting the cervical or occipital region (as with all adjustments during pregnancy), the motion segments adjust easily due to the effects of relaxin, pregnanediol, and estriol. If too much force is used, hypermobility of the motion segments, instability of the joints, pain, and early arthritic changes may result. The thrusts should be of low force, very high velocity, low amplitude, and performed in the open-pack position.

CONCLUSIONS

Chiropractic physicians may find it useful to develop a conceptual model of the pathophysiology and the pathobiomechanics responsible for the patient's condition prior to instituting adjustive care, particularly with the unique considerations that may affect women. Treatment procedures should be chosen based on affected tissues. Depending on the cause of the restriction of motion or the static misalignment of a motion segment, a non-thrust procedure may be the technique of choice such as trigger point therapy, Logan basic, therapeutic exercises, or passive mobilization procedures. The same thrusting procedures may be used, with some modifications, when treating female patients regardless of age or pregnancy. The doctor should always be aware of the unique considerations when treating female patients and modify his or her thrusting procedures accordingly. Every attempt should be made to make the chiropractic treatment procedures as tissue- and effect-specific as possible.

REFERENCES

1. National Board of Chiropractic Examiners. *Job Analysis of Chiropractic.* Greeley, Colo: National Board of Chiropractic Examiners; 1993.
2. Bredkjaer SR. Musculoskeletal disease in Denmark. *Acta Orthop Scand.* 1991;62(suppl 241):10–12.
3. McPoil TG, Knecht HG, Schmidt D. A survey of foot types in normal females between the ages of 18 and 30 years. *J Orthop Sports Phys Ther.* 1988;9(12):406–409.
4. Rothbart BA, Estabrook L. Excessive pronation: a major biomechanical determinant in the development of chondromalacia and pelvic lists. *J Manipulative Physiol Ther.* 1988;11:373–379.
5. Morscher E. Etiology and pathogeneses in leg length discrepancies. *Prog Orthop Surg.* 1997;1:9–19.
6. Okun SH, Morgan JW, Burns MJ. Limb length discrepancy. *J Am Podiatr Med Assoc.* 1982;72:595–599.
7. Beech RA. The fundamentals of the short leg syndrome. *Ann Swiss Chiro Assoc.* 1965;3:7–36.
8. Bluestein S, D'Amico J. Limb length discrepancy. *J Am Podiatr Med Assoc.* 1985;75:200–206.
9. Schwab WA. Principles of manipulative treatment: the low back problem: XV statistics and summary. *J Am Osteopath Assoc.* 1934;33:286–288.
10. Kerr H, Grant J, McBain R. Some observations on the anatomical short leg in a series of patients presenting themselves for treatment of low back pain. *J Am Osteopath Assoc.* 1943;42:437–440.
11. Giles LGF, Taylor JR. Low back pain associated with leg length inequality. *Spine.* 1981;6:510–521.
12. Gerow G, Matthews B, Jahn W, Gerow R. Compartment Syndrome and shin splints of the lower leg. *J Manipulative Physiol Ther.* 1993;16(4):245–252.
13. Nichols PJR. Short leg syndrome. *Br Med J.* 1960;1:1863–1865.
14. Janse J. Clinical biomechanics of the sacroiliac mechanism. *J Am Chiro Assoc.* 1978;12:51–58.
15. Giles LGF. Leg length inequalities associated with low back pain. *J Can Chiro Assoc.* March 1976:25–32.
16. Vernon H, Bereau J. A radiographic study of the incidence of low sacral base and lumbar lateral curvature related to the presence of an apparent short leg. *J Can Chiro Assoc.* 1983;27:11–15.
17. Mahar RK, Kirby RL Macleod DA. Simulated leg length discrepancy: its effect on mean center of pressure position and postural sway. *Arch Phys Med Rehabil.* 1985;66:822–834.
18. Giles LGF, Taylor JR. Lumbar spine structural changes associated with leg length inequality. *Spine.* 1982;7:159–162.
19. Papaioannou T, Stokes I, Kenwright J. Scoliosis associated with limb length inequality. *J Bone Joint Surg.* 1982;64A:59–62.
20. Gibson PH, Popaioannou T, Kenwright J. The influence of the spine on leg-length discrepancy after femoral fracture. *J Bone Joint Surg.* 1983;65B:584–587.
21. Stoddard A. *A Manual of Osteopathic Technique.* London, England: Hutchinson Medical Publishers; 1980.
22. Ingelmark BE, Lindstrom J. Asymmetries of the lower extremities and pelvis and their relation to lumbar scoliosis. *Aeta Morphol Neer-Scand.* 1963;5:221–234.
23. Pawels P. A correlation between disc degeneration and short leg. *J Clin Chiro.* 1978;2:3–11.
24. Giles LGF. Lumbosacral facetal "joint angles" associated with leg length inequality. *Rheum Rehabil.* 1981;20:233–238.

25. Gofton JP, Trueman GE. Studies in osteoarthritis of the hip: part II. Osteoarthritis of the hip and leg length disparity. *Can Med Assoc J.* 1971;104:791–799.
26. Gofton JP, Trueman GE. Studies in osteoarthritis of the hip: part IV. Biomechanics and clinical considerations. *Can Med Assoc J.* 1971;104:1007–1011.
27. Subotnick SI. Limb length discrepancies of the lower extremities. *J Orthop Sports Phys Ther.* 1981;3:11–15.
28. Murphy JP. Short leg and sciatica. *JAMA.* 1979;242:1257–1258.
29. Beal MC. The short leg problem. *J Am Osteopath Assoc.* 1977;76:745–751.
30. Gleeson PB, Pauls JA. Obstetrical physical therapy: review of literature. *Phys Ther.* 1988;68:1699–1702.
31. Fligg DB. Biomechanical and treatment considerations for the pregnant patient. *J Can Chiro Assoc.* 1986;30:145–147.
32. Zink GJ, Lawson WB. Pressure gradients in the osteopathic manipulative management of the obstetric patient. *Osteopath Ann.* 1979;7:41–49.
33. Smith LK, Weiss EL, Lehmkuhl LD. *Clinical Kinesiology.* 5th ed. Philadelphia, Pa: F.A. Davis; 1996.
34. Norkin C, Levangie P. *Joint Structure & Function: A Comprehensive Analysis.* Philadelphia, Pa: F.A. Davis; 1990.
35. Gatterman MI, Hansen DT. The development of chiropractic nomenclature through consensus. *J Manipulative Physiol Ther.* 1993;17(5):302–309.
36. Kessler R, Hertling D. *Management of Common Musculoskeletal Disorders.* New York: Harper & Row; 1990.
37. Bartol KM. The use of generic nomenclature of chiropractic treatment procedures in chiropractic publications. *Chiro Educ.* 1993;7:29–34.
38. Bartol KM. *Foundations of Chiropractic: Osseous Manual Thrust Techniques.* St Louis, Mo: Mosby; 1995.
39. Bergmann T, Peterson D, Lawrence D. *Chiropractic Technique.* New York: Churchill-Livingstone; 1993.
40. Magee DJ. *Orthopedic Physical Assessment.* Philadelphia, Pa: W.B. Saunders; 1987.
41. Sullivan MS, Dickinson CE, Troup JDG. The influence of age and gender on the lumbar spine sagittal plane range of motion. *Spine.* 1994;19:682–686.
42. Kapandji IA. *The Physiology of the Joints.* New York: Churchill-Livingstone; 1987; III.
43. Larsson L, Baum J, Mudholkar G, Srivastava D. Hypermobility: prevalence and features in a Swedish population. *Br J Rheum.* 1993;32:116–119.
44. Rauterberg J. Age-dependent changes in structure, properties, and biosynthesis of collagen. In: Platt D, ed. *Gerontology, 4th International Symposium.* New York: Springer-Verlag; 1989.
45. Hoefner VC. Osteopathic manipulative treatment in gerontology. *Osteopath Ann.* 1994;10:546–549.
46. Culham EG, Jimenez AI, King CE. Thoracic kyphosis, rib mobility, and lung volumes in normal women and women with osteoporosis. *Spine.* 1994;19:1250–1255.
47. Willow JR, Carrington, ER. The chemistry and biochemistry of progesterone and relaxin. In Zuckerman S, Mandl AM, Eckstein P, eds. *Obstetrics and Gynecology.* St. Louis, Mo: Mosby, 1987.
48. Golightly R. Pelvic arthropathy in pregnancy and the puerperium. *Physiotherapy.* 1982;68:216–220.
49. Mahan LK, Escott-Stump S. *Food, Nutrition, and Diet Therapy.* Philadelphia, Pa: W.B. Saunders; 1996.
50. McCarthy KA. Management considerations in the geriatric patient. *Top Clin Chiro.* 1996;3:66–75.
51. Riggs BL. Overview of osteoporosis. *West J Med.* 1991;154:63–77.
52. Haldeman S, Rubinstein SM. Compression fractures in patients undergoing spinal manipulative therapy. *J Manipulative Physiol Ther.* 1992;15:450–454.
53. Dodson D. Manipulative therapy for the geriatric patient. *Osteopath Ann.* 1979;7:114–119.
54. Bergmann TF, Larson L. Manipulative care and older persons. *Top Clin Chiro.* 1996;3:56–65.
55. Phillips CJ, Meyer JJ. Chiropractic care, including craniosacral therapy, during pregnancy: a static-group comparison of obstetric intervention during labor and delivery. *J Manipulative Physiol Ther.* 1995;18:525–529.
56. Diakow PRP, Gadsby TA, Gadsby JB, Gleddie JG, Leprich DJ, Scales AM. Back pain during pregnancy and labor. *J Manipulative Physiol Ther.* 1991;14:116–118.
57. Fast A, Shapiro D, Ducommun EJ, Freidmann LW, Bouklas T, Flowman Y. Low back pain in pregnancy. *Spine.* 1987;12:368–371.
58. Melzack R, Schaffelberg D. Low back pain during labor. *Am J Obstet Gynecol.* 1987;156:901–905.
59. Esch S, Zachman Z. Adjustive procedures for pregnant chiropractic patients. *Chiro Tech.* 1991;3:66–71.

14

Partner Abuse: Recognition and Intervention Strategies

Dorrie M. Talmage

Partner abuse is a rising epidemic in North America as well as worldwide. It is unclear whether this rise is due to an increase in abuse or an increase in reporting of abuse. Abuse first arrived on North American shores with the Puritans whose early American laws were based on the old English common law doctrines that permitted wife beating for the purpose of correcting behavior deemed inappropriate by husbands. One such law in effect until the end of the 19th century, known as the Rule-of-Thumb law, permitted a husband to beat his wife with a stick no larger than the circumference of his thumb.[1] This concept was struck down by the Massachusetts Supreme Court in 1871.[2] In the 1870s, an old Pennsylvania town ordinance prohibited a husband from beating his wife after 10:00 PM or on a Sunday.[1] It was not until the late 1960s and early 1970s that partner abuse was recognized as a growing problem. The first shelter for battered women appeared in London in 1971.[2]

Partner abuse occurs in every economic, racial, ethnic, religious, educational, intellectual, and social stratum, as well as all geographic areas. Both sexes are abused by their partners, but women tend to be the victims of abuse more often than men primarily because of strength and economic issues.[3] Violence against women has recently been recognized by the United Nations as a fundamental abuse of women's human rights.[4] The form in which the abuse manifests ranges from psychologic and sexual to physical abuse. Definitions of physical abuse vary in different societies and cultures. Physical abuse may be classified as slapping, biting, punching, kicking, beating with a blunt instrument, knifing, or shooting. Primary health care providers need to be alert for signs of abuse as well as become knowledgeable about the interventions available. The goal of this chapter is to review the prevalence, cycles of family violence, identification of victims of partner abuse, tactics for intervention, and legal responsibilities.

SCOPE OF THE PROBLEM

The exact prevalence of partner abuse is not known. Confusion as to what constitutes partner abuse, as well as the reluctance of the victim to disclose the abuse due to feelings of self-blame, shame, loyalty to the abuser, or fear, confounds prevalence data. Moreover, women in many cultures are socialized to accept physical and emotional chastisement as part of the husband's marital prerogative, making them less likely to self-identify as abused persons.[4]

Current prevalence data indicate that nearly 30% to 35% of all couples report at least one episode of violence (slapping, hitting, biting, and so on) during their marriages.[4-7] The danger lies in the fact that when this physical boundary has been crossed once, it is more likely to occur again when tensions mount or conflict arises.[4-7] However, the prevalence of abuse may be underestimated and is thought to affect between 50% and 60% of all couples.[5] A study by McFarlane and associates[8] reports the prevalence of physical or sexual abuse during pregnancy to be 17%. Long[9] estimates that 25% to 45% of women are abused during pregnancy. Gazmararian and coworkers[10] report that violence may be a more common problem for pregnant women than pre-eclampsia, gestational diabetes, and placenta previa, conditions for which pregnant women are routinely screened and evaluated.

The Federal Bureau of Investigation and the American Medical Association have estimated and reported a number of statistics associated with partner abuse in the United States.[1,6] These statistics are presented in Table 1.

Table 1. Prevalence issues

- A women is beaten every 18 seconds; almost 4 million women are beaten annually.
- 21% of all women who use emergency departments are battered women.
- Almost half of all injuries suffered by women seen in emergency departments are due to battering, yet only 4% are "recognized" as such by health care workers and are offered appropriate treatment.
- 30% of all women who are murdered are murdered by their husbands, boyfriends, or ex-partners.
- Battering is a cause of one out of four suicide attempts by all women.
- Domestic violence costs $5 to $10 billion each year in health care, lost productivity, and criminal justice intervention.
- Women are more often the victims of domestic violence than they are of burglary, muggings, or other physical crimes combined.

CYCLES OF FAMILY VIOLENCE

The phrase "cycles of abuse," first described by Lenore Walker,[3,5,11-13] is typically characterized by three distinct phases: the tension building phase, the violent (acute battering) phase, and the honeymoon phase.

Tension-building phase

In this initial phase, verbal and emotional abuse begin. Typically victims feel as though they must "walk on egg shells," and they often try extra hard to please the abuser. Minor abuse may occur over housekeeping or cooking complaints, but victims frequently try to accept their partner's behavior passively, hoping to avoid escalation to violence. Victims often perceive that efforts to please are not good enough in the abuser's opinion, so self-esteem erodes further and isolation increases. Some victims may passively provoke a violent episode as a result of increased fear and psychologic stress that an acute battering episode may be imminent. For example, a woman may fail to return an abusive partner's telephone calls or not meet expectations by not preparing an anticipated meal on time, or returning home when expected. Some victims may feel that the outbreak of violence is better than walking a tightrope in order to avoid the beatings.[14]

Violent phase

Following the tension-building phase an acute battering episode usually occurs. This phase typically includes a physical beating; however, such actions as verbal abuse, threats, throwing or breaking things, or sexual abuse may also occur. The violent phase is distinguished from the tension-building phase by its greater intensity and destructiveness. It cannot be controlled or accurately predicted.

Honeymoon phase

Following an acute battering or violent behavior, the abuser may apologize, promise to change, and act lovingly or contrite. Promises that the abuse will never happen again are also characteristic. Abusers may seek to make amends through gifts and offering assurances that lead their victims to believe they have the power to get concessions or change behaviors. As a result abused individuals may feel things are better and not seek help or leave the relationship. Frequently, following a short period of time, the abuser may begin to shift blame for the incident back to the victim, minimizing the severity of an episode or even denying that a battering took place.

IDENTIFYING A VICTIM OF SPOUSAL ABUSE

Domestic violence is both a public health and criminal issue. Identification of abuse victims can often be difficult for providers, and an enhanced insight into clinical clues and strategies for interventions is necessary. In 1986, the surgeon general recommended that the training of all health care professionals include methods to identify patients who are battered and helpful intervention strategies.[15]

In an attempt to accomplish this goal the Joint Commission on Accreditation of Healthcare Organizations (Joint Commission) recommended that accredited emergency departments have policies, procedures, and training in place to guide staff in the treatment of battered adults.[16] It is also recommended that physicians enhance their understanding and empathy for the effects of violence on women's lives through first-person accounts in literature or audiovisual materials. Examples of such materials can be found in books such as Fraser's *My Father's House* and Bass and Davies' *The Courage to Heal*, or films such as "After the Montreal Massacre."[17]

Despite increased awareness and the recommendations of clinical opinion leaders, government agencies, and domestic abuse groups, health care practitioners seldom recognize injuries resulting from partner abuse.[15] Yet failure to recognize these signs can result in serious harm and even lethal consequences for victims.

Victims may often experience a syndrome similar to post-traumatic stress disorder. Features of this syndrome appear to be anxiety-related symptoms in response to stress, evidenced by physical and psychologic problems. Psychologic effects of abuse can include any or all of the following: chronic depression, low self-esteem, relationship difficulties, sleep disorders, sexual dysfunction, obsessive-compulsive disorders, anxiety disorders, somatization disorders, dissociative phenomena and disorders, and alcohol and substance abuse.[18] Physical complaints that may be encountered in the chiropractic setting may be vague or nonspecific complaints such as myalgias; arthralgias; malaise; headaches; gastrointestinal symptoms; or chest, pelvic, and back pain. The patient may also demonstrate more obvious signs of acute battering, such as bruises, fractures (mandible or nasal), missing teeth, burns, whiplike bruises, choke marks on the neck, wounds on the back of the head (usually covered by hair), areas on the head where hair has been pulled out, or perforated tympanic membranes.

Repeated batterings to the head may cause the patient to develop dementia pugilistica (punch drunk syndrome), which is characterized by damage to the pyramidal, extrapyramidal, and cerebellar systems and by progression from affective disturbance and memory loss, through psychosis, to progressive dementia.[19] Physical injuries caused by battering are more likely to occur in a central pattern (head, neck, breasts, chest, abdomen) than peripherally.[15,20] However, defense-type injuries may be noted on the upper extremities such as grab or scratch marks on the upper arms or contusions on the lower arms when raised in defense.[15,20]

Other indicators of abuse may also occur that can serve as clues to a provider. A victim may frequently cancel or reschedule appointments. Behavioral changes may also be noticed including withdrawal, anxiety, nervousness, depression, panic attacks, suicidal ideation, or a history of suicide attempts. A victim may worry about the length of time an appointment is taking and about getting home late. If any of these subtle indicators occur, there may be a basis for suspecting abuse. It is then critical to pursue a careful history and examination, which may uncover more substantive indicators of domestic violence. Algorithm 1 sorts through clinical clues to spousal abuse.

HISTORY

A victim of suspected abuse should be interviewed in a private, safe setting where confidentiality is assured and a potential abuser is unable to stay with the victim during history and examination. An abuser who is present during a clinical encounter may act overly solicitous, overly affectionate, may try to explain away the injuries, and may try to prevent the victim from relaying accurate details to the clinician.[21]

Clinicians should record all patient statements regarding a history of abuse in the victim's own words.[22] Victims may feel ashamed, embarrassed, evasive, hesitant, jumpy, or anxious and frequently may not openly admit that abuse has occurred. For this reason, it is important for a provider to remain patient and gain the victim's trust by showing empathy, care, and a supportive, nonjudgmental demeanor. It can be helpful for a clinician to identify and confront his or her own feelings of disgust, anger, anxiety, helplessness, or disbelief regarding a patient's disclosure of abuse. Recognition of one's own feelings can assist in remaining helpful and empathic, rather than succumbing to inappropriate rationalization of a situation. For example, if a physician feels disgust, it may be easy to become distant or detached, minimize the abuse, or, in some instances, even blame the victim. If feelings of helplessness are produced, the physician may take on the role of rescuer, which may further disempower the victim.[17] Some clinicians are afraid to question the victim about suspected abuse for fear it will open "Pandora's box" and get them involved in something that they are not mentally or psychologically equipped to handle.[23]

During the history the clinician must avoid questions that label the victim (eg, "Are you a victim of family violence?") because the victim may be unable to accept that type of self-description. If a victim discloses information, it is likely that this individual is ready to receive help. General questions that may be helpful in the office setting are listed in Table 2.[24,25]

Once a patient has been identified as a victim of abuse, the clinician should acknowledge the abuse by saying something along the lines of "Your safety is important to me. You do not deserve to be hurt. There is help for you." This type of response indicates to the victim that the clinician cares and focuses on a high priority, the patient's safety.[13]

Richard F. Jones III, MD, of the American College of Obstetrics and Gynecology states, "The patient needs to know that the doctor understands the issue and cares about her as a person. She needs affirmation that she doesn't have to live like this if she chooses not to, and that the physician, or clinic, or hospital, or whatever her health care provider system is, is eager to be supportive of her and what she chooses to do to be safe."[26(p1224)] The clinician should avoid questions or statements that blame (eg, "Why did you let it go on for so long?") or minimize (eg, "You say that this experience is in the past and that you have coped with it. Why don't we move on, then, to the concerns you have today?").[27]

For complete documentation, the clinician should get a detailed description of the abuse, quoting the victim, using phrases in the patient's chart such as "suspected abuse," "appears to be," "suspicion of" as opposed to a direct label. Utilizing this information, the clinician should try to determine if the victim is in immediate danger. If so, the patient should be discouraged from returning home. In addition, all injuries need to be completely documented in case this information is needed in a criminal investigation.

PHYSICAL EXAMINATION

The physical examination is also important in documenting abuse. The examination procedures should be thoroughly explained to the victim, and the intent behind each procedure

Table 2. Questions for the victim interview

1. Has anyone at home ever hurt you, threatened you, or otherwise treated you badly? In what ways?
2. How were you hurt? How badly have you been hurt?
3. Has anyone threatened or abused your children?
4. Have you ever been in an abusive relationship?
5. Has anyone ever destroyed things that you cared about or taken things without asking?
6. Have you ever been forced to have sex when you did not want to?
7. Have you ever been forced to take part in activities that make you uncomfortable?
8. Are you afraid of anybody at home? If so, who?
9. All families fight. What happens when there is an argument at your house?
10. Does anyone in the family use drugs or alcohol? How does that person behave at those times?
11. Do you have guns or other weapons in your home? Has anyone ever threatened to use them on you?
12. Has anybody prevented you from getting medical care when you needed it?
13. I notice you have a number of bruises. Tell me how you were bruised. Did someone hit you? Who? When did the abuse first begin and when did this episode occur?
14. Who else lives in the home? (signs of child or older person abuse)
15. Are the children in danger? Have they been hit? If so, how badly?
16. Have you told anyone before? If so, who?
17. Have you protected yourself? If so, how?
18. Have you ever called the police? If yes, when and what was the outcome?
19. Have you tried to press charges?
20. Have you been threatened? Did the abuser attempt to kill you?
21. Are you afraid to go home?
22. Have you ever called a shelter or hotline? If yes, which? What was the outcome?

should be understood. Also, due to self-esteem and modesty issues, it is preferable if a female is present during the examination. If the victim has acknowledged abuse or injuries are inconsistent with the history, the clinician's suspicions should be charted as an opinion. As the examination is being performed, the clinician should be especially aware of bruises of differing colors (old versus new abuse) and bilateral injuries (defense wounds). The clinician should move slowly and start the examination distally on extremities, usually hands, so that the patient may feel as comfortable as possible.

The clinician should thoroughly document any injuries as to location, shape, size, number, color, stages of healing, and type. If possible, the practitioner should document an opinion as to the probable cause in the chart. Optimally, photographs of the patient's injuries should be obtained. They may be useful if future criminal proceedings occur. The photographer should sign and date each photograph, and the pictures should be stored in a secure location. As additional evidence, a signed consent form explaining why the photographs were taken should be placed in the patient's file. Radiographs may be necessary to document new fractures and demonstrate the varying stages of healing injuries.[2,12,22]

It is also important to note that women who are abused often shy away from male doctors, feeling that men generally may be unsafe to them. If the physical examination shows evidence of possible abuse, more information regarding the abuse may be more readily obtained from a physician of the same gender.

INTERVENTION

To identify abuse and intervene appropriately, health care professionals need to optimize their effectiveness in dealing with partner abuse. The following considerations can assist doctors in navigating this difficult and emotionally laden clinical terrain[28]:

- Be aware of your own attitudes. Strive to be nonjudgmental and evaluate prejudices.
- Know personal limits of time and energy. If your practice is too busy to allow adequate time to care for the victim, then refer the patient to an appropriate person.
- Realize that there may be a high level of frustration inherent in dealing with victims of abuse. The victim may not be emotionally, physically, or mentally equipped to follow advice immediately. Be patient and supportive, and avoid conveying frustration or irritation with the patient's coping strategies.
- Be alert for health problems that an abuse victim may be reluctant to reveal.
- Become familiar with domestic violence. Horror stories should not be allowed to scare or overwhelm the doctor and subsequently the victim.

A number of barriers to effective management may need to be overcome by clinicians unfamiliar with effective management strategies in working with abused individuals[3,29]:

- Sanctity of the family. Health care professionals may be reluctant to intervene in family privacy issues.
- Rationalization. The professional may view the problem as the victim being unable or unwilling to fulfill duties. Abuse may also be viewed as normal by the doctor in that family's lifestyle or culture.
- Definition of violence. The definition of violence varies from person to person. Therefore, what one individual views as normal another may view as abuse.

- Blaming the victim. The professional may have the belief that a patient "asked for it." In some sectors of the population this view can still be a major issue.
- Factors related to the battered person. The victim may be unwilling to seek help or get out of the abusive relationship for personal reasons.
- Professional inadequacy. A clinician may not have the necessary training or experience to deal effectively with abuse situations.
- Overreaction. The professional may be overwhelmed and therefore overreact to the signs of abuse. This response frightens the victim into silence.
- Excusing the assailant. The clinician may see the abuser's apologetic behavior and encourage the couple's reconciliation.

Certain goals have been established to help clinicians implement appropriate intervention in spousal abuse cases (Table 3). *Healthy People 2000*[30] sets a national goal of reducing physical abuse directed at women by male partners to no more than 27 cases per 1,000 couples (baseline, 30 per 1,000 in 1985). In order to help realize these goals, clinicians should suggest and encourage the use of resources available for victims of abuse. Table 4 contains a list of hotline numbers that can be made available to patients who are or appear to be victims of abuse. Other resources can be used to reassure and provide effective support for victims (such as brochures on physical abuse, sexual abuse, and harassment placed in waiting rooms). It also is recommended that providers reinforce the idea that patients do not deserve to be abused (Table 5). Brown and colleagues state, "The clinician should try to empower the victim by supporting her within her relationship over a period of time, . . . try to work on self-esteem issues and help her gain some insight into why they are there, . . . get her strong enough to either leave or to come to terms with the abuse and stay."[31(p187)]

Clinicians should attempt to identify whether or not it is safe for a suspected victim to return home. If the decision is to return home, the victim should be given a safety plan and an exit plan that provide specific actions that can be taken to help cope with an acute abusive episode and safely get away from the partner. Some of the features of a safety plan include the following[13]:

- If a battering is imminent, do not go into a kitchen (too many potential weapons) or bathroom (little opportunity for escape).
- Do not go into rooms containing weapons and do not threaten the abuser with a weapon.
- Know all escape routes from the house and get out if you feel threatened.
- Find a "safe house" (eg, shelter, friend's, or relative's house).
- Prepare an exit plan and have all items ready to go.
- Find a neighbor who would allow the use of a telephone in the case of an emergency.
- Inform others about the violence (eg, friends, relatives, coworkers).
- Remind the children that the violence is not their fault.
- If an attack is imminent, faint, vomit, or fake a seizure (or other serious illness). This action may deter the abuser.

An exit plan should include the following:

- Copies of car license and ownership papers; bank account numbers; driver's license (victim and abuser); social security numbers (victim, abuser, and children);

Table 3. Goals of intervention

1. Let the victim know help is available. Help the victim set up a safety and an exit plan.
2. Give specific information about resources available.
3. Document the battering with accurate medical records.
4. Acknowledge the victim's experiences in a supportive manner and offer reassurance that regardless of what decision is reached about the abuse the victim is always welcome at your clinic.
5. Respect the victim's right to make personal decisions.

Table 4. Hotlines

National Domestic Violence Hotline
  (800) 799-SAFE
National Organization of Victim Assistance
  1575 Park Road, NW
  Washington, DC 20001
  (800) TRY-NOVA
National Coalition Against Domestic Violence
  P.O. Box 18749
  Denver, CO 80218
  (303) 839-1852
National Resource Center on Domestic Violence
  6400 Flank Drive
  Suite 1300
  Harrisburg, PA 17112
  (800) 537-2238
American College of Obstetricians and Gynecologists
  409 12th Street, SW
  Washington, DC 20024-2188
  (202) 863-2518
Women's Transitional Living Center
  P.O. Box 6103
  Orange, CA 92667
  (714) 992-1931

Table 5. Providing effective support

1. Let victims know you believe them.
2. Let victims express their feelings.
3. Express your concern for the safety of the victim and the safety of any children.
4. Let victims know that help is available.
5. Reinforce the idea that nobody deserves to be beaten.
6. Realize that the victim may be embarrassed and humiliated about the abuse.
7. Be aware of the effects of isolation and control through fear.
8. Assure victims that you will not betray their trust.
9. Document the battering with specific information in the medical record.
10. Remember that victims may have other problems that demand immediate intervention.

---

health records; copy of last income tax statements (state and federal); and proof of custody of the children (if from previous marriage and applicable).

- Addresses and telephone numbers of doctors, lawyers, friends, relatives, and abuse hotlines.
- Extra cash, credit cards, extra car and house keys, clothing, diapers (if applicable), food and water, and medicine (if applicable).

In addition to the safety and exit plans, encourage victims to call the police if they feel threatened. In a 1983 Minneapolis study,[1] police arrests were shown to be the best deterrent to recurrence. A Miami program[1] noted that arrested batterers who had little experience with the law and spent a night in jail appeared positively affected by this experience. They began constructive introspection about their behavior. The clinician should neither encourage the victim to return to the abuser nor encourage couples therapy. This form of therapy may put the victim at greater risk and does not hold the abuser solely responsible for the violence.[32] The clinician's knowledge of the abuse needs to empower the victim to get help, not to change the abuser. The clinician may also advise the victim about getting a job, appropriate legal counsel, housing assistance, education, and child care.[20]

The last important aspect of intervention is to maintain contact with the victim. Follow-up visits will increase the trust the victim has in others and increase the likelihood that a safe environment will be sought or that the relationship will be left completely.

CLINICIAN'S LEGAL RESPONSIBILITIES

Domestic violence laws differ from state to state. It is important that all health care professionals become familiar with their state's laws and the mechanisms for reporting abuse. Lower prevalence rates may be due in part to the lack of clinician knowledge regarding reporting abuse. For example, in the state of California every health practitioner employed in a health facility, clinic, or physician's office must immediately make a telephone or written report to the police when partner abuse is suspected.[33] Failure to make the report may result in up to 6 months in jail and/or a fine of $1,000. The *American Journal of Public Health*[34(p460)] reports that "at least one other state (Kentucky) requires the reporting of adult domestic violence, and several other states have laws mandating that health care providers report injuries resulting from criminal acts including assaults."[15(p16)] In cases of partner abuse, it is also imperative that clinicians remember that any children in the home need to be observed for possible signs of child abuse. Federal law mandates reporting of all suspected cases of child abuse.

CONCLUSIONS

Partner abuse is a major health problem, and chiropractors need to recognize and intervene to prevent further abuse and possible death. There is a mnemonic ABCDES[24] that can be used to recall all pertinent areas:

A—Acknowledge that the patient feels *Alone*.
B—State your *Belief* that violence is always wrong and never the fault of the victim.
C—Reassure the patient as to the *Confidentiality* of patient records.
D—*Document* all evidence of abuse.
E—*Educate* yourself as to the available resources for your patients.
S—Assess the patient's *Safety* prior to sending her home.

Partner abuse is largely a secret malady that influences a victim's physical and mental health. Physicians are more likely to have contact with the victim than anyone else and are called upon to be observant.[24] It is important that clinicians include a routine screening history of abuse assessment of all female patients. A question such as "Are you now, or have you ever been, in a relationship where someone has abused you physically, emotionally, or sexually?" should be a routine component of history taking. Health care providers should recognize the importance that the doctor-patient relationship can play in facilitating a safer future for those entwined in abusive relationships.

REFERENCES

1. Dickstein LJ. Spouse abuse and other domestic violence. *Psychiatr Clin North Am.* 1988;11(4):611–628.
2. Dym H. The abused patient. *Dent Clin North Am.* 1995;39(3):621–635.
3. *Spouse Abuse.* Assoc for Adv Training; 1992.
4. Heise LL, Raikes A, Watts CH, et al. Violence against women: a neglected public health issue in less developed countries. *Soc Sci Med.* 1994;39(9):1165–1179.
5. Kornblit AL. Domestic violence—an emerging health issue. *Soc Sci Med.* 1994;39(9):1181–1188.
6. American Medical Association. 4 million American women abused annually. *Hosp Health Netw.* Dec 1994:15.
7. Candib LM. Moving on to strengths. *Arch Fam Med.* 1995;4:397–400.
8. McFarlane J, Parker B, Soeken K, et al. Assessing for abuse during pregnancy. *JAMA.* 1992;267(23):3176–3178.
9. Long T. Invited commentary. *Phys Ther.* 1996;76(1):18–19.
10. Gazmararian JA, Lazorick S, Spitz AM, et al. Prevalence of violence against pregnant women. *JAMA.* 1996;275(24):1915–1920.
11. Steiner RP, Vansickle K, Lippmann SB. Domestic violence—do you know when and how to intervene? *Postgrad Med.* 1996;100(1):103–116.
12. Olsen EA. Identifying and responding to the battered woman. *J Neuromusculoskel Syst.* 1996;4(2):45–51.
13. Wilson JS. Guidelines for the care of abused women. *Home Healthcare Nurse.* 1994;12(4):47–53.
14. Williams LS. Failure to pursue indications of spousal abuse could lead to tragedy, physicians warned. *Can Med Assoc J.* 1995;152(9):1488–1491.
15. Clark TJ, McKenna LS, Jewell MJ. Physical therapists: recognition of battered women in clinical settings. *Phys Ther.* 1996;76(1):12–19.
16. Centers for Disease Control and Prevention (CDC). Emergency department response to domestic violence—California 1992. *JAMA.* 1993;270(10):1174–1176.
17. Archer LA. Empowering women in a violent society—role of the family physician. *Can Fam Physician.* 1994;40:974–985.
18. Saunders BE, Villeponteaux LA, Lipovsky JA, et al. Child sexual assault as a risk factor for mental disorders among women. *J Interpersonal Violence.* 1992;7:189–204.
19. Roberts GW, Whitwell HL, Acland PR, et al. Dementia in a punch-drunk wife. *Lancet.* 1990;335:918–919.
20. American College of Obstetricians and Gynecologists (ACOG). Issues Technical Bulletin on Domestic Violence. *ACOG Technical Bulletin 207.* American Family Physician. 1995;52(8):2387–2389.
21. Newberger EH, Barkan SE, Lieberman ES, et al. Abuse of pregnant women and adverse birth outcome. *JAMA.* 1992;267(17):2370–2372.
22. McDowell JD, Kassebaum DK, Stromboe SE. Recognizing and reporting victims of domestic violence. *J Am Dent Assoc.* 1992;123:44–50.
23. Sugg NK, Inui T. Primary care physicians' response to domestic violence—opening Pandora's box. *JAMA.* 1992;267(23):3157–3160.
24. Brandt EN, Hadley S, Holtz HA. Family violence: a covert health crisis. *Patient Care.* 1996:138–166.
25. McLeer SV, Roth B. *Structured Interview for Battered Women.* Emergency Medicine Department of the Medical College of Pennsylvania. 1979–80. Unpublished.
26. Randall T. Domestic violence hot line's demise: what's next? *JAMA.* 1993;269(10):1223–1225.
27. Draucker CB. *Counseling Survivors of Childhood Sexual Abuse.* Sage; London, England; 1992.
28. Domestic violence training for medical providers. Adopted from Why does she stay by Women's Center of San Joaquin County.
29. Council on Ethical and Judicial Affairs, AMA. Physicians and domestic violence—ethical considerations. *JAMA.* 1992;267(23):3190–3193.
30. US Department of Health and Human Services. *Healthy People 2000: National Health Promotion and Disease Prevention Objectives.*
31. Brown JB, Lent B, Sas G. Identifying and treating wife abuse. *J Fam Pract.* 1993;36:185–191.
32. Segal-Evans K. The dangers of traditional family therapy when intervening in domestic violence. *Calif Ther.* July/Aug 1991:1–5.
33. CAL Ch 992 (AB1652). Spousal and Domestic Violence Reporting Laws, 1993.
34. 9211(PP): Domestic violence. *Am J Public Health.* 1993;83:458–463.

Algorithm 1

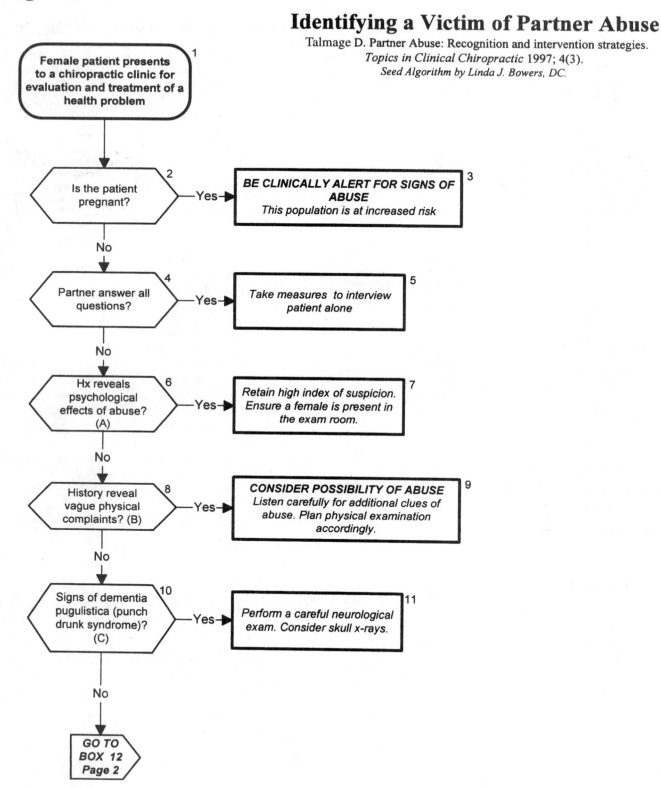

Identifying a Victim of Partner Abuse

Talmage D. Partner Abuse: Recognition and intervention strategies. *Topics in Clinical Chiropractic* 1997; 4(3). *Seed Algorithm by Linda J. Bowers, DC.*

Algorithm 1, continued

Identifying a Victim of Partner Abuse - Page 2

Talmage D. Partner Abuse: Recognition and intervention strategies.
Topics in Clinical Chiropractic 1997; 4(3).
Seed Algorithm by Linda J. Bowers, DC.

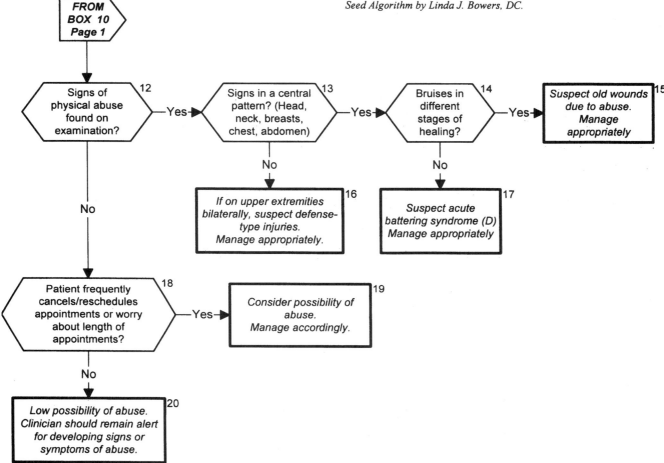

Annotations:
(A) Chronic depression. low self-esteem, relationship difficulties, sleep disorders, sexual dysfunction, obsessive/compulsive disorder, anxiety, somatization, alcohol/substance abuse, suicidal ideation, panic attacks.
(B) Myalgias, arthralgias, malaise, headaches, gastrointestinal symptoms, chest/pelvic/back pain.
(C) Memory loss, psychosis, progressive dementia.
(D) Bruises, fractures (mandible, nasal), missing teeth, burns, whiplike bruises, choke marks on the neck, wounds on the back of the head covered by hair, areas of hair pulled out, perforated tympanic membrane.

Appendix II-A

A Guide to Women's Health Resources

GENERAL HEALTH

Institute for Research on Women's Health
1616 18th Street, NW
Suite 109B
Washington, DC 20009
(202) 483-8643

Jacobs Institute of Women's Health
409 12th Street SW
Washington, DC 20024-2188
(202) 488-4229

Melpomene Institute for Women's Health Research
1010 University Avenue
St. Paul, MN 55104
(612) 642-1951

National Black Women's Health Project
1211 Connecticut Avenue, NW
Suite 310
Washington, DC 20036
(202) 833-8709

National Women's Health Network
514 10th Street, NW
Suite 400
Washington, DC 20004
(202) 347-1140

National Women's Health Resource Center
2425 L Street, NW
3rd Floor
Washington, DC 20037
(202) 293-6045

Society for the Advancement of Women's Health Research
1920 L Street, NW
Suite 510
Washington, DC 20036
(202) 223-8224

World Health Organization
20 Avenue Appia
Geneva 27, Switzerland
41-22-971-2111

AIDS

CDC National AIDS Clearinghouse
P.O. Box 6003
Rockville, MD 20849
(800) 458-5231

National Association for People with AIDS (NAPWA)
1413 K Street, NW
7th Floor
Washington, DC 20005
(202) 898-0414

National Resource Center on Women and AIDS
Center for Women Policy Studies
2000 P Street, NW
Suite 508
Washington, DC 20036
(202) 872-1770

BREAST CANCER/DISEASE

National Alliance of Breast Cancer Organizations
9 E 37th Street
10th Floor
New York, NY 10016
(800) 719-9154

Susan G. Komen Breast Cancer Foundation
5005 LBJ
Suite 370
Dallas, TX 75244
(800) IM-AWARE (463-9273)

Y-ME National Breast Cancer Organization
212 W Van Buren
5th Floor
Chicago, IL 60607
(800) 221-2141

continues

CANCER

American Cancer Society
1599 Clifton Road, NE
Atlanta, GA 30329
(800) ACS-2345

National Coalition for Cancer Survivorship
1010 Wayne Avenue
5th Floor
Silver Spring, MD 20910
(301) 650-8868

R.A. Bloch Cancer Foundation
4410 Main Street
Kansas City, MO 64111
(816) 932-8453

CARDIOVASCULAR

American Heart Association
7272 Greenville Avenue
Dallas, TX 75231
(800) AHA-USA1

CHILDBIRTH

Childbirth Education Foundation
P.O. Box 5
Richboro, PA 18954
(215) 357-2792

International Cesarean Awareness Network
P.O. Box 152
Syracuse, NY 13210
(315) 424-1942

International Childbirth Education Association
P.O. Box 20048
Minneapolis, MN 55420
(612) 854-8660

La Leche League International
Box 4079
Schaumburg, IL 60168
(847) 519-7730

Midwives Alliances of North America
P.O. Box 175
Newton, KS 67114
(316) 283-4543

National Maternal and Child Health Clearinghouse
8201 Greensboro Drive
Suite 600
McLean, VA 22102
(703) 821-8955

EATING DISORDERS

American Anorexia/Bulimia Association
418 E 76th Street
New York, NY 10021
(212) 734-1114

Anorexia Nervosa and Related Eating Disorders
P.O. Box 5102
Eugene, OR 97405
(503) 344-1144

National Association of Anorexia Nervosa and Associated Disorders (ANAD)
Box 7
Highland Park, IL 60035
(847) 432-8000

ENDOMETRIOSIS

Endometriosis Association
8585 N 76th Place
Milwaukee, WI 53223
(414) 355-2200

FAMILY PLANNING

Adoptive Families of America
3333 Highway 100 N
Minneapolis, MN 55422
(612) 535-4829

Choice
1233 Locust Street
3rd Floor
Philadelphia, PA 19107
(215) 985-3300

Planned Parenthood Federation of America
810 7th Avenue
New York, NY 10019
(800) 230-7526

FERTILITY

The American Fertility Society
1209 Montgomery Highway
Birmingham, AL 35216
(205) 978-5000

RESOLVE, Inc.
1310 Broadway
Somerville, MA 02144
(617) 623-0252

GYNECOLOGICAL

American Academy of Family Physicians
8880 Ward Parkway
Kansas City, MO 64114
(816) 333-9700

Association of Professors of Gynecology and Obstetrics
409 12th Street, SW
Washington, DC 20024
(202) 863-2507

Interstitial Cystitis Association
Box 1553
Madison Square Station
New York, NY 10159
(212) 979-6057

National Association for Continence
Box 8310
Spartanburg, SC 29305
(803) 579-7900

Vulvar Pain Foundation
Drawer 177
Graham, NC 27253
(910) 226-8518

HYSTERECTOMY

Hysterectomy Educational Resources and Services (HERS) Foundation
422 Bryn Mawr Avenue
Bala Cynwyd, PA 19004
(610) 667-7757

MENOPAUSE

The North American Menopause Society
Box 94527
Cleveland, OH 44101
(212) 844-8708

continues

MENTAL HEALTH

National Mental Health Association (NMHA)
1021 Prince Street
Alexandria, VA 22314
(800) 969-NMHA

NUTRITION

American Dietetic Association (ADA)
216 W Jackson Boulevard
Suite 800
Chicago, Il 60606
(312) 899-0040

OSTEOPOROSIS

National Osteoporosis Foundation
1150 17th Street, NW
Suite 500
Washington, DC 20036
(202) 223-2226

PHYSICAL FITNESS

American Fitness Association
P.O. Box 410
Durango, CO 81301
(303) 247-4109

Women's Sports Foundation
Eisenhower Park
East Meadow, NY 11554
(800) 227-3988

SELF-HELP

American Self-Help Clearinghouse
St. Clares–Riverside Medical Center
Denville, NJ 07834
(201) 625-7101

National Self-Help Clearinghouse
City University of New York Graduate Center
25 W 43rd Street
Room 620
New York, NY 10036
(212) 354-8525

SEXUAL HEALTH

American Social Health Association
Box 13827
Research Triangle Park, NC 27709
(919) 361-8425

Sex Information and Educational Council of the US
130 W 42nd Street
Suite 2500
New York, NY 10036
(212) 819-9770

SUBSTANCE ABUSE

Al-Anon Family Groups
1600 Corporate Landing Parkway
Virginia Beach, VA 23454
(800) 356-9996

Alcoholics Anonymous World Services
475 Riverside Drive
New York, NY 10163
(212) 870-4300

Alcoholism Center for Women
1147 S Alvarado Street
Los Angeles, CA 90006
(213) 381-8500

Do It Now Foundation
P.O. Box 27586
Tempe, AZ 85285
(602) 491-0393

Women for Sobriety (WFS)
P.O. Box 618
Quakertown, PA 18951
(215) 536-8026

Part III

Geriatric Health

15

Normal Aging

Thomas Souza and Shahihaz Soliman

The older patient is often viewed with some degree of ambivalence. Often, signs and symptoms are attributed to the normal aging process. It is logical that normal aging does result in some decreases in function, however, the distinction between this process and other disease processes is not always readily evident. Being cognizant of the effects of normal aging may facilitate a more focused examination, improving the examiner's ability to interpret "normal" and identify "abnormal." Unfortunately, working off the assumption that all decreases in function are age-related may delay intervention or allow a misdiagnosis that seriously restricts a patient's lifestyle, which in turn may compound his or her problems.

The first solution to this overgeneralization is not to look at all older persons as the same. Shephard[1] suggests dividing the older population into the following functional categories:

- Young old—Patients who have maintained a level of fitness that allows participation in recreational and daily activity requirements.
- Middle old—Patients who are independent with daily activities, however, they need assistance with more demanding tasks.
- Old old—Disabled patients who require nursing care.

These three categories often correspond to the age categories of 65–75, 75–85, and older than 85, respectively. Generally, classifying a patient as being an older person is based largely on social and political events that take place when a person reaches the age of 65.[2]

Second, it is important to understand those changes expected with aging and those that are the result of disuse or misuse (ie, modifiable aspects). With this anticipation, the patient may also be educated as to what is normal and what is pathologic and perhaps become a more responsible partner in health care. An educated patient and doctor may decrease the number of unnecessary visits and therefore heighten the doctor's concern with an older patient's complaint.

The aging process involves the gradual loss in reserve capacity of organs and systems; thus there is a progressive decline in the ability of the body to respond to the stresses of the environment. Aging processes are defined as having the following four characteristics:

1. They must be deleterious to the organism.
2. They must be progressive over a period of time.
3. They must be intrinsic to the organism and not modifiable by environmental factors.
4. They must be universal, occurring in all members of the species.

Age-related diseases, such as cancer and cardiovascular disease, show striking increases with advancing age. However, in any age-related finding, longitudinal studies must be done to discover if the finding is an inevitable conclusion of aging or a result of an external or internal stress to the body over time.

Last, it is important to consider the end-stage effects of various chronic problems or illnesses such as diabetes and atherosclerosis. Moreover, modifiable factors (eg, weight, diet, and exercise; smoking; and alcohol and drug usage) act to accelerate the aging process in many patients.

THEORIES OF AGING

There are many theories of aging, however, they can be organized into two main groups: (1) genetically determined, and (2) accumulated damage to key cellular processes. It seems clear that there are certain cultures in which age is independent of environment and must therefore have a strong genetic component. This finding has also been demonstrated with simple organisms; however, the degree to which it is evident in humans is unknown.

There are generally three theories put forth regarding accumulated damage with aging. The first theory focuses on the damage caused by oxidative metabolism with the production of superoxide and hydroxyl free radicals (also hydrogen peroxide). The transcription of genes encoded for protective enzymes (eg, superoxide dismutase, catalase) decreases with age. This finding has led some nutritionists to recommend supplementation of these enzymes.

The glycation theory postulates that glucose reactions with certain proteins and nucleic acids generate glycoadducts called advanced glycosalation end-products (AGEs). Through either cross-linkage or other modifications, molecules are altered reducing certain key physiologic functions. Prevention of AGE formation has been demonstrated to retard the aging process in animals.[3]

The theory of cellular aging is based on a concept of limited capability for cell proliferation. The doubling capacity of some cultured cells is inversely proportional to a donor's age. The system is inherently finite. There is some caution warranted about extrapolating from cultured, in vitro findings to in vivo processes.

EFFECTS OF THE AGING PROCESS

All body systems exhibit effects associated with aging. Although the aging process itself is normal and unavoidable, there are a number of physiologic changes that may have significant clinical consequences necessitating a clinical management strategy. Table 1 provides examples of changes that occur in major body systems and the clinical relevance these changes may have.

MORPHOLOGY OF AGING OF THE CENTRAL NERVOUS SYSTEM

Anatomy and structure

Macroscopic aging of the nervous system includes fibrosis of the meninges (with or without calcifications). The blood vessels may appear to be atherosclerotic with associated shrinkage of the cerebral sulci and enlargement of the gyri, especially in the frontal region. This shrinkage leaves the older person more susceptible to a subdural hematoma from a minor head trauma.

With aging comes a decrease in cerebral blood flow and an associated loss of neurons. Neuron loss occurs primarily in the cerebral and cerebellar cortices, with 45% of neurons lost.[4] In areas where degeneration does not occur, accumulation of lipofuscin, an aging pigment, creates a creamy, yellow tinge. The cerebral ventricles increase in size with the appearance of granulations.[5]

Some neurons in the normal senescent brain will show accumulation of so called neurofibrillary tangles within their cell bodies. They are composed of abnormal cellular protein. When these changes are rampant throughout the cortex, they represent the pathologic license plate for Alzheimer's disease. Other neurons may be lost completely in many brain regions with senile plaques accumulating in the hippocampus and limbic cortex. These plaques appear to be formed by degeneration of neuronal dendrites.[6]

Recently, the relationship of aging to the length of the spinal cord and to the cross-sectional area at the level of C-6 and L-3 were studied. The investigation[7] revealed a significant decrease in the cross-sectional area after the age of 80, particularly at the level of C-6, however, the length of the spinal cord was found to have no correlation with aging. Another study[8] revealed that the gray matter of the lumbar cord in bed-ridden patients also showed a significant decrease in size.

Neurophysiologic changes

General physiologic features of central nervous system aging include the following[9]:

- Depletion of neurotransmitters, including dopamine.
- Reduction in the concentration of enzymes and coenzymes (eg, tyrosine hydroxylase) and catecholamine precursors.
- Alteration in the regulation, formation, and degradation of acetylcholine with resultant loss of dopamine, norepinephrine, and acetylcholine receptors, which will eventually lead to death of the neurons.

CLINICAL PICTURE OF NORMAL AGING AND THE NERVOUS SYSTEM

Sensory

Sensory signs of aging are characterized by impairment of position sense, light touch reception, and pain, more obviously in the toes and feet. These changes account for poor navigation in dimly lit environments and explain why accidents and falls are more common in older persons. Multiple sensory impairment can overcome the normal adaptive ability of the visual, vestibular, and proprioceptive systems to maintain balance.

Hearing often decreases with age. Significant hearing loss occurs in 25% of patients over the age of 65.[9] The most common diagnosis is presbyacusis, a distinct clinical entity presenting as bilateral hearing loss with specific loss of higher

Table 1. Consequences of "normal" aging

Structure	Changes	Clinical consequence
Spine		
Intervertebral disc	Dry, fibrocartilaginous islands of hyaline cartilage, little or no proteoglycans; after age 40 virtually no nucleus pulposus	Disc herniation not likely in the older person
Uncinate processes	Become flat and project bone laterally and posterolaterally	Prevent disc herniation
Dural root sleeves	Become fibrotic and rigid	More prone to stretch injury
Spinal canal	Hypertrophied ligamentum flavum and osteophytes compromise canal space	Cord compression more likely than in younger patients
Zygapophysial joints	Menisci have tendency to proliferate as a fibrous pannus	Joints less mobile
Cardiovascular		
Blood vessels	Some degree of artherosclerosis and thickening, which creates aortic stiffening	Increase in blood pressure
Heart	Ventricular thickening in response to increased peripheral resistance	Decrease in stroke volume
	Decrease in pacemaker cells	
	Decreased response to sympathetic stimulation	Decreased response to pressure changes
Baroceptors	Decreased sensitivity	
Respiratory		
Chest wall	Stiffening	Increases work of breathing
Lungs	Decrease in elastic tissue, destruction of alveolar septa, loss of capillaries, and calcification of bronchi	Reduction in various measures of air flow with an increase in residual volume
Gastrointestinal		
Esophagus	Diminished peristalsis amplitude and decreased lower sphincter tone	Slower transit time to stomach Reflux and hiatal hernia
Stomach	Decrease in acid production and hyposecretion of intrinsic factor	Digestion less effective B_{12} deficiency more common
Small intestine	Absorption functions decreased, particularly calcium	Decrease in vitamins B_{12} and C Decrease in vitamin D
Liver	Slower biotransformation of lipid-soluble drugs Decrease in albumin production	Relative increase in drug bioavailability Serum concentrations of albumin decreased (liver function tests are normal)
Pancreas	Usually unimpaired	
Colon	Transit time is usually normal	Constipation is not necessarily a result of aging unless associated with diabetes or other disorders
Genitourinary		
Kidney	Shrinkage with loss of almost half of the glomeruli	Decreased excretion function (significant with drugs)
Bladder	Bladder capacity and bladder and urethral elasticity are reduced (combined with decrease in central nervous system inhibition)	Nocturia and frank incontinence increase with age
Endocrine		
Female	Ovarian secretion of estrogens and progestins ends	Atrophic changes in uterus, vagina, and mammary glands
Male	Increased prostatic binding of dihydrotestosterone	Prostatic hypertrophy
Blood sugar	Decreased peripheral response to insulin (pancreatic function of insulin secretion is usually normal)	Fasting blood sugar increases 5 mg/dL per decade after age 50 (do not confuse with diabetes)
Thyroid	Thyroid function should not decline with age, however, the thyroid may migrate down toward manubrium	Thyroid function tests are normal Palpate lower for thyroid in older persons

continues

Table 1. (*continued*)

Structure	Changes	Clinical consequence
Musculoskeletal		
Bone	After age 40, bone mass decreases by 5% to 10%/decade (faster in women until seventh decade)	Osteopenia more likely leading to susceptibility to compression fractures of the spine and hip fractures
Muscle	Decrease in muscle mass (increase in fat)	Gradually declining strength; may be more susceptible to injury
Tendons/ligaments	Decreased extensibility	Decrease flexibility; more strain on muscles
Nervous		
Brain	Shrinkage of cerebral sulci and enlargement of gyri with fibrosis of meninges; 20%–25% loss of cerebral and cerebellar neurons; lipofuscin accumulates	More susceptible to subdural hematoma with minor head trauma
Peripheral nerves	Slower transmission; velocity decreases by 10%	Decreased reaction time and adaptive responses

frequencies. There is some degree of presbyacusis in approximately 60% of individuals over the age of 65. The different subcategories reflect possible normal aging processes:

- sensory—degeneration of the hair cells of the organ of Corti,
- neural—degeneration of cochlear neurons,
- strial—atrophy of the stria vascularis, and
- mechanical—stiffness of the basilar membrane.

Beyond the direct effects, there are significant social disabilities and handicaps related to hearing loss including depression, decreased physical activity, and increased social and emotional isolation.

Vision loss is also evident in older persons, with one in six individuals between the ages of 75 and 84 affected, and one in four over the age of 85 affected. Most individuals over the age of 50 develop some degree of opacification of the ocular lens known as cataracts. The degree to which the cataract impairs vision is variable, but it may result in the need for surgery. Although not considered "normal aging" in all older persons, age-related macular degeneration is common. Degeneration of Bruch's membrane (layer between the choriocapillaries and retinal epithelium) cascades into ingrowth of colloidal vessels and subsequent leakage of fluid and blood into the macular area causing loss of central vision. Most age-related changes such as impaired accommodation or corneal abnormalities can be managed with corrective lenses.

Some other examples of cranial nerve deterioration include an absence of the upward conjugate gaze and convergence and deterioration in pupillary constriction in response to light and slow, irregular movements of the eye. Other changes may include absence of Bell's phenomenon (upward deviation of the eyes on closure of the lid), impaired accommodation, and sluggish corneal reflex.

Motor

The slow movement of an older subject might be attributed to the 10% to 15% reduction in conduction velocity of peripheral nerves. This decrease could be due to segmental demyelination with a decrease in the action potential of these nerves. The number of motor units decline with advancing age with selective decreases of type II muscle fibers. These findings led to the concept of denervation atrophy of skeletal muscles as one of the major proposed mechanisms of muscle degeneration in old age.[10] However, it should be emphasized that the extent of age-related changes varies from muscle to muscle and from one person to another. Motor signs of aging may reveal decreased speed of movement and impaired coordination with or without tremors.

Sleep

With advancing age, there is an increase in the number of times the subject wakes during the night and in the proportion of the night spent awake. On average the typical older person sleeps several hours less than someone 20 to 30 years younger. Specifically, there are decreases in the time spent in stages 3 and 4. Subsequent to age 70, stage 4 sleep is nonexistent, with some residual amounts of stage 3 still evident. Proportionally, there is a greater time spent in "light sleep."

Nine out of 10 older persons complain about their sleep patterns. How much is attributable to normal aging and how much is modifiable? Recent studies[11] suggest that melatonin may be a factor. There appears to be a decrease in production of melatonin associated with aging. Lower melatonin levels seem particularly evident in those seniors with sleeping difficulties. Melatonin, which is produced by the pineal gland, is believed to play an important role in regulating the sleep-wake cycle. Studies[11] have shown that even small doses of melatonin taken at night have a significant effect on sleep efficiency.

The mental function changes of a healthy older person are expressed as mild benign forgetfulness and slowing in the speed of thinking. Confusion in stressful situations may become apparent. These changes are due in part to the loss of neurons and a decrease in the amount of certain neurotransmitters.

Neurologic changes may also affect reaction time. Reaction time involves many factors. The individual must perceive that an event has occurred, decide what to do about the event, and carry out the decision. Simple reaction time (responding to one stimulus) involves a decision time and a motor time. The most noticeable change with aging occurs in the decision time component. Reaction times with more complex stimuli (driving a car) take greater time as age increases. Thus, older adults are at a disadvantage in situations demanding rapid response, especially when the decision to be made is complex and difficult.

NORMAL AGING OF THE MUSCULOSKELETAL SYSTEM

Studies[12] have shown that until humans are 60 to 70 years old, age-related changes in muscle function and structure are relatively small. After age 70 these alterations are accelerated considerably. Factors responsible for the aging of skeletal muscles are complex and include intrinsic biochemical changes in muscle metabolism, changes in the distribution and size of muscle fibers, and a general loss of muscle mass. In addition, other factors such as neural control and the influence of exercise, immobility, and nutrition may also contribute to age-related muscle function.[13] Psychologic disorders such as depression may be manifested by a decrease or, at the very least, a sense of decreased motor ability.

It would be wrong to assume that a decrease in muscle mass results in an inability to gain strength with exercise. Studies[2,14] indicate that there is a training effect with exercise that increases strength values for older males. However, while the strength gains in younger populations have to do with muscle hypertrophy in older adults the gains seem to be associated with an increased neural efficiency with increasing recruitment of additional muscle units.

Muscular wasting in older adults is characterized by a decrease in the number and bulk of muscle fibers, particularly in the small muscles of the hands, which become thin and bony with deep interosseous spaces. Thin, flabby arm and leg muscles with a mild degree of weakness are often evident and are usually out of proportion to the degree of muscle wasting. Other findings may include increased muscular rigidity, which can be manifested clinically by increased resistance to passive movement.[15] This finding may be difficult to differentiate from Parkinson's disease.

Older people have less lean body mass, specifically muscle mass, and are thus less able to tolerate trauma.[16] They also recover more slowly when compared with younger patients experiencing similar trauma. Thus it is important to emphasize that manipulation of an older patient should be performed with caution.

There is a proportional increase in fat deposition in the older adult. Other than the obvious health-related issues, it is clinically important because lipophilic drugs have more uptake potential and, in essence, prolonged pharmacologic action.

The posture of an older person is usually flexed with the head and neck held forward and the dorsal spine becoming kyphotic. The upper limbs are bent at the elbows and wrists, and the hips and knees are also slightly flexed. These changes occur as a result of ankylosis of ligaments and joints, shrinkage and sclerosis of tendons and muscles, and degenerative changes in the extrapyramidal nervous system. Sudden onset of a kyphosis is suggestive of a compression fracture. The fracture is often accompanied by significant pain, however, the patient may recall minor or no trauma. In the older adult, a pathologic fracture should also be considered due to the higher incidence of cancer.

The movements of the older person, as mentioned before, are characteristically slow. At times, a resting tremor may be present. This tremor may be attributable to degeneration of the extrapyramidal system. A recent hypothesis[10] suggests that impairment of growth hormone secretion may contribute to the age-related changes of membrane electrical properties of skeletal muscle. This condition may play a role in the impairment of muscle function experienced as a person ages.

Examination of a geriatric patient may reveal decreased deep tendon and abdominal reflexes. There may be difficulty in eliciting the plantar response mainly due to deformities of the feet. These deformities include valgus or equinovalgus deformities of the great toe, stiffness or ankylosis of the first metatarsalphalangeal joint, and hardening of the sole. Other clinical features of aging of the musculoskeletal system may include muscular fasciculations, cramps, rest pain of the legs, and changes in muscle mass.

Fat pad syndrome

Fat pads provide shock absorption for the heels. Age and activity-related thinning of the fat pad results in a condition called fat pad syndrome. It is characterized by heel pain that is central (plantar fasciitis is more medial) and responds to a firm heel counter and heel cups, which act to restrict thinning of the fat pad on weight bearing.

Spontaneous muscular fasciculations

Spontaneous muscular fasciculations are termed myokymia and could be a manifestation of slowly progressive degeneration of anterior horn cells, cranial motor nerves or, less often, nerve roots. Fasciculation occurs commonly at the eyelids, hands, calves, and feet.[17]

Muscle cramps

Muscle cramps are sustained involuntary and painful contractions of muscle, usually occurring in one muscle group of the calf, foot, thigh, hand, or hip following unusual muscular effort and usually at night. Causes of muscle cramps in the older person may include peripheral vascular insufficiency, hyponatremia, uremia, hypocalcemia, and hypoglycemia. Rarely, cramps may be due to toxins such as tetanus bacillus, a black widow spider bite, and anterior horn cell or peripheral nerve disease. Muscle cramps also occur in association with certain muscle disorders including stiff man syndrome, McArdle's syndrome, congenital myotonia, myotonic dystrophy, hypothyroid myopathy, and paroxysmal myoglobinuria.

Resting pain in the legs is usually in the form of paresthesias, which usually occur at rest and are relieved by movement of the leg. The cause is sometimes obscure, but in some cases it can be due to diabetic neuropathy, lumbar osteoarthritis, hypoglycemia, hypocalcemia, or alkalosis.

NORMAL AGING OF THE BONES, JOINTS, AND CONNECTIVE TISSUE

Certain changes in the structure and behavior of cartilage and its components have been found to occur with normal aging. There is a decline in the concentration of dehydrolycinoleucine (a reducible cross-linking compound), with a corresponding increase in a 3-hydroxy pyridinum compound, which forms stable, nonreducible cross-linkages. The bone mineral content and compressive strength of trabecular bone also decrease with aging. Although at age 70 this loss may be gender blind (senile osteoporosis), females must contend with a gender-specific problem of postmenopausal osteoporosis. Starting at age 50, men lose on the average 0.4% bone mass per year, whereas females lose 0.75% to 1% per year starting between the ages of 30 and 35.[18] Bone loss may equal 2% to 3% of total bone mass per year during the first 5 years of menopause. A woman may lose up to 30% of her total bone mass by age 70. This decrease is preferential to trabecular and endosteal bone. The sparing of cortical bone is generally a function of metabolic rate. Trabecular bone has a higher metabolic rate, remodeling approximately 25% each year compared to only 2% to 5% for cortical bone. The increased loss of bone is primarily due to a slowed rate of remodeling that is, in part, hormonally dependent. The female dilemma is complicated by an increased susceptibility to vertebral compression fractures and hip fractures. An additional complicating factor is the decrease in calcium absorption seen in older adults.

The spine

There are some significant changes in the human spine with aging.[19] The nuclei pulposi are virtually nonexistent in the older person. Uncinate processes in the cervical region are flattened, and an osteogenic extension laterally and posterolaterally supports the disc, however, decreases intervertebral foramina space. Other changes include a fibrosis of the dural root sleeves and spinal nerve exit, thickening of the ligamentum flavum, and proliferation of a pannus-like material replacing the facet joint menisci of the younger individual.

Changes in the spine may influence patient presentation. Whereas in a younger population a herniated disc is a possible cause of leg pain, acquired stenosis and tethering of fibrous root sleeves would be more likely in the older patient. Clinically, this condition is demonstrated by a decrease in positive straight-leg raise (nerve tension) tests for leg pain and possible signs of neurogenic claudication.

Temporomandibular joint

At the temporomandibular joint (TMJ) level, several studies[20] revealed that the various components of this joint undergo degenerative alterations with age such as osseous remodeling, erosion, and articular disc perforation. Clinically these changes can be manifested by pain, tenderness, swelling, limited movement, and clicking.

NORMAL AGING OF THE CARDIOVASCULAR SYSTEM

The general cardiovascular performance of older people is determined by inherent changes of the cardiovascular system that develop with age. Delay of degenerative changes in some subjects is probably due to genetic factors, optimal physical activity, and a proper diet. Acquired diseases, particularly arteriosclerosis and hypertension, have a significant accelerating effect.[21] Sclerotic changes occurring in the valves of the heart lead to nodular thickenings that occur along the closure lines of the valves. The mitral and aortic valves are most affected. Aortic valve sclerosis leads to the systolic ejection murmur frequently heard in older patients. Also, both the mitral and aortic valves may develop mucoid degeneration, which can lead to insufficiency murmurs.

The aging pigment lipofuscin is deposited in the myocardium. An age-associated reduction in the number of pacemaker cells with an increase in the number of fibrous tissue and fat, together with the loss of Purkinje fibers (in the bundle of His and in the major right and left branches), may result in different kinds of cardiac dysrhythmias and heart block in older persons.

Clinical features of aging of the cardiovascular system

Heart rate at rest is not markedly affected by age. Variation in sinus rate with respiration, however, diminishes with advancing age. As a result of degenerative changes of the vascular wall, systolic blood pressure rises with advancing age in men and women.

The left ventricular wall thickness and cardiac mass increase with age, while the left ventricular end diastolic dimensions do not change significantly in the healthy older person. The afterload or impedance to ejection is moderately increased at rest. There is also an increase in aortic volume that occurs with age. Prolonged duration of cardiac contraction relative to that in the younger patient is about 15% to 20% longer in the older adult. The ventricular filling rate in the 60- to 80-year age group is about half that observed in the 25- to 44 age group, with age-related alterations in passive and active left ventricular stiffness during early diastole. This change results in greater cardiac compromise in older individuals when confronted with tachycardia or ischemic stress. There is a high prevalence of asymptomatic carotid artery atherosclerosis among the very old. The association between risk factors and carotid atherosclerosis is less pronounced in older patients than in younger subjects.[22]

Age changes in cardiovascular response to exercise in normal humans

With exercise, there are no age-associated decreases in cardiac output, but there are age-associated decreases in heart rate. In the older person, the heart rate during exercise is about 140 beats per minute, which is much less than that of a younger person (about 175 beats per minute) when compared at the same exercise level.[23] There is sufficient increase in myocardial function in the older person due to augmentation of stroke volume above that seen in younger individuals as exercise progresses. A recent study[24] attributed the limitation of exercise ability in older subjects to decreased skeletal muscle function and pulmonary or motivational factors rather than to cardiovascular disorders.

HEMATOLOGIC ALTERATIONS WITH AGE

Hemoglobin concentration in males decreases after the age of 65, probably related to a decrease in androgen production.[25] While it decreases little, if at all, in older females, when it does, it is due mainly to cessation of menstruation, which makes iron deficiency anemia a less frequent occurrence in postmenopausal women. The effect of age on iron absorption and excretion appears to be small. By 75 years of age, maximum oxygen flow will be 50% of that present at 20 years of age owing to an age-related decrease in cardiac and pulmonary functions. As a result there is an increased hazard of hypoxia, which occurs with aging. On the other hand, the blood volume is unchanged in the older person. However, there is a reduced capacity to redistribute blood flow in cases of hypoxia associated with bleeding, anemia, cardiac failure, and some other cardiovascular disease processes.

Aging is associated with increased susceptibility to infections. One of the causes of this liability is the decline in the formation and development of leukocytes. The neutrophils count does not change by age, but there is a limitation in their rate of response to infections and limitations in the rate of their recovery after infections or chemotherapy. Other changes that take place with age can be in the form of eosinophilia due to allergies or occult malignancies. Also basophilia in older individuals could be due to myeloproliferative disorders (eg, polycythemia vera or myeloid leukemia). The T cell function declines as well; therefore, there is an increase in susceptibility to infections for this reason. There is a very significant age-related increase in the frequency of individuals having increased quantities of homogeneous IgG immunoglobulins in their blood. This condition is recognized clinically as idiopathic paraproteinemia.

NORMAL AGING OF THE KIDNEYS

The kidneys are the second most common organ after the lungs to show dramatic changes with aging in normal humans.[25] Aging is characterized by progressive decline after maturity in the glomerular filtration rate and proximal tubular functions. Renal threshold for glycosuria increases with age, thus glucose may appear in the urine of a young patient with diabetes at a lower blood glucose level than in an older patient with diabetes. Reduced function of the aged kidney reduces the individual capacity to respond to a variety of physiologic and pathologic stresses.

Drug excretion by the kidney is markedly altered by age. One of the main factors that must be considered with advancing age is the excessive intake of medications. Older persons are often prescribed medications from various sources. These prescriptions are often not coordinated into a coherent plan, thereby running the risk of drug interactions and complications. Due to decreased excretion, there is an increased possibility of toxicity and relative overdose at levels that are safe for a younger population. Drug adjustment is, in part, based on creatinine clearance.

Adaptive mechanisms responsible for maintaining a constant volume level and composition of the extracellular fluid are impaired in older persons. Thus, with acute illness, geriatric patients with normal renal function may be complicated by derangement in fluid and electrolyte balance thereby delaying recovery and possibly prolonging hospitalization. Also there is a blunted renal response to acute reduction in salt intake in older persons. This finding indicates that older patients are capable of decreasing urinary sodium losses and reaching salt balance with dietary restriction of sodium.

Their response is very slow compared with younger adults. Other changes in the renal function of the older person may include a decline in renin-angiotensin system response by about 30% to 50%. This change will decrease the levels of plasma aldosterone by the same percentage (30% to 50%). Therefore, older people can easily develop dehydration when faced with salt and water deprivation. Older persons, when faced with an acute salt load as a result of inappropriate intravenous fluid, dietary indiscretion, or sodium-rich radiographic contrast agents such as intravenous pyelogram, are at risk of developing sudden expansion of their extracellular fluid volume, which can predispose them to acute heart failure with or without previous myocardial disease. The capacity of older individuals to conserve water and produce a concentrated urine is blunted, when compared with younger adults. Therefore, impaired renal response to antidiuretic hormone occurs with aging.

NORMAL AGING OF THE BLADDER

Bladder capacity and elasticity decrease with age.[25] These changes, combined with a decrease of the normal inhibitory cortical control of the bladder, lead to a decreased ability to control voiding. Thus, incontinence occurs in as many as 20% to 40% of individuals over the age of 65, and nocturia occurs in as many as 60% to 70% of older individuals.[25] Generally, younger patients void daily fluid before 9 PM, whereas older patients void daily fluid after 9 PM.

NORMAL AGING OF THE PULMONARY SYSTEM

As a result of the continuous exposure to environmental pollutants throughout life, the lung is the most likely organ to develop structural and functional deterioration with aging.[25] The older lung has a decrease in base-to-apex length and an increase in anteroposterior diameter. Aging is associated with a reduction in the elastic recoil of lung tissue, which reduces expiratory air flow rates. The alveolar ducts are enlarged, and the alveoli are flattened with advancing age.

The chest cage can become rigid with age, along with a lowered diaphragm and a loss of abdominal tone. The total lung capacity does not change appreciably with normal aging, however, airway narrowing and dynamic compression elevate the residual volume of the lungs. The vital capacity is decreased in older persons due mainly to the increase in the closing and residual volume. The normal level of arterial P_{CO_2} is unchanged with age, while the arterial P_{O_2} does decrease progressively with age, particularly in the supine position.

NORMAL AGING OF THE GASTROINTESTINAL TRACT

Due to a decreased peristaltic response of the esophagus, dysphasia and food regurgitation are very common in older persons.[25] The lower esophageal sphincter often becomes incompetent, leading to reflux esophagitis and a corkscrew esophagus (presbyesophagus). It occurs from prolonged contraction of ring-like segments of the distal two thirds of the esophagus. The stomach shows decreased motility and secretion of acid and pepsin leading to impairment of absorption of vitamins B_{12} and D. Atrophy and fibrosis of the small intestine lead to a broader, shorter intestine, which can lead to subclinical degrees of malabsorption.

The weight and size of the liver decrease with a concomitant decline in its capacity to metabolize various medications. With advancing age, there is a decreased number of hepatic cells and mitochondria. Their activity and volume are increased, although their regeneration is weak with rapid exhaustion.[26] While there are no liver diseases specific to advanced age, the presentation, clinical course, and management of liver diseases in older persons may differ in important respects from younger individuals. For example, alcoholic liver disease presents at a more advanced stage. Drug-induced liver disease and viral hepatitis may also be more severe. A recent study[27] described an age-related decrease in total bile flow with similar reductions in 14 C erythritol clearance, suggesting a decreased canalicular bile flow with aging.

CONCLUSION

It is apparent that normal aging processes may result in different responses to the demands of infection, drug therapy, and other external factors. These normal processes may also manifest as an adjusted norm with standard examination procedures. With the knowledge of normal processes, examiners may better focus their examination to common decreases or variations of function in the older adult. Management concerns are governed by the knowledge of these variations and are heightened when these variations are not evident or are excessive. It is important to instill in the older person the concept of adaptive functioning. Often, through intellectual compensation the older person with dysfunction may still be productive. It is also important to point to hope as an essential need in older persons for adaptation to their illness and to transcend the limitations of aging. Hope generates energy that enables individuals to cope with numerous problems and losses, overcome obstacles, and continue functioning.[28]

REFERENCES

1. Shephard RJ. Physical training for the elderly. *Clin Sports Med.* 1986;5:515–533.
2. Andres R, Bierman EL, Hazard WR. *Principles of Geriatric Medicine.* New York, NY: McGraw-Hill; 1985.
3. Lee AT, Cerami A. Role of glycation in aging. *Ann NY Acad Sci.* 1992;21:63–70.
4. Finch CE, Hayflick L, eds. *Handbook of the Biology of Aging.* New York, NY: Van Nostrand Reinhold; 1985.
5. Timiris PS, ed. *Physiological Basis of Geriatrics.* New York, NY: Macmillan; 1988.
6. Jucker M, Walker LC, Schwarb P, Hengemihle J, Kuo H, Snow AD. Age-related deposition of glia fibrillar material in brains of 57BL/16 mice. *J Neurosci.* 1994;60:875–889.
7. Sasaki A, Mizutan T, Takasaki M, et al. Morphometric study of age-related changes of the spinal cord. *Nippon Ronen Igakkai Zasshi.* 1994;31:462–467.
8. Harris GJ, Schlaepfer J, Peng LW, Lee S, Federman FB, Pearlson GD. Magnetic resonance imaging evaluation of the effects of aging on grey-white ratio in the human brain. *Neuropathol Appl Neurobiol.* 1994;20:290–293.
9. Reichel W. *Clinical Aspects of Aging.* Baltimore, Md: Williams & Wilkins; 1989.
10. Grimby G, Saltin B. The aging muscle. *Clin Physiol.* 1983;3:209–218.
11. Garfinkel D, Laudon M, Nof D, Zisapel N. Improvements of sleep quality in elderly people by controlled release melatonin. *Lancet.* 1995;346:541–544.
12. Carmeli E, Reznick AZ. The physiology and biochemistry of skeletal muscle atrophy as function of age. *Poc-Soc Exp Biol Med.* 1994;20:103–113.
13. Lewis CB. *Aging: The Health Care Challenge.* Philadelphia, Pa: F.A. Davis; 1990.
14. Annianson A, Gustafaaon W. Physical training in elderly men with special reference to quadriceps muscle strength and morphology. *Clin Physiol.* 1981;1:87–98.
15. Calkins E, Davis PJ, Ford AB. *The Practice of Geriatrics.* Philadelphia, Pa.: W.B. Saunders; 1986.
16. Villareal DT, Morley JE. Trophic factors in aging. *Drug Aging.* 1994;41:492–509.
17. Hodkinson HM. *An Outline of Geriatrics.* New York, NY: Grune & Stratton; 1981.
18. Smith EL. Exercise for prevention of osteoporosis. A review. *Phys Sportsmed.* 1982;10:72–83.
19. Bland JH. Cervical and thoracic pain. *Curr Opin Rheumatol.* 1991;3:218–225.
20. Reider CE, Martinoff JT. The prevalence of mandibular dysfunction: part II. Multiphasic dysfunction profile. *J Prosthet Dent.* 1983;50:237–44.
21. Hradec J, Petrasek J. Old age from the view point of cardiologist. *J Cas Lek Cesk.* 1994;133:397–400.
22. Fabri SF, Zanocchi M, Bo M, Fonte G, Poli L, Bergoglio I. Carotid plaque, aging and risk factors. *Stroke.* 1994;25:1133–1140.
23. Poulin ML, Cunningham DA, Paterson DH, Rechnitzer PA, Eclestone NA, Koval JJ. Ventilatory response to exercise in men and women 55 to 86 years of age. *MJ Crit Care Med.* 1994;149(2 pt 1):408–415.
24. Stanford BA. Exercise and the elderly. *Exerc Sport Sc Rev.* 1988;16:341–376.
25. Arking R. Biology of aging: observations and principles. Englewood Cliffs, NJ: Prentice Hall; 1991.
26. Kroll J. The mitochondrial ATPase and the aging process. *Med Hypotheses.* 1994;42:395–396.
27. Mahon NM, James OF. Liver diseases in the elderly. *J Clin Gastroenterol.* 1994;18:330–334.
28. Forbes SB. Hope, an essential need in the elderly. *J Gerontol Nurs.* 1994;20:5–10.

16

Clinical Assessment of Geriatric Patients: Unique Challenges

Linda J. Bowers

The aging of America assures that every physician involved in primary care will become increasingly involved in geriatric health care. Between 1989 and the year 2030, the number of individuals over age 65 is projected to double, with the number of women over age 65 continuing to increase to a greater degree.[1] At age 65, the average man will live an additional 14.5 years and the average woman an additional 18.6 years.[2] An estimated 9.5 million noninstitutionalized individuals presently experience difficulty in performing basic life activities such as walking, self-care, and home management activities.[3]

Comprehensive geriatric assessment (CGA) provides the physician with an individualized care plan for at-risk older patients with complex health problems. It should be considered whenever there is any evidence of decline in physical or mental function or any question of the patient's ability to live alone.[4] The data collected can then be used to generate a current medical and functional problem list followed by development of a management plan tailored for the individual patient. The basic components of CGA are a history and physical examination, as well as an evaluation of mental, functional, and social/economic health,[5-8] nutritional status,[9-14] and pertinent risks.[4] Notably, the US Preventive Services Task Force (USPSTF) recommends an annual office visit for patients age 65 and older to review screening needs, conduct counseling, deliver health education, promote healthy lifestyles, identify immunization needs, and discuss the use of chemoprophylactic agents (eg, estrogen replacement therapy).[2]

INTRODUCTION

Traditionally, geriatric assessment has been performed when a patient becomes sick enough to be admitted to a hospital where a team of professionals work over a long period of time to determine an appropriate care plan for the patient. Although ideally this assessment is performed by a team of professionals from a variety of disciplines, the primary care physician may perform a limited version in the office and then make appropriate referrals for further evaluation as necessary. A computer-assisted comprehensive geriatric assessment has been developed with a goal of a preventive approach to health care.[6]

Geriatric patients usually require extra time and diligence to assess and track their health problems. An older patient often tires during a protracted session; thus, the initial evaluation may need to be divided into two or more sessions.[15] A comprehensive geriatric assessment, organized on a one-page, easily updated checklist can be used to generate a medical as well as a functional problem list and risk assessment.[4] Unlike the routine patient evaluation, geriatric assessment stresses functional status and quality of life, attempting to identify any reversible illness or disability.[5] The purpose of the assessment is to keep the patient healthy and living independently as long as possible.[8] It includes diagnosing illness early to prevent disability, detecting disability when it does occur, arranging necessary support systems, and monitoring and upgrading those supports as needed. To meet the challenge of performing a comprehensive geriatric assessment, the clinician must prioritize, persist, employ patience, and practice. Assessment of a geriatric patient is provided in Algorithm 1.

Adapted from *Top Clin Chiro* 1996; 3(2): 10–22
© 1996 Aspen Publishers, Inc.

HEALTH HISTORY

General considerations

A full history remains the primary investigative tool. Although the health history in the average adult may approach a diagnostic yield of 90%, its utility in geriatric patients is often much lower.[16] Older patients tend to underreport illness, present with disease in an atypical fashion, have lengthy medical histories, and may suffer from conditions that decrease effective communication such as aphasia, dementia, or sensory loss. An older patient's health history will often need to be augmented by a caregiver (spouse, family member, home health aide), especially for cognitive and functional assessments.[4] The clinician should be aware that there is a tendency for the spouse to underestimate cognitive loss.[15]

The format for the health history is similar in the geriatric patient but certain caveats hold true. For example, older patients often have several illnesses that may interact as well as present atypically. In fact, disease in older patients can often present as a functional decline rather than as a chief complaint or constellation of signs and symptoms indicative of a certain condition. They may suddenly stop eating or drinking, become incontinent or confused, or lose weight. The physician should ascertain the general reason for the visit (eg, check-up, wellness care, health complaint, or the need for advice) and not focus entirely on the chief complaint. In older patients, disease symptoms are frequently nonspecific, and thus symptom complexes often overlap.[1] For reasons not clearly understood, pain due to illness or trauma that would be expected in a younger individual is often minimal or absent in the older person.[7] For example, a myocardial infarction is commonly pain-free, and the patient may present with shortness of breath or a nonspecific illness rather than chest pain. Studies[7] in general practice show that an older patient has, on average, at least three disabilities, and, for every one known to the primary care practitioner, there is another that is not. Typically, incontinence, difficulty in walking, painful feet, dementia, and depression often go unreported.

The tempo at which symptoms develop is particularly important. Forgetfulness that has been gradually increasing over 2 or 3 years suggests senile dementia of the Alzheimer's type (SDAT), whereas a sudden onset of confusion over a day or two indicates a toxic confusional state (delirium). The latter requires a search for underlying physical problems such as an infection or myocardial infarct.[7] A sudden onset of headaches or a recent change in bowel or bladder habit is never normal in old age. However, gradually failing hearing and vision may be normal and might be remedied by a hearing aid or new eyeglasses.

If older patients are not able to give the health history themselves, an alternate source must be found (relative, neighbor, social worker, spouse). However, a study[17] comparing the effects of the presence of a third person during interviews between a physician and an older patient concluded that a third person changes the interactional dynamics between physician and older patient and may influence the development of a trusting and effective physician–older patient relationship. Previous health records are important sources of information and should usually be obtained.

In addition to the chief complaint and history of present illness, the history should review *significant* surgeries, illnesses, and accidents. Asking an older patient to list every childhood illness and malady is usually a waste of time. Rather, the practitioner should ask questions regarding major illnesses or injuries that caused the patient to lose a lot of time from school or work and common chronic diseases such as tuberculosis, diabetes mellitus, rheumatic fever, or atherosclerotic vascular disease. The doctor should document important life events and work experiences and have the patient describe a typical day to reveal problem areas. The doctor should also document use of community resources by the patient and caregivers.

While the family history remains relevant with aging, the emphasis changes. Diseases such as Alzheimer's disease, Huntington's chorea, and breast and bowel cancer have a hereditary component.[4] Although a family history of dementia or senility is useful to know in a patient with dementia, a detailed family history to review genetically based disease is of little relevance in the geriatric patient.[16] However, the physician should determine the presence of social supports, especially in high-risk groups such as persons over age 85, those living alone or living with a chronically ill spouse, those recently bereaved, and those with dementia.

In addition to the usual laundry list of symptoms asked in the review of systems (ROS), the physician should focus on problems that interfere with function such as confusion, memory loss, falls, incontinence, immobility, insomnia, dysphagia, and sensory loss. Vague symptoms of apathy, anorexia, fatigue, self-neglect, and weight loss are often associated with depression though they can also represent manifestations of organic disease as well. Depression is very common in older patients and asking a screening ROS question such as "Do you often feel sad or depressed?" is useful.

Falls

Falls are the leading cause of death due to injury in older persons.[1] There is a dramatic increase in falls after age 85.[1] One third of adults over age 65 report one or more falls annually, and the risk of serious injury increases substantially with age.[18] Twenty percent to 40% of adults aged 70 and above who are community dwelling fall each year[1] causing an inordinate amount of pain, immobility, loss of self-confidence, isolation, health care costs, and premature nursing home placement. On average, women fall twice as often as men.[1]

The changes in posture and gait that come with advancing age tend to follow an essentially extrapyramidal pattern resulting in a stance of general flexion with increased muscle tone, poverty of movement, and bradykinesia. With increasing age the first change in balance detected in normal persons is increased sway; there is also a change in gait resulting in a shorter step length and slower walking.[7] An important contribution to postural control of balance is provided by the activity of mechanoreceptors in the apophysial joints of the cervical spine. They exert a reflex influence on the activity of neck and limb muscles, and damage to this mechanism—typically from cervical spondylosis—can cause a feeling of unsteadiness during movements, often worse on turning the head.[7] Cervical spondylosis probably only becomes important if there are also visual problems or vestibular defects.[7]

The first step in the examination of the patient with falls is a good history, because it allows the differentiation between a straightforward trip or accident and a spontaneous fall.[7] The acronym SPLAT (symptoms associated with the fall, prior falls, location of the falls, activity at the time of the fall, and time of day falls occur) provides further diagnostic information as to the possible cause of falls.[16] The Get-up and Go test (GUGT)[1] is a useful test for general mobility and a semiquantitative approach to identification of individuals at risk for balance and mobility problems. The patient is observed and timed while he or she rises from an arm chair, walks 3 meters, turns, walks back, and sits down again. Table 1 indicates potentially correctable risk factors for falling.

Incontinence

Office evaluation of urinary incontinence includes a thorough history as well as a patient voiding record.[19] The voiding record is a simple hourly record kept for a week that includes each normal void without incontinence and each occurrence of urine leakage. Physical examination procedures of a digital rectal examination as well as a pelvic examination in women should follow. Patients (and their families) need to be educated that incontinence is not a normal, natural consequence of aging, that there is nothing to be ashamed about, and that much can be done to lessen the condition.[1] For urinary incontinence, it is important to inquire about the volume of urine loss as well as the frequency because volume predicts the social consequences better than frequency.[1]

Lifestyle factors

The physician should ask about recommended health promotion and disease prevention measures and assess the patient's current health status. Tables 2 and 3 present a checklist that can be used to determine immunization status and screening tests recommended for older patients. Such information may assist in determining the cause(s) of the patient presentation. For example, if a patient presents with a fever and cough, it is useful to know if he or she has had an annual influenza shot or received the pneumococcal vaccine.

As with any patient, counseling regarding lifestyle matters is important. Lifestyle choices affect both health and independence. A recent survey demonstrated that the lifestyles of many older adults places them at risk for injury or disease: 16% smoke, 12% drink 10 to 12 alcoholic beverages every 2 weeks, 71% are sedentary, 20% are overweight, 41% sleep less than 7 to 8 hours per night, 50% do not use seat belts regularly, and 11% complain of stress affecting their health.[2] Fries'[20] compression of morbidity theory suggests that preventive interventions might allow better management of old age by delaying the onset of these morbid conditions to a "compressed" time period at the end of an otherwise set life span.

Older persons differ from younger in their susceptibility to the adverse effects of deconditioning, which appear earlier, are more severe, and take longer to reverse.[18] The reported health benefits of an active lifestyle that incorporates regular aerobic exercise include reduced risk of coronary artery disease and hypertensive cardiovascular disease, reduction in the decline of maximum aerobic capacity, increased muscle strength and efficiency, reduced diastolic blood pressure, increased bone mineral density, improved joint flexibility, reduced body fat, improved mental health, and a modest in-

Table 1. Risk factors for falling

Difficulty with balance, gait, and transfers
Foot problems
Lack of outdoor activity
Living alone
Muscular weakness
Polypharmacy
Postural hypotension (systolic blood pressure <110 mm Hg)
Use of sedatives

Table 2. Immunizations

	Date
Pneumococcal vaccine	_____
Influenza vaccine	_____
Tetanus booster vaccine	_____

Table 3. Screening tests

	Date/result
Blood pressure reading	_____
Breast examination	_____
Cholesterol test	_____
Dental examination	_____
Eye examination	_____
Flexible sigmoidoscopy	_____
Glaucoma check	_____
Hearing test	_____
Mammogram	_____
Pap smear/pelvic examination	_____
Rectal/prostate examination	_____
Stool guaiac test	_____

crease in longevity.[18] Regular exercise improves flexibility, strength, cardiovascular fitness, and glucose tolerance, even in the frail older person.[5] The American Heart Association and the American College of Sports Medicine have formulated lists of problems that represent contraindications to exercise programs.[18]

Older patients who smoke should be encouraged to quit, as they have a 52% higher risk of coronary heart disease and death than nonsmokers. This risk declines rapidly after smoking cessation, resulting in a life expectancy increase of 2 to 4 years.[4] The USPSTF recommends that Pap smears be done every 1 to 3 years for women without previous documented screening in which smears have been consistently negative.[2] Approximately 45% of new breast cancers are detected after age 65.[2] Annual clinical breast examination and mammography every year after age 50 until age 75 is recommended.[2] After age 75 annual mammography screening may be discontinued, unless pathology is detected.[21]

Many older patients are taking numerous medications, making the medication history of paramount importance. The clinician should be sure to include questions regarding the use of vitamins and mineral supplements, laxatives, minor pain medications, nonprescription sleep aids, cold and flu remedies as well as prescription medications.[15] Factors to consider are the total number of medications, potential interactions among drugs, whether each medication is needed at all, whether a more benign drug would do as well, and the proper dosage of each medication. The prevalence of adverse drug effects increases markedly above five daily medications.[1] It is useful to ask the patient to bring along a bag containing every medicine and health product in use.[8]

Older persons are more sensitive to the effects of alcohol,[1,4] and alcohol abuse is higher among older individuals than previously suspected.[8] The suggested prevalence ranges from 6% to 53%.[22] One out of three chronic alcoholics develops the problem after the age of 60.[23] Alcoholism is underrecognized among older individuals.[15] Alcohol-related problems can occur in older adults even without a change in lifelong drinking habits. Alcohol abuse can contribute to insomnia, anxiety, falls, and a decline in cognitive functions. Useful questionnaires such as the CAGE, HALT, FATAL DT, or BUMP may help to determine any problems or concerns with alcohol.[24] According to the USPSTF, physicians should routinely ask all adults to describe their use of alcohol.[2] Table 4 describes techniques that may facilitate history taking in an older patient.

PHYSICAL EXAMINATION

Because of the multiplicity of disorders often found in an older patient, it might appear that an extensive and detailed examination of every system is required. Such an approach may exhaust a frail patient, and the results of a prolonged neurologic examination is likely to frustrate and confuse the doctor.[7] However, with practice, the examination can be thorough, informative, and relatively quick if the clinician focuses on screening for and identifying disabilities and assessing loss of function. When examining a geriatric patient, the clinician should strive to avoid patient discomfort, maintain patient dignity, and distinguish signs of disease from changes that occur with normal aging.[21] Table 5 describes a comfortable and safe environment for examining older patients. For diagnostic utility, aspects of the standard physical examination are modified for older patients. Special attention is paid to problems that interfere with function such as gait disorders, incontinence, and hearing and visual loss.[21]

Vital signs

Serial measurements of height and weight should be obtained and recorded. Stable weight may reflect not only caloric balance but also the opposing effects of malnutrition

Table 4. Techniques for geriatric interviewing

Schedule more than one visit for the initial patient history.
Schedule midmorning or early afternoon times.
Send a preprinted history form prior to visit and/or previous records.
Ask patient to bring in all current medications including over-the-counter medications and vitamin and mineral preparations.
Maximize office set-up for geriatric patients (adequate lighting, large printing, decreased ambient noise level).
For patients with hearing deficits, have them speak into a stethoscope.
Speak slowly and clearly while facing the patient.
The patient should wear dentures, eyeglasses, and hearing aids to facilitate both verbal and nonverbal communication.

Table 5. Examination techniques to maximize patient comfort and safety

Keep the room quiet and at a comfortable temperature (about 75°) to avoid chilling a disrobed older patient.
Use chairs that have arm rests and that are of adequate height to allow for easy rising.
Place a pillow under the patient's head.
Make sure examining gowns are short enough to prevent tripping and have easy closures to facilitate ease of dressing.
Plan the examination to avoid excessive position changes (eg, standing, seated, prone, supine).
Assist the patient on and off the examining table.
Keep the room clear of rugs and other items that could trip a patient.
Use a wide sturdy footstool to facilitate transfers.
Never leave an older patient alone, because a fall from the examining table could be devastating.
Allow the patient extra time to disrobe and gown and get on the table.

(weight loss) and fluid retention (weight gain). Loss of height is a late sign of osteopenia.[15] Thermoregulatory responses are impaired as one ages due to disordered autonomic function.[7] Baseline measurements of temperature improve the recognition of fever. Important temperature elevations may include any rise of 1.33°C (2.4°F) over baseline.[15] If the oral temperature is less than 98°F, it should be rechecked with a low-reading rectal thermometer to rule out hypothermia.[21]

Because blood pressure fluctuates considerably, multiple measurements under resting conditions are required to diagnose hypertension. Because postural hypotension is common in older patients, their blood pressure and pulse should be measured both while they are seated and standing. A rise of less than 10 beats per minute with a drop in blood pressure suggests a baroreceptor reflex impairment.[21] A rise in pulse rate of greater than 16 beats per minute upon standing upright indicates orthostatic tachycardia.[15] Orthostatic hypotension consists of a drop in systolic blood pressure of at least 15 mm Hg, or a fall in diastolic blood pressure of at least 10 mm Hg, on being seated after a supine measurement, or on standing after a seated measurement.[15] Postural hypotension with an unchanging pulse rate indicates autonomic dysfunction. A seated blood pressure greater than 160/90 mm Hg in an older patient is considered elevated.[7] Performing Osler's maneuver may distinguish hypertension from pseudohypertension due to nonelastic, stiff atherosclerotic arteries.[1,15,21] Osler's maneuver is performed by feeling the pulse, then occluding the artery proximal to the pulse with a blood pressure cuff or finger. If the distal artery can still be felt unchanged, even after the pulse is obliterated, the patient has sufficient arteriosclerosis to produce some degree of pseudohypertension.

The normal respiratory rate in the aged is 12 to 20 breaths per minute.[15] A rate above 22 breaths per minute suggests the possibility of a lower respiratory tract infection, even prior to the appearance of other clinical signs and before the emergence of a previously undifferentiated respiratory problem.[15]

Vision and hearing tests

Visual and auditory disabilities are common in older persons and can seriously interfere with independent daily function.[19] Almost 8% of older Americans are severely visually impaired so it is imperative that clinicians check visual acuity using a Snellen eye chart or a hand-held Jaeger chart.[19,21] A newer instrument, the Activities of Daily Vision Scale, has been devised to evaluate visual function.[8] Visual impairment can cause problems for older patients, including isolation and increased risk for frequent falls.[1] Arcus senilis is not of pathologic significance. The USPSTF does not recommend routine performance of tonometry by primary care physicians as a screening test for glaucoma but advises periodic referral to an ophthalmologist for glaucoma testing.[21]

Impaired hearing increases with age and can contribute to poor health, social isolation, depression, and paranoid psychosis.[7] About 30% of older individuals regard themselves as having a hearing impairment but audiometric testing reveals a 60% prevalence in persons over 70 years of age.[7] Considering the prevalence of hearing loss in the geriatric population and its effect on psychosocial function, routine use of hearing examinations in the office is recommended.[19] Valid, reliable screening may be performed with a hand-held audioscope[19,21] although a hearing evaluation using whisper tests in a quiet room has been shown to approximate the results of a full audiometric examination.[1] Weber and Rhinne tests also may be performed to localize bone and air conduction hearing loss. Examination of the eardrums for wax should be routine. Important components of the geriatric physical examination may be found in Table 6.

MENTAL HEALTH STATUS ASSESSMENT

Cognitive impairment is a failure of the brain to function properly.[25] Dementia, depression, and delirium are the most common mental health problems for older patients.[5,26] About 5% of noninstitutionalized Americans older than 65 and approximately 20% of those older than 75 have some degree of clinically detectable impairment of cognitive function.[25] The Canadian Task Force on the Periodic Health Examination reported in 1979 that there was fair evidence to support the inclusion of screening for manifestations of progressive mental

Table 6. Important aspects of the physical examinaton of older patients

Area	Pathology screen	Examination
Eyes	Acuity (far/near vision)	Snellen eye chart, normal print
	Macular degeneration	Grid matrix
		Peripheral fields by confrontation
	Cataracts	Lens opacification
	Glaucoma	Funduscopic (increased cupping)
Head	Temporal arteritis	Palpate temporal arteries for tenderness, nodularity, and pulsations, scalp tenderness and nodules
Ears	Hearing	Hand-held audioscope
		Free-field voice testing at 0.6 m (eg, "What is your first name?" is a simple question even for the individual with cognitive impairments)
		Weber, Rhinne tests
		Hearing Handicap Inventory for the Elderly
Mouth	Gingivitis	Inspect for erythematous, edematous gingiva, bleeding gums, loose teeth, exposure of the root surfaces of the teeth
	Dentures	Check fit, food debris, bacterial plaque
	Oral cancers	Inspect for persistent erythroplasia
Neck	Decreased mobility	Range of motion, observe dizziness
	Thyroid disease	Palpate thyroid for nodules or enlargement
	Jugular venous pulse	Check on right side of neck
	Carotid artery stenosis	Bruits
Thorax	Chronic obstructure pulmonary disease	Chest expansion
	Lung disease	Auscultation
Cardiovascular	Orthostatic hypotension	Measure blood pressure supine and upright (a drop of 20 mm Hg or more systolic and 10 mm Hg or more diastolic)
Breasts	Breast cancer	Annual clinical breast examination
Back	Vertebral compression fracture	Spinous percussion
	Osteoporosis	Kyphosis
Abdomen	Osteoporosis	Skin bunched into folds from collapse of multiple vertebra
	Urinary retention	Percussion of suprapubic area
	Aortic aneurysm	Lateral or anteroposterior pulsatile mass, bruit
	Constipation	Palpable mass
Prostate	Cancer	Palpable, hard nodule
	Benign prostatic hypertrophy	Enlarged, smooth, soft prostate
Gynecologic	Stress incontinence	Pad test (have patient cover urethral area with a small pad and cough forcefully three times in the standing position to check for leakage of urine)

continues

Table 6. (continued)

Area	Pathology screen	Examination
Extremities	Decreased mobility	Range of motion
	Arterial insufficiency	Peripheral pulses, temperature, ulcers
	Diabetic foot	Ulcers, fungal infections
	Falls	Check for proper footwear
Skin	Hydration status	Check skin turgor
	Senile purpura	Dorsum of hand and forearm
	Actinic keratosis	Sun-exposed areas of skin
	Physical abuse	Unexplained bruising
	Melanoma	Lesion larger than 6 mm across, deep black areas, irregular borders and shape
Neurologic	Balance	Push gently with eyes open, then closed
	Range of motion	Seated: Place hands behind head and back, touch toes (if normal, has adequate range of motion to allow normal grooming and dressing)
	Gait and mobility	Ask patient to sit and then rise from armless chair, ask patient to walk across room, turn 180°, and return to chair
	Gait	Normal older female: Waddling, narrow-based, decreased arm swing
		Normal older male: Wider-based, smaller-stepped, decreased arm swing
	Parkinsonism	Short steps, shuffling feet, stooped trunk, decreased arm swing, festination, tendency to fall backward
	Pernicious anemia	Sensory ataxic gait (wide based)
	Motor tone	Check for spasticity, lead pipe stiffness, paratonia
	Tremor	Check for Parkinson's disease, cerebellar dysfunction, hyperthyroidism, or essential tremor
	Vibratory sense	Normal decrease (especially in lower extremities)
	Primitive reflexes	Normal release (snout, glabella, palmomental)

health status incapacity in the periodic health examination of older people.[27]

The onset of symptoms and the rate of progression are particularly important. An insidious onset of cognitive decline in the absence of early motor signs and progression to severe dementia suggest SDAT whereas stepwise, irregular, decrements in cognitive functions favor a diagnosis of multi-infarct dementia. The sudden onset of cognitive impairment should prompt a search for delirium. Reversible causes of cognitive impairment account for a significant percentage of patients who present with dementia and, therefore, diagnosis is important.

The evaluation of cognitive status focuses primarily on the clinical syndromes of delirium and dementia and the more benign age-associated memory impairment. Age-associated memory impairment is defined as a patient at least 50 years old, with a subjective sense of memory changes, and performing at least one standard deviation below the mean on standardized memory tests.[26] There are data to show that age-associated memory loss may be indicative of dementia in 15 to 20 years.[26]

Dementia is characterized by deterioration of intellectual functions of sufficient severity to interfere with the individual's ability to cope with daily life.[28] This disorder affects 5% to 10% of persons over age 65 and at least 20% of those over age 80.[25] The most common diseases causing dementia are SDAT (50% to 60%) and stroke (10% to 20%).[25,28] Alzheimer's disease is a clinical diagnosis based on the typical presentation and supported by excluding other disorders[23] approximating a diagnostic accuracy of 80% to 90%.[25] As originally described by the German neurologist Alois Alzheimer, SDAT is progressive and is characterized by prominent aphasia, amnesia, and cognitive impairment, but relatively intact motor functions until the final stages.[29] Definitive diagnosis can be made only at autopsy or by brain biopsy. Because neither of these are practical to obtain, the National Institute of Neurological and Communicative Disorders and Stroke and the Alzheimer's Disease and Related Diseases Association have developed criteria for diagnosing probable SDAT.[29]

Mental status can be difficult to assess, and the patient may try to hide deficits. The Mini-Mental State Exam (MMSE),[1,8,19,29,30] the Short Portable Mental Status Questionnaire (SPMSQ),[19] the Blessed Dementia Rating Scale, and the Short Blessed[1] are often used to screen for cognitive impairment. Of these, the SPMSQ and the MMSE fulfill acceptable methodologic criteria and are practical to use.[27] The MMSE checks memory, reading, writing, naming, calculations, and spatial relationships. As a screening tool, it is an excellent validated instrument; however, it tests for very specific areas of cognition (eg, orientation, recall, and praxis), but it does not test for abstract thinking and judgment. It is more sensitive in measuring left hemispheric damage than right.[18] It is insensitive to mild cognitive impairment (a "ceiling" effect), so that patients in the very early stages of dementia may obtain scores in the normal range. It is also somewhat insensitive to severe cognitive impairment (a "floor" effect). The MMSE may be the most valuable test in monitoring disease progression over time, because it is well validated, can be administered in a short period of time, and yields a readily calculated score ranging from 0 to 30.[19,28] A value that distinguishes between normal and pathologic is 17 or less for those with 8 or fewer years of education, and a score of 23 or less for those with 9 or more years of education.[1] An example of a more sensitive cognitive instrument is the Wechsler Memory Scale, an age-normed instrument that allows comparisons of a patient's score to that of others who are his or her age.[5]

Clock drawing can be a useful assessment procedure for spatial abilities.[28] The Draw-a-Clock test is used for rapid assessment of nonverbal cognitive function. It consists of handing the patient a paper with a circle on it, and giving the following directions, "First, draw a clock with all the numbers on it. Second, put hands on the clock to make it read 11:15." Scoring criteria and interpretation are published elsewhere.[15]

Three specific serologic tests considered part of the standard dementia evaluation are thyroid function studies, serum vitamin B12 levels, and tests for syphilis.[19] Supplemental information can be obtained by a few additional tests that are listed in Table 7.

Delirium is an acute, reversible brain dysfunction associated with almost any physical ailment[15]; it is especially common in older persons, occurring in 35% or more of hospitalized patients.[25] Its detection carries enormous prognostic and therapeutic implications. Delirium evaluation encompasses more than the mental status examination, but begins with this assessment. Currently, although delirium is common, more often than not it is either overlooked or misdiagnosed. The assessment of delirium is a relatively new area of research, and the best screening approach has not yet been clarified. Some leading choices are the Global Accessibility Rating, the Delirium Rating Scale, the Confusion Assessment Method, and the Brief Psychiatric Rating Scale.[1] Probably the most important diagnostic tool for delirium is a high index of suspicion in the proper setting. Even after removal of the inciting cause, delirium can take 3 weeks or longer to clear.[1]

Table 7. Mental status assessment supplemental tests

Deficit tested	Method of testing
Spatial relationship defects	Drawing a clock face
Abstract reasoning	Proverbs and word similarities
Language fluency and information categorization	Word generation (eg, "In 60 seconds how many things can you name that one can buy at a grocery store?")
Judgment	Problem-solving questions (eg, "What would you do if the smoke detector alarm sounded?")

Older persons actually suffer less affective illness than do younger patients although this finding may be due to the atypical presentation of depression in older persons.[1] However, depression is dangerous for older individuals, and thus early recognition is crucial. Studies[1] indicate that older women experience depressive symptoms more frequently than men. The two best assessment scales are the self-reported Beck Depression Inventory and the Geriatric Depression Scale (GDS), both of which identify nearly 90% of patients with depression[1] and can easily be performed by trained office personnel.[19] The GDS provides an efficient way to discover low mood; it is filled out by the patient and takes 10 to 15 minutes. The short (15 item) version (GDS15) has been recommended by the Royal College of General Practitioners as the depression screening instrument of choice.[31] The Beck Depression Inventory, which is filled out by a patient in 5 to 10 minutes, is reliable and valid for screening purposes.[8] The DSM-III-R contains criteria for diagnosing dementia, delirium, and depression.[25] Jarvik and Wiseman[32] recommend the use of the mnemonic FICS'M (**f**amily, **i**ntellectual status, **c**ontinence, **s**leep, and **m**obility) to address treatable problems associated with dementing illnesses. A mental assessment protocol is provided in Algorithm 2.

FUNCTIONAL ASSESSMENT

The chronologic age of an older patient may bear little relation to his or her functional age.[7] When assessing an older patient it is generally more useful to think in terms of functional ability than to place emphasis on the underlying pathology. The pathologic conditions producing ill health in older individuals are largely irreversible, whereas some degree of functional improvement is nearly always possible.[7] Functional assessment is the cornerstone of a geriatric assessment and a crucial component of the health history of older patients. Changes in functional status are usually significant.[4] To a geriatric patient, improving function is probably a more important result than any that can be achieved by medical or chiropractic intervention. Functional assessment may be determined via either a questionnaire or a health professional's observation.

The clinician should be aware that patients sometimes falsely report that they can perform an activity because they fear the repercussions or simply cannot remember. A combination of asking the patient, asking the family, and observing the patient may improve the assessment. Traditionally, in gerontologic research two types of functions are usually addressed: instrumental activities of daily living (IADL) and activities of daily living (ADL).[5,16] The focus of a functional assessment is the ability to perform self-care. The questionnaires are usually based on self-assessment in the form of questions such as "Can you do?" or "Do you usually do?" Recently, there has been a trend toward broadening assessment at the healthier end of the scales and reconceptualizing them as basic, intermediate, and advanced ADL functions.[1]

Instrumental activities of daily living

The IADL scale operates on a more sophisticated level and should be used with active individuals living in the community. Poor scores on the IADL scale provide the first sign that independence is being eroded and should be periodically reviewed in patients with chronic musculoskeletal problems. IADL questionnaires assess the skills needed to live independently in the community whereas ADL questionnaires assess more basic skills such as toileting and feeding. People living in the community who are unable to perform IADL generally are unable to function well at home.[5] In addition to identifying patients at risk, the IADL scale pinpoints specific areas in which a patient is having problems, thereby targeting possible intervention strategies as well. Some authors claim that if patients are independent in all IADL functions, a review of ADL function is unnecessary.[16]

Activities of daily living

The ADL Index is one of the most familiar and easiest to use, requiring as little as 2 to 4 minutes of interviewer time.[8] Although all ADL functions are important, the ability to self-transfer is particularly crucial.[1] An easily remembered mnemonic—ABCDFTT—regarding ADL can be used (**a**mbulation, **b**athing, **c**ontinence, **d**ressing, **f**eeding, completing one's **t**oilet, and **t**ransfers).[4] It is hierarchical in nature in that those who can bathe can usually perform all the other tasks. People unable to feed themselves will likely be dependent in other areas. Patients with impaired ADL scores are probably already dependent in most of their IADL functions and at great risk for nursing home placement, long hospital stays, and death.[5] A patient's ADL score should periodically be checked for any changes. The ADL score is a more powerful predictor of health care outcomes than the single medical diagnosis[5] and has been shown to be a powerful predictor of those individuals who will do poorly following discharge from a hospital or emergency department.[1]

A study[33] comparing self-administered, interviewer-administered, and performance-based measures of physical function suggests that these instruments are not measuring the same construct. It concluded that the measurement of physical function is complicated and may be best assessed by multiple methods. Selection of a particular instrument should be guided by the underlying purpose, sensitivity and specificity, and with the realization that the assessment may not be entirely accurate or comprehensive in nature in determining an older person's physical functional status. Table 8 depicts activities of daily living.

NUTRITIONAL ASSESSMENT

Though nutrition surveys have shown a marked decrease in energy requirements and intakes of nutrients with increasing age,[7] malnutrition is common among older persons.[4,19] A survey[7] of older people living at home found that 3% were suffering from malnutrition in most cases the result of some underlying medical problem. However, social factors are likely to be important causes of subclinical malnutrition. Older people are generally identified as being at particular risk of poor dietary intake and nutritional problems and are thus a high-priority target group for nutrition education.[34] In general, the people most at risk are frail older persons with significant physical and mental health problems and few or

Table 8. Activities of daily living (ADL)

Basic ADL	Intermediate ADL	Advanced ADL
Bathing	Cooking	Strenuous physical activities
Dressing/grooming	Housekeeping	
	Laundry	Heavy work around the house
Toileting	Telephone use	
Self-feeding	Transportation use/driving	
Mobility level		Walk 1 mile or longer without rest
Continence (bowel/bladder)	Money management	
Transfers	Self-medication	Walk ¼ mile without rest
	Shopping	

no social and environmental supports.[10] Nutritional problems are usually due to poorly fitting dentures, difficulties with shopping or meal preparation, and problems with swallowing or digestion.[4] It usually goes unrecognized and, even when recognized, treatment is infrequently administered.[1] Nutrition is a critical determinant of immunocompetence and of the risk of infection-related illness in old age.[35] It is likely that the correction of nutritional deficiencies will result in improved immune responses. Warning signals and risk factors of malnutrition have been developed to help caregivers and providers who are in contact with older people.[9–12]

Because early nutritional intervention has been shown to improve the functional outcome of at-risk older persons, it is crucial to search for early forms of malnutrition in older adults.[1,19] It is important to realize that undernutrition is more dangerous for older persons than is overweight.[1] Weight loss in an older patient may be a manifestation of disease or a reflection of depression, unavailability of food, or feeding difficulty. Though no single factor adequately screens for malnutrition, several have been developed. The Nutrition Screening Initiative (NSI), an interdisciplinary project of the American Academy of Family Physicians, the American Dietetic Association, and the National Council of the Aging, Inc, highlights the need to consider the nutritional aspects of health care.[36]

The NSI focuses on malnutrition-related causes of disability in older Americans, with an emphasis on disease prevention and health promotion through proper nutrition.[14] The NSI suggests an adaptable, tiered approach to screening for poor nutritional status in older Americans. The first level of screening is a checklist to be completed by the older individual or caregiver. This checklist describes the warning signs of poor nutritional status. Also included are two screening tests designed to help clinicians detect poor nutritional status or risk factors for poor nutrition. The level I screen is to be completed by a social service or health care professional; the level II screen focuses on additional information to be obtained by a physician.[13] Given the potential consequences of nutrition-related health problems in older patients, nutritional assessment should be a routine part of office practice.[14] The American Dietetic Association has a position statement regarding geriatric nutrition that urges comprehensive nutrition services for older persons as an integral component of the continuum of health care and recommends continued research, education, and development of national policy in the area of geriatric nutrition.[37]

The clinician should inquire about the patient's eating habits; ability to chew and swallow; use and fit of dentures; ability to afford high-quality nutritious food; and access to a grocery store, kitchen facility, meals on wheels, or a senior center that serves hot meals. A 24-hour dietary recall is less reliable in older persons than in younger patients, but it still may help to determine typical dietary patterns.[16]

Gross assessment of nutrition status includes height, weight, and percent body fat; dentition; and dietary assessment.[19] The components of nutritional assessment have been summarized into the mnemonic ABCD (**a**nthropometric measurements, **b**iochemical parameters, **c**linical evaluation, **d**ietary history).[14,38] Techniques for performing a nutritional assessment have been reviewed and are largely applicable to the geriatric population.[38]

Visceral protein status can be measured by serum albumin; the most useful concentration of albumin that indicates risk of malnutrition-related adverse events appears to be approximately 4 g/dL or less.[1] A cholesterol of approximately 160 mg/dL or less indicates serious undernutrition in older patients.[1] Table 9 provides the mnemonics SCALES or DETERMINE, which are useful in recognizing malnutrition in older patients.[1]

Dichter[38] suggests that based on the total number of older people projected in the near future, consideration should be given to designing foods for this group of individuals. Examples include easy-to-open containers, large print, and formulations that are "protective" in nature such as heart healthy or cancer-fighting foods.

DIAGNOSTIC TESTING

In the routine management of older patients, the usual objective of diagnostic testing is to prevent the loss of independence when chronic disorders interfere with activities of daily living.[19] In selecting diagnostic tests, clinicians must weigh the alternatives based on patient needs, cost-effectiveness, accuracy, applicability, and the availability of testing. A few questions should be considered: Does the patient have the physical and mental capacity to benefit from a proposed treatment? Will the test result be likely to influence manage-

Table 9. "Scales" and "Determine"—Undernutrition mnemonics

Scales	Determine
Sadness	Disease
Cholesterol	Eating poorly
Albumin	Tooth loss/mouth pain
Loss of weight	Economic hardship
Eating problems	Reduced social contact
Shopping and food preparation	Medications/drugs
	Involuntary weight loss/gain
	Need assistance with self-care
	Elder years (>80 years of age)

Source: Miller DK, Kaiser EE. Assessment of the older woman. *Clin Geriatr Med.* 1992;9:1–31.

ment in useful ways? Will the investigation establish a diagnosis that affects the prognosis significantly?

The impact of age-associated physiologic changes on interpretation of laboratory data has only recently been elucidated.[39] Although laboratory values change minimally in the healthy geriatric patient,[4] interpreting laboratory data is confounded by the multiple disease states, polypharmacy, and atypical disease presentations commonly found in this population. The truly significant differences are between sick older patients and younger patients. However, laboratory tests very often provide a vital assessment tool in geriatric health care in differentiating the causes of the atypical presentation of disease in the older person. Though baseline values (hematology, biochemistry, and urinalysis) are useful, routine blood analysis should remain discretionary.[4] The USPSTF has recommended four tests as part of initial screening for an asymptomatic patient over age 65 with no other risk factors: nonfasting total blood cholesterol, dipstick urinalysis (to check for hematuria, bacteriuria, and proteinuria), mammography (up to age 75 and then if otherwise indicated), and thyroid function tests (in females).[8,40] Recommended for certain high-risk groups are an electrocardiogram, fasting plasma glucose, fecal occult blood test, sigmoidoscopy or colonoscopy, Pap smear, and tuberculin skin test.[8]

There are a number of confounding factors regarding laboratory data in the geriatric population: reference ranges for laboratory tests in older individuals are lacking; data concerning the effect of age on laboratory values are generally lacking, especially in patients over the age of 75; atypical disease presentation is common; there is a multiplicity of diseases; and there is a high frequency of drug use in older persons.[41]

The erythrocyte sedimentation rate (ESR) increases with age and has been quantified as an increase of 0.22 mm/hour/year from age 20 onward.[40,41] Clinical findings of an elevated ESR in an older patient can be problematic because it may or may not suggest the presence of an underlying pathology. Generally, an elevated ESR of less than 50 mm/hour has little importance unless a clinical correlation can be made. However, ESRs of greater than 80 mm/hour are almost always associated with an underlying neoplasm, infection, or rheumatic disease.[41]

Musculoskeletal disorders

Musculoskeletal problems are a potentially significant cause of decreased function in the older population, and accurate diagnosis may play an important role in successful management. Four areas to consider for diagnostic testing are osteopenia, degenerative joint disease, inflammatory arthropathies, and systemic inflammatory disease.[19] Measurements of serum calcium, phosphorus, and alkaline phosphatase are helpful in patients with suspected osteopenia.[19]

Plain radiographs are usually sufficient for evaluation of joint abnormalities.[19] Basic blood testing can usually be limited to an ESR and a serum uric acid level; rheumatoid factor and antinuclear antibody tests are performed only when a systemic inflammatory process is suspected.[19]

Cardiopulmonary disorders

Cardiovascular disease is responsible for the greatest number of deaths and significant disability in older persons, especially in the young old.[19] Diagnostic testing for cardiac disease is perhaps the most sophisticated in health care. In-office electrocardiograms are available but their value is limited to providing information on conduction disturbances, scars from previous infarcts, and simple rhythm disturbances.[19] Furthermore, interpretation of an ambulatory electrocardiogram can be problematic, because asymptomatic rhythm disturbances are not uncommon in the older population.[19]

The two pulmonary conditions of particular concern in the older population are chronic bronchitis and emphysema. Pulmonary function testing can easily be performed in the office at relatively low cost using desktop spirometers.[19]

Endocrine and metabolic disorders

Common disorders in this category that affect older individuals include glucose intolerance, hypothyroidism, and hyperthyroidism.[19] Decreasing glucose tolerance with age is well documented, as is the increased incidence of diabetes mellitus.[7,41] Age-related changes in blood glucose values make the diagnosis of diabetes mellitus or impaired glucose tolerance more difficult.[4] However, it is still useful to screen for abnormally high levels because early intervention can prevent progression. For initial diagnosis, the use of oral glucose tolerance tests (OGTTs) can largely be discarded in favor of a fasting blood glucose or 2-hour postprandial blood glucose measurement. As a general rule of thumb, a 2-hour postprandial blood sugar should not exceed 140 mg/dL in patients under age 40 and should not exceed 100 plus the patient's age in patients over the age of 40.[41]

Total cholesterol level increases by 30 to 40 mg/dL in men by age 55 and age 60 in women.[40] High-density lipoprotein (HDL) level increases by 30% in men between the third and eighth decades and decreases by 30% in women during this same period.[41] Hypercholesterolemia is a risk factor for coronary heart disease in older persons, but screening and treatment to lower serum cholesterol level have not been shown to improve morbidity or mortality.[1,4] If both total cholesterol and HDL are normal when tested after age 65, additional screening is unnecessary.[2] Care must be exercised in trying to extrapolate data that currently exist only for younger, middle-aged individuals for use in older individuals.

Changes in both thyroid function and structure occur with age; the size of the gland and follicles decreases, and the size of interfollicular tissue increases.[41] Because thyroid disease may be subtle and an unrecognized cause of depression in the older person a high index of suspicion and clinical intuition needs to be maintained. Although routine screening for thyroid disease is not recommended by some authors,[4] thyroid-stimulating hormone (TSH) is an adequate single measure for hypothyroidism and may be warranted as a useful screen of thyroid function.[1,19] When hyperthyroidism is suspected, an ultrasensitive TSH test is indicated.

SUMMARY

Studies of successful aging have identified personal qualities shared by older adults who maintain active and healthy lifestyles. These characteristics include intellectual growth, productivity and creativity, ongoing community involvement, intergenerational communication, altruism, optimism, spiritual faith, and love of life.[2] The comprehensive geriatric assessment is within the capability of every family physician and will improve the quality of geriatric care[4] in order to attain and maintain these successful aging qualities. The effort and time involved may be minimized by collecting information efficiently over several office visits. Six percent of Medicare reimbursements are directly attributable to elevated health risks from smoking, hypertension, hypercholesterolemia, elevated serum glucose level, body mass index, heart rate, and alcohol consumption,[2] indicating that preventive geriatrics can be cost-effective as well as improve the function of older adults. The extra time, effort, and ingenuity required for a comprehensive assessment of the older patient will be richly repaid by enhanced diagnosis, functional ability, and patient health outcomes. And, most important, they will bring about an improved quality of life for all older persons.

REFERENCES

1. Miller DK, Kaiser FE. Assessment of the older woman. *Clin Geriatr Med.* 1992;9:1–31.
2. Kligman EW. Preventive geriatrics: basic principles for primary care physicians. *Geriatrics.* 1992;47:39–49.
3. Harada N, Chiu V, Damron-Rodriguez J, Fowler E, Siu A, Reuben DB. Screening for balance and mobility impairment in elderly individuals living in residential care facilities. *Phys Ther.* 1995;75:462–469.
4. Pereles LRM, Boyle NGH. Comprehensive geriatric assessment in the office. *Can Fam Physician.* 1991;37:2187–2194.
5. Fillit H, Capello C. Making geriatric assessment an asset to your primary care practice. *Geriatrics.* 1994;49:27–33.
6. DeVore PA. Computer-assisted comprehensive geriatric assessment in a family physician's office. *South Med J.* 1991;84:953–955.
7. Souhani RL, Moxham J, eds. *Textbook of Medicine.* New York, NY: Churchill-Livingstone; 1990.
8. Beck JC, Freedman ML, Warshaw GA. Geriatric assessment: focus on function. *Patient Care.* Feb 1994:10–32.
9. Davies L, Knutson KC. Warning signals for malnutrition in the elderly. *J Am Diet Assoc.* 1991;91:1413–1417.
10. Rauscher C. Malnutrition among the elderly. *Can Fam Physician.* 1993;39:1395–1403.
11. White J. Risk factors for poor nutritional status in older Americans. *Am Fam Physician.* 1991;44:2087–2097.
12. Ham RJ. Indicators of poor nutritional status in older Americans. *Am Fam Physician.* 1992;45:219–228.
13. Lipschitz DA, Ham RJ, White JV. An approach to nutrition screening for older Americans. *Am Fam Physician.* 1992;45:601–608.
14. Dwyer JT, Gallo JJ, Reichel W. Assessing nutritional status in elderly patients. *Am Fam Physician.* 1993;47:613–620.
15. Schneiderman H. Physical examination of the aged patient. *Conn Med.* 1993;57:317–324.
16. Fields SD. History-taking in the elderly: obtaining useful information. *Geriatrics.* 1991;46:26–35.
17. Greene MG, Majerovitz SD, Adelman RD, Rizzo C. The effects of the presence of a third person on the physician–older patient medical interview. *J Am Geriatr Soc.* 1994;42:413–419.
18. Means KM, Currie DM, Gershkoff AM. Geriatric rehabilitation. 4. Assessment, preservation, and enhancement of fitness and function. *Arch Phys Med Rehabil.* 1993;74(5):s417–s420.
19. Ochs M. Selecting routine outpatient tests for older patients. *Geriatrics.* 1991;46:39–50.
20. Fries JF. Aging, natural death, and the compression of morbidity. *N Engl J Med.* 1980;303:130–135.
21. Fields SD. Special considerations in the physical exam of older patients. *Geriatrics.* 1991;46:39–44.
22. D'Archangelo E. Substance abuse in later life. *Can Fam Physician.* 1993;39:1986–1993.
23. Butler RN, Lewis MI, Sherman FT, Sunderland T. Aging and mental health, part 2: diagnosis of dementia and depression. *Geriatrics.* 1992;47:49–57.
24. Bowers LB. Back to basics: the patient's story. *Top Clin Chiro.* 1995;2:1–12.
25. Wang AM, Ramsdell JW. Diagnosis and management of diseases causing cognitive dysfunction. *Compr Ther.* 1992;18:17–23.
26. Aging and mental health: primary care of the healthy older adult. *Geriatrics.* 1992;47:54–65.
27. Canadian Task Force on the Periodic Health Examination. Periodic health examination, 1991 update: 1. Screening for cognitive impairment in the elderly. *Can Med Assoc J.* 1991;144:425–431.
28. Mungas D. In-office mental status testing: a practical guide. *Geriatrics.* 1991;46:54–66.
29. Spooner MA. Is it really Alzheimer's? *Can Fam Physician.* 1994;40:1141–1145.
30. Folstein MF, Folstein SE, McHugh PR. "Mini-mental state." A practical method for grading the cognitive state of patients for the clinician. *J Psychiatr Res.* 1975;12:189–198.

31. Mullan E, Katona P, D'ath P, Katona C. Screening, detection and management of depression in elderly primary care attenders. II: detection and fitness for treatment: a case record study. *Fam Pract.* 1994;11:267–270.

32. Jarvik LF, Wiseman EJ. A checklist for managing the dementia patient. *Geriatrics.* 1991;46:31–40.

33. Reuben DB, Valle LA, Hays RD, Siu AL. Measuring physical function in community-dwelling older persons: a comparison of self-administered, interview-administered, and performance-based measures. *J Am Geriatr Soc.* 1995;43:17–23.

34. Horwath CC. Nutrition goals for older adults: a review. *Gerontologist.* 1991;31:811–821.

35. Chandra RK. Nutrition and immunity in the elderly. *Nutr Rev.* 1992;50:367–371.

36. *Report of Nutrition Screening I: Toward a Common View.* Washington, DC: Nutrition Screening Initiative; 1992.

37. Position of the American Dietetic Association: nutrition, aging, and the continuum of health care. *J Am Diet Assoc.* 1993;93:80–82.

38. Bowers LB. Back to basics: assessment of nutritional status. *Top Clin Chiro.* 1995;2(4):1–12.

39. Cavalieri TA, Chopra A, Bryman PN. When outside the norm is normal: interpreting lab data in the aged. *Geriatrics.* 1992;47:66–70.

40. Dichter CR. Designing foods for the elderly: an American view. *Nutr Rev.* 1992;50:480–483.

41. Duthie EH, Abbasi AA. Laboratory testing: current recommendations for older adults. *Geriatrics.* 1991;46:41–50.

Algorithm 1

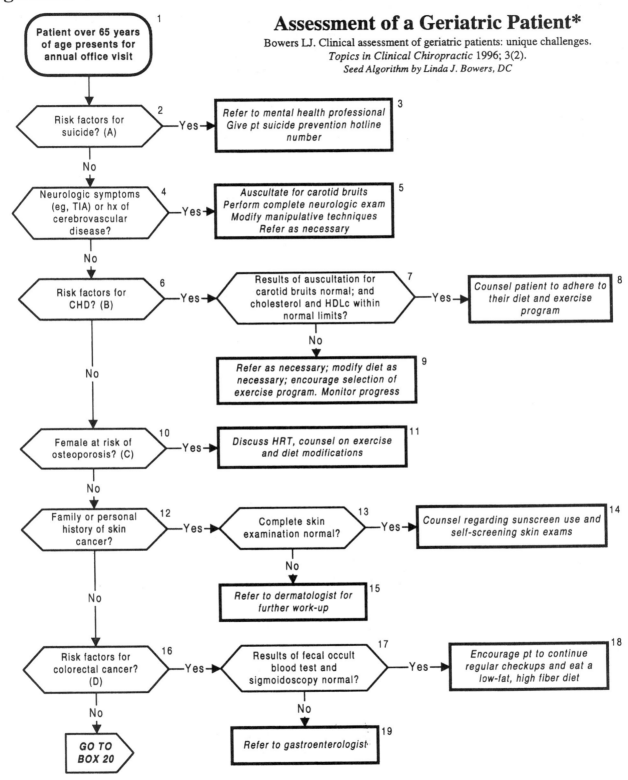

Assessment of a Geriatric Patient*

Bowers LJ. Clinical assessment of geriatric patients: unique challenges.
Topics in Clinical Chiropractic 1996; 3(2).
Seed Algorithm by Linda J. Bowers, DC

* Based in part on *The Periodic Health Examination: ages 65 and over*, from Report of the US Preventative Services Task Force: Guide to Clinical Preventative Services. Baltimore, MD, Williams & Wilkins, 1989.

Algorithm 1, continued

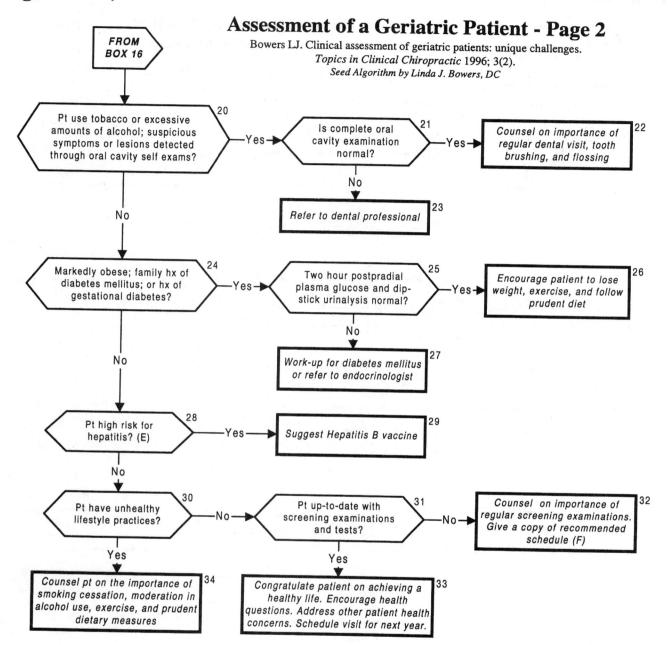

Assessment of a Geriatric Patient - Page 2
Bowers LJ. Clinical assessment of geriatric patients: unique challenges.
Topics in Clinical Chiropractic 1996; 3(2).
Seed Algorithm by Linda J. Bowers, DC

Annotations:
(A) E.g., recent divorce, separation, unemployment, depression, alcohol or other drug abuse, serious medical illnesses, living alone, or recent bereavement.
(B) E.g., hypertension, smoking, diabetes mellitus, coronary artery disease, hypercholesterolemia.
(C) E.g., white, low bone mineral content, bilateral oophorectomy before menopause, early menopause, slender build.
(D) E.g., first degree relative with colorectal cancer; a personal history of endometrial, ovarian, or breast cancer; a previous diagnosis of inflammatory bowel disease, adenomatous polyps, or colorectal cancer.
(E) Homosexually active men, intravenous drug users, recipients of some blood products, persons in health-related jobs with frequent exposure to blood or blood products.
(F) Annual clinical breast examination, annual influenza vaccine, mammogram every 1-2 years for women until age 75, thyroid function tests for women, Papanicolaou smear every 1-3 years, Tetanus-diphtheria booster every 10 years.

Algorithm 2

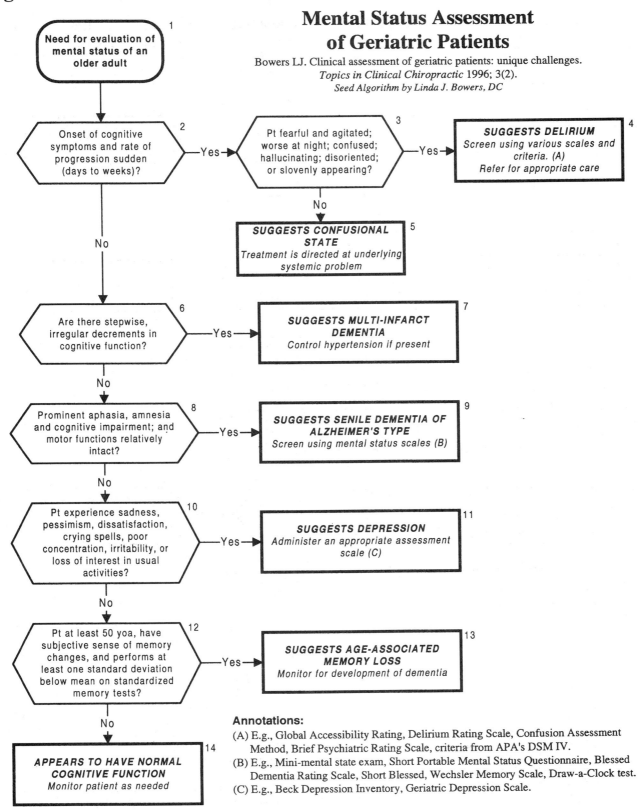

17

Management Considerations in the Geriatric Patient

Kevin A. McCarthy

Chiropractic practice provides abundant opportunities for managing geriatric patients. An understanding of normal aging, the pathology of common conditions, and methods of assessment is essential in developing an effective treatment program. Definitive treatment protocols are difficult to find in the literature, and the art of practice is put to the test in caring for the geriatric patient. It can be said that aging is nothing more than the effect living life has on the human body, and that the practice of geriatrics is the clinician's challenge of discovering how life's traumatic, behavioral, and work experiences have affected the patient's aging process. Many issues must be considered in developing appropriate treatment plans for the geriatric patient. Key issues in general management and strategies in providing ongoing management focus on minimizing and reducing morbidity, as well as optimizing opportunities for activity and function.

LIVING ARRANGEMENTS AND FAMILY RELATIONSHIPS

Are most older patients living in a "home" of some type? Are most isolated and kept away from their family? In reality, only about 5% of persons 65 years of age or older live in nursing homes, and those who do tend to be older, female, white, and to have limitations in one or more activities of daily living. In 1988, 67% of the older noninstitutionalized population lived in a family setting, while 30% were living alone.[1] However, even these numbers can be misleading. Older men are more likely to live with their spouses, while older women are more likely to live alone. Disabled older persons are more likely to live with others.

Despite the acknowledged mobility of the American family, most older persons live within close proximity to at least one of their children and maintain close contact with their families.[2] Three out of every four older people with children either live in the same household as one of their children or live within 30 min driving distance of a child. Of equal importance is that while the proportion of households shared by parents and children has declined, the proportion of older people living within a 10-min drive of a child increased.

Many believe that the large number of social programs provided for older people act as a net and provide for this population's needs. The truth is that despite the development of numerous health and social service agencies, families provide the overwhelming majority of long-term care services to older family members. A national survey[2] shows that 75% to 80% of older persons with disabilities living outside of institutions rely solely on informal care given by family and friends. Therefore, the clinician must ensure adequate communication exists with the patient, and with family members or friends who may provide assistance.

MORBIDITY—HEALTH AND FUNCTIONAL DISABILITY

Measuring years spent without major infirmity and disabling conditions provides meaningful information for health care providers. As an individual ages, the likelihood of onset of disease, followed by a period of disability and ultimately death, increases. Rowe and Kahn[3] have proposed that human aging be classified into two categories: usual and successful. They feel that the study of so-called normal aging is erroneous and actually represents that which "usually" occurs in the older population. They describe a population of older persons who, although they do not escape the eventuality of disease, disability, and death, are able to decrease their

Adapted from *Top Clin Chiro* 1996; 3(2): 66–75
© 1996 Aspen Publishers, Inc.

overall morbidity and delay the onset of disability. Their success has been attributed not only to "intrinsic" factors such as heredity but also to extrinsic factors such as stress, diet, and exercise.

This concept is an important one for the chiropractic physician who, by the unique nature of practice, seeks to limit or halt a vicious cycle of "disease-disability-new incident disease." The degree to which disease and disability can be compressed and postponed until the later years of life has been a source of great controversy. While some may argue that such forms of assisted adaptation are possible, the work of Guralnik and others[4] seems to indicate that those dying at the oldest ages had more disability than those dying at younger ages. Thus, if more older people die at older ages, they are likely to experience even greater functional deterioration for more years prior to their deaths than if they had died at younger ages.

The work of Olshansky and others[5] argues that there will be an expansion of morbidity as medical technology improves the likelihood of survival from previously fatal diseases, without a parallel improvement in quality of life. Thus, they argue that older persons will have traded death at an earlier age for more years spent with one of the nonfatal diseases of aging and its associated disability prior to death.

The 10 most prevalent diseases for those over 65 years of age are (in increasing order of prevalence): tinnitus, visual impairment, diabetes, deformity or orthopedic impairment, cataracts, chronic sinusitis, heart disease, hearing impairment, hypertensive disease, and arthritis.[6] The most serious disorders (ie, those leading to hospitalization) are heart and circulatory disease, diseases of the digestive and respiratory systems, and cancer. Heart disease, cancer, and stroke are the leading causes of mortality among older persons, accounting for 75% of deaths.[6]

In most studies it is noted that age has a substantial effect on disability. Whereas 85% of older persons between the ages of 65 and 69 experienced no difficulty in self-care activities or walking, only 66% of older persons between 80 and 84 and 51% of elders over 85 could report similar levels of well-being.[6] It should be noted, however, that there is also some evidence that some older persons are able to maintain a high level of function. In a longitudinal study of physical ability of the oldest-old, Harris and associates[7] found that one third of those over age 80 reported no difficulty in walking a quarter of a mile; lifting 10 lb; climbing 10 steps without resting; or stooping, crouching, and kneeling.

Older persons are also disproportionately prone to depression and, as an age group, have the highest suicide rates in the population. This fact is principally accounted for by older white males, whose suicide rate in 1986 was five times the national average.[6] This finding is of particular importance because of the large number of secondary depressions arising from organic illness and medication effects and interactions.

CHANGES IN HEALTH CARE STRATEGIES

Developments affecting the demand for health care services appear to be increasingly influencing many clinical management strategies. Examples include growing public skepticism toward new therapies and drugs; increasing emphasis on patient autonomy and other indications of willingness by the public to assume greater responsibility for personal health; changing relations between income, education, and health care use; the aging of the population and the rise in chronic conditions; and alterations in structure and size of the American family. There appears to be a leveling off of acute hospital care, even apart from external financial constraints, and a rising demand for preventive services as well as primary and long-term care. Butler,[3] founding director of the National Institute on Aging, feels that as much as 80% of the degenerative disease that older people suffer could be prevented or postponed if health care systems were more effectively attuned to age-related diseases and their prevention.

UNIQUE ASPECTS OF GERIATRIC HEALTH CARE

The geriatric patient can be a unique health care consumer for many reasons. Although individual pathophysiologic processes themselves may have much in common regardless of the age at which they occur, potential combinations of pathologies, atypical presentations, and changes in the speed and robustness of healing, along with propensity toward a higher incidence of iatrogenic effects of medications, can significantly alter the clinical picture.

Multiple pathologies

Older patients usually have at least two coexisting problems, and oftentimes they have more. An example might be the patient with severe degenerative joint disease (DJD) who is also taking anti-inflammatory medication and developing gastric irritation and is referred for mid-thoracic pain. Medical overspecialization frequently becomes a source of frustration when a doctor does not look deep enough to identify problems with other systems. A doctor of chiropractic might inquire about an older patient's concurrent medical care and learn that he or she regularly goes for blood pressure monitoring. Such a patient may know that his or her spine and heart are well cared for, however, he or she may be gradually falling victim to cataracts and hearing loss that are having a significant effect on lifestyle and ability to function.

Atypical presentations

Many problems of the geriatric patient are known for their slow onset and progression. Because of this fact the patient may accept some loss of function as being a "part of aging."

A survey[8] of "healthy" geriatric patients presenting to a clinic found that 14% of these healthy individuals had congestive heart failure, 4% had postural hypotension, and 10% had painful untreated arthropathy. Many doctors are also not familiar enough with the atypical presentation of some illnesses in this group. Occurrences of pneumonia without fever and vertebral fractures without trauma are not uncommon.

Drug-related symptoms

Drug-induced illness is a serious concern in older persons.[9] As the number of chronic diseases per person increases with age, older persons are at risk from the effects of multiple medications. Advancing age with improved economic status correlates positively with increased use of prescription drugs. Almost 77% of the older population are taking medications, and almost 40% must take at least one drug per day to accomplish the activities of daily living. As many as 70% use self-selected medications, usually without discussing them with their physician.[9]

Polypharmacy, the excessive and unnecessary use of medication, can occur in older persons for a number of reasons. In particular, physicians may rely on drug therapy to accomplish goals that could be achieved from nonpharmacologic methods. In addition, the patient may contribute to the problem by obtaining prescriptions from multiple physicians or receiving medications from friends or family members who want to share the benefits of their prescription. Others may use over-the-counter or self-help remedies that interact with other agents.

Common adverse drug reactions of which the clinician should be aware are listed in Table 1.[10] While not all-inclusive, this list provides information on common adverse reactions and their causes.

Response to therapy

The Arndt-Schultz principles[11] address the normal changes found in the geriatric patient and how these changes affect the patient's response to therapy. These principles should be kept in mind, especially when judging physical response to therapy. They include the following:

- Older persons require a higher level or a longer period of stimulation before the threshold for initial physiologic response is reached.
- The physiologic response in older persons is rarely as big, as visible, or as consistent as is noted in younger groups.
- Similar to the young, once threshold is reached, the more stimuli provided the greater the response.
- In older persons the range of safe therapeutic stimulation is smaller than for the young.

EXERCISE IN AGING

Individuals put forth much effort to alleviate the effects of aging, however, none has been studied more, nor has been found to be more effective, than exercise. Introducing exercise into the normal activity of all older patients is an essen-

Table 1. Common adverse drug reactions in older persons

Adverse reaction	Example	Common causes
Sedation	Drowsiness and sleepiness	Sedative-hypnotics, narcotic analgesics, anti-psychotics
Confusion	Disorientation, delirium	Antidepressants, narcotic analgesics, anticholinergic drugs
Depression	Intense sadness and apathy	Barbiturates, antipsychotics, alcohol, antihypertensive agents
Orthostatic hypotension	Dizziness or syncope when assuming an upright position	Antihypertensives, antianginal agents
Fatigue and weakness	Strength loss and inability to perform normal activities	Muscle relaxants, diuretics
Dizziness	Loss of balance and falling	Sedatives, antipsychotics, narcotic analgesics, antihistamines
Anticholinergic effects	Confusion, nervousness, drowsiness, dry mouth, constipation, urinary retention	Antihistamines, antidepressants, certain antipsychotics
Extrapyramidal symptoms	Tardive dyskinesia, pseudoparkinsonism, dystonias	Antipsychotic medications

tial part of managing health care in the aging patient. It is important to consider how activity levels of the older patient affect different body systems. Tables 2 and 3 review exercise issues for older patients.

Cardiovascular changes and exercise

A progressive increase in exercise intensity will be accompanied by a progressive increase in oxygen consumption in older persons. However, if the cardiovascular dynamics are the same during submaximal exercise, then why does it seem harder for older persons to perform even light exercise? First, the older individual may have to perform less external work to reach the same heart rate as the younger person. In addition, older persons generally exercise at a higher percentage of that individual's maximum exercise capacity than the young.

The gold standard for defining an individual's ability to exercise is maximum oxygen consumption. A higher maximum oxygen consumption gives the individual a greater ability to exercise. The maximum ability of the body to use oxygen during exercise declines with age by approximately .45 mL/kg/min/year.[12] The rate of decline amounts to a 9% reduction in aerobic capacity per decade after the age of 25 in sedentary healthy men.[12] Factors that contribute to this decline are changes in the maximum heart rate, maximum stroke volume, and maximum arteriovenous oxygen difference.

The maximum heart rate or the highest heart rate during exercise also declines with age. The maximum heart rate for the 25 year old is approximately 195 beats per minute, whereas the healthy 75 year old can be expected to reach a heart rate of around 165 beats per minute.[13] The clinical implication of this difference is that older persons have a lower exercise capacity and can reach a more intense level of exercise at lower pulse rates than a younger person. A pulse rate of 125 in an older person in response to assisted ambulation may indicate considerable cardiovascular stress.

Exercise affects cardiovascular function in a number of ways. Resting and submaximal exercise oxygen consumption levels do not change as a result of an exercise training program

---

Table 2. Safe exercise program information

EXERCISE SAFELY

Never
- Try to progress too quickly.
- Exercise or walk when you don't feel well.
- Exercise within 1 hour after eating or after drinking alcohol.
- Take an extremely hot bath or shower after exercising.
- Exceed your target heart range (see below).

Always
- Keep a record of exercise sessions.
  — Record: date, time, minutes of exercise, distance walked, pulse, breathing
  — Note: any pain, fatigue, weakness, sweating that occurs
- Exercise and walk on a regular basis.
- Whenever you miss a week or more of exercise, reduce the amount you do when you start and work up to your prior level.

Stop exercising immediately if you experience
- Tightness or severe pain in your chest, arms, or legs
- Severe breathlessness (can only speak one or two words at a time)
- Lightheadedness or dizziness
- Nausea or vomiting

CHECK PULSE RATE AND BREATHING

Pulse
- Increased heart rate is normal with exercise.
- Take your resting pulse before beginning warm-up exercises and walking. Count your pulse for 10 seconds and multiply by 6.
- Take your pulse immediately after you finish walking and 5 minutes after you finish cool-down exercises. Your pulse should be within 6 beats of your initial resting pulse. Monitor the time until it reaches the resting level. If there are any irregularities, ask your doctor or exercise therapist.

Breathing
- Some shortness of breath is expected after exercise unless you are highly trained.
- By 10 minutes after exercise, your breathing should be comfortable again at a rate of 12 to 16 breaths per minute.

Target Heart Rate Zone

	60% of Max		70% of Max	
Age	Male	Female	Male	Female
50	126	130	137	141
55	123	127	134	138
60	120	124	130	134
65	117	121	127	131
70	114	118	123	127
75	111	115	120	124
80	108	112	116	120
95	105	109	113	117

Data from Karnash AR. The golden key club. *Focus on Geriatric Care & Rehabilitation.* 1991;5(1):1–8. Reynolds P. Focus on exercise program information and guidelines. *Focus on Geriatric Care & Rehabilitation.* 1991;4(8). Copyright © 1991, Aspen Publishers, Inc.

Table 3. Warm-up and cool-down exercises

WARM-UP EXERCISES

Warm-ups prepare the muscles for exercise and decrease the possibility of injury by gradually increasing blood flow and heart rate.

1. Chin tucks: Sit upright on a chair, tuck chin in as if the back of your head is being pulled toward the ceiling. Hold for 10 seconds and breathe normally. Repeat five times.
2. Chicken wing: Sit on a chair with your back straight and feet flat on the floor:
   - Bend your elbows and hold them at your sides. Push your forearms out as far as possible then return to the starting position. Repeat 10 times.
   - Lock your hands behind your head with elbows pointing straight out in front of you. While deeply inhaling, gently extend your elbows backward, then as you exhale, return to the beginning position. Repeat 10 times.
3. Trunk extensions:
   - Lie on your stomach with a bed pillow or folded blanket under your abdomen. Push yourself up slowly, arching your back. Repeat 10 times.
   - While standing, place your hands on your hips and gently bend backward from the waist. Hold for 10 seconds. Repeat 5 times.
4. Wall push-ups: Face a corner (or flat wall). Place your hands on the wall and do push-ups against the wall. Repeat 10 times.
5. Windmills: Stand with your feet shoulder width apart. Extend arms out at shoulder level. Bend forward and reach as far as possible trying to touch your left foot with your right hand. Stand erect. Bend and repeat with your left hand to right foot. Repeat 10 times.

COOL-DOWN EXERCISES

Cool-down exercises help prevent blood flow from becoming stagnate in your extremities, and improve joint and muscle flexibility following exercise.

1. Hip extensors: Hold the back of a chair and extend one leg backward with knee bent. Do not bend forward at the waist. Do five repetitions on each leg with knee bent, then do five more on each leg with knee straight.
2. Leg stretcher: Sit on the floor or on a mat with legs straight and open at a comfortable distance. Reach both hands toward one foot and hold for 30 seconds. Repeat for the other leg.
3. Hip stretcher: While lying on your back, bend one knee and bring it to your chest, hold it with your hands while keeping the other leg straight. Alternate 5 to 10 repetitions with each leg.
4. Pelvic rock: Sit on a chair with your back straight and your feet flat on the floor. Rock your pelvis backward and press the small of your back firmly against the chair. Return to the resting position. Repeat 10 times.

Data from Reynolds P. Exercise and walking: a health promotion initiative. *Focus on Geriatric Care & Rehabilitation.* 1991;4(8):1–8. Copyright © 1991, Aspen Publishers, Inc.

---

in older persons. There is no change in resting heart rate, stroke volume, or cardiac output. There is, however, some decrease in the submaximal heart rate to a standard level of exercise.

Older people are able to increase their maximum oxygen consumption between 10% and 20% through regular endurance exercise. In addition, the rate of V_{O_2} decline can be lowered from 9% per decade to 5% per decade if a high level of training is maintained.[14] Thus, sustained endurance training allows one to improve functional capacity to peak performance. In many instances, though, the goal for exercise may not be to improve functional capacity to such a degree. A moderate level of exercise has been shown to elicit results of increasing aerobic capacity and thus improving tolerance for daily activities with less fatigue, dyspnea, and perceived exertion.[15]

Pulmonary function

A discussion of pulmonary function is different from that of the cardiovascular system in that although there are changes, these changes typically have less of an impact on the ability of an individual to function. There is an overall decrease in the functional ability of the lung to move air in and out as people age. Loss of elastic recoil leads to a decrease in vital capacity and an increase in residual volume. Thus, less of the air breathed is contributing to blood oxygenation. Also, changes in the rigidity of the rib cage and declining strength of the respiratory muscles with aging contribute to an increase in the work of breathing. Loss of efficiency in breathing and greater work of breathing mean that the older person must have more ventilation for the same oxygenation than the younger person.[16]

An aerobic exercise program that lasts 3 months can significantly change ventilatory function in 60 to 70 year olds.[17] As a result of interval-type training for 1 hour three times per week changes could be found. Ventilation decreased significantly during submaximal exercise. A decrease in the carbon dioxide production and the respiratory exchange ratio, a ratio of the carbon dioxide produced to the oxygen consumed, occurred with the decreased ventilation. The blood lactate level also declined. These changes suggest that the exercise training improved the efficiency of the muscle metabolism by producing fewer metabolic byproducts in response to exercise. Exercise training also increases the maximal ventilation during exercise. These changes will reduce the breathlessness experienced by older persons, the sense of exertion, and the percentage of maximal ventilation used during exercise.

Musculoskeletal performance

There is a decline in muscle strength as people age. Strength declines take place beyond the age of 60 and accelerate in individuals 80 years of age or older. Despite the loss of fiber numbers and size, there does not appear to be a decrease in the enzymes related to energy metabolism. Consequently, the capacity for both aerobic and anaerobic metabolism in skeletal muscle does not seem to decline with age.[18]

Isometric and progressive resistive exercise regimens that are of sufficient intensity and that take place over a period of 6 to 25 weeks produce a significant increase in strength in older people. The strength changes found after resistance training are better than a walk/jog exercise program designed to increase general exercise endurance. Significant increases in strength can occur in frail, institutionalized 80 and 90 year olds.[19]

Skeletal changes

Bone is a tissue that is constantly being broken down and rebuilt. If the balance between bone turnover degenerates, then more bone can be broken down than is replaced, thus leading to bony loss. Low dietary calcium, reduced calcium absorption, and hormonal changes such as reduced postmenopausal estrogen levels have all been implicated in bone loss. Exercise can decrease bone loss as people age. Both aerobic-type activities, such as walking and jogging, and strengthening activities that are pursued for at least 9 months to 1 year will influence bone density.

CONNECTIVE TISSUE, STIFFNESS, AND DEGENERATION

One cannot assume that the disease of osteoarthritis is purely a mechanical result of aging. If that were true, then it would be reasonable to expect all older persons to develop osteoarthritis. However, they do not. Genetic, biochemical, traumatic, and morphologic factors may also be interrelated with the effects of aging and development of osteoarthritis.

Age-related research[20] suggests that ligaments and tendons increase in stiffness and demonstrate a decrease in the maximal length at which rupture occurs. A mechanism to account for the increase in stiffness in age-related periarticular connective tissue may be the fact that aged collagen has increased numbers of cross-links between adjacent molecules. Increased rates of cross-linking would increase the mechanical stability of collagen and may explain the increased stiffness in the tissue.[20]

Hyaline cartilage lines articular ends of bone and protects the joint from damaging transarticular forces. It contains a small population of chondrocytes widely dispersed in a relatively dense extracellular matrix. The matrix is chiefly composed of water, collagen fibers, and long branching proteoglycan macromolecules. Histologic observation of healthy articular cartilage in the aged adult shows that the density of chondrocytes and the amount of collagen within the extracellular matrix remain essentially unchanged. The water content in the tissue, however, does reduce with advanced age. Dehydrated articular cartilage may have a reduced ability to dissipate forces across the joint. This feature renders the cartilage susceptible to mechanical failure, causing fragmentation and weakening, and thus localized structural disintegration.[21] These areas are often referred to as "fibrillated cartilage."

The literature tends to support the notion that some amount of fibrillation in articular cartilage is normal and a natural age-related process. Fibrillated cartilage does not tolerate compression and tensile forces nearly as well as intact aged cartilage. The cumulative mechanical wear of advanced age may cause, or is strongly associated with, a weakening of articular cartilage.

The loss of passive range of motion in older persons is often progressive and subtle, occurring usually at the extremes of a joint's potential movement. Healthy adult men and women tend to have their greatest joint mobility in their twenties, with a gradual decrease thereafter. The loss is highly variable across joint and subject. Females tend to lose range of motion at a slower rate than males, and joints of the upper extremities remain more flexible than the joints of the lower extremities.[22] Several factors may impede full active or passive range of motion in older persons. Age-related changes may occur in the joint from previous injury, occupation, or poor posturing. Subsequent excessive joint wear may predispose osteophyte formation and incongruities at the articular surfaces. These factors, in conjunction with increased viscosity of the synovium, calcification of articular cartilage, and increased fatigability of muscle, could all interfere with full joint motion.

The link between range of motion and overall health is worthy of note. One study[23] of 1,000 subjects found that over 50% of the subjects over age 75 could not actively abduct their shoulders up to 120°. Also, the mean shoulder abduction range of 75 year olds was about 30° less than a group of subjects with an average age of 39. From a practical point of view, a maximal range of 120° of shoulder abduction should be considered a significant impairment, because many functional activities that require the hand to be brought overhead would be limited. In this study, Bassey and colleagues found that the amount of shoulder motion deficit was positively correlated with an index of the subject's health. Of interest was a statistically significant correlation between 10% loss of mean shoulder abduction for women and the presence of arthritis, lack of mobility overall, and incontinence.

It is important to realize that not all older individuals lose significant range of motion as they age. When exceptions are found, reasons for such losses should be analyzed as clues for effective treatment. The literature does report cases of very athletic older individuals who have significantly greater range of motion than younger or more sedentary persons. In addition, significant increases in range of motion can be gained in older individuals through regular stretching programs.[24]

Effects of whole body posture on ability to perform and on early degeneration must also be considered. Postural changes can cause long-standing pressure on joints and the supportive ligamentous base. These pressures over a period of time can lead to ligaments that become more "plastic" than elastic, and lead to joint deformity. In addition, the joint becomes less effective in performing an action through an entire range of motion, therefore work becomes less efficient, requiring greater effort and causing more fatigue.

PREVENTING "FRAIL" HEALTH

Disabilities that may arise from normal aging, chronic conditions that result from illness or injury, or those that come from disuse or abuse, may, if left without modification, lead to the development of the frail geriatric patient. Frailty is a poorly defined term that generates the image of the geriatric patient lacking physiologic reserves to meet the demands of daily living or who becomes unable to be involved in any social context within society. This individual may therefore become dependent, suffer psychologically, and ultimately be associated with dramatic health care costs.

Causes of frail health

Disuse (inactivity) induces or accelerates loss of capacity or reserve in each of the systems associated with frail health. It has been suggested that there are four types of limitations on physical activity: restricted neuromuscular activity, physical immobilization, static positioning in relation to gravity, and sensory deprivation.

The rates of loss of aerobic capacity are greatly accelerated by bedrest. Full immobilization, such as complete bedrest, results in a loss of aerobic capacity on the order of 1% per day; 1 day of bedrest causes the same loss in capacity as 1 year of sedentary lifestyle. In addition, losses in strength of approximately 3% a day, or 18% to 20% per week, have been recorded.[16] Although strength and endurance may be the most obvious victims of immobility, other major systems, such as the skeletal, cardiovascular, respiratory, and nervous systems, also suffer deleterious effects.

Bedrest studies[16] in middle-aged adults show that the effects of bedrest on muscle strength, aerobic capacity, and other cardiovascular indicators are eliminated virtually as rapidly as they occur, simply by resuming normal activities. Remarkably, there is some evidence that exercise may not accelerate the recovery from bedrest and resumption of full activities may be sufficient for full physiologic recovery. Obstacles or blocks to the resumption of usual activities may account for recovery failures. A few of the obstacles are discussed in the text that follows.

The rest dogma

A crucial obstacle to recovery that has received the greatest attention over the last 5 years is the deeply rooted misconception that rest facilitates recovery from illness. This misconception has influenced classic medical care for years. The rest dogma is slowly being discredited and replaced by the perspective from sports medicine that appropriate, graduated physical activity facilitates recovery whereas insufficient or abusive activity can impede recovery.

Despite numerous efforts, the general public (well meaning family members) and many caregivers continue to facilitate the rest dogma. Driven by a fear of recurrence or re-injury, these individuals take an extremely conservative course and often influence further deterioration in functional status. Concerns about malpractice may also motivate health care providers to take an extremely conservative approach for fear that activity-related accidents may occur.

Lack of knowledge about exercise

In general, healthy older adults generally acknowledge the importance of staying active in order to preserve good health, however, they have little concept of how to best stay active. A study[25] of injuries in older athletes found that most injuries were due to overuse, and the rate of overuse injuries was much higher in older than in younger athletes. Underactivity is still more of a problem than overactivity. Unfortunately, many older persons who feel that they are sufficiently active are not. Research[25] on perceived exertion may partly explain this situation. Compared with younger adults, many older individuals perceive even mild exercise as involving high levels of exertion. Thus many older individuals feel that their minimal activity is capable of maintaining conditioning, instead they are allowing continued deterioration. Muscle must be taxed beyond its ordinary activities in order to increase strength. Older adults often feel lost about how to sustain exercise when they can no longer exercise in their accustomed way and do not readily seek new avenues for activity.

Activity inhibitors

Common inhibitors to activity in older adults include falls, medications, stressful life events, and depressive illness. One third or more of community-dwelling older individuals fall each year. After a fall, older adults tend to reduce activity, even if they were not injured, and fear of falls may become paralyzing to the older adult.

There is a strong association between depression and functional disability. Causal pathways are complex because depression may be a cause or a consequence of disability. Depressed adults appear to be more sedentary than normal adults, and often they have associated weight loss due to decreased consumption, often accompanied by further muscle wasting.

Removing obstacles to recovery

Perhaps the greatest obstacle to effective recovery is the health care system as it now functions. There currently exists no model for effective team management of the geriatric patient. In general, the current health care system is managed by medical professionals who rarely exhibit an emphasis or interest in prevention. The health care reimbursement system provides no ability to provide counseling and yields no motivation for the clinician to practice wellness and preventive health care.

From the chiropractic perspective, the tremendous limitation brought about by the number one illness of the geriatric population, arthritis, should lead the clinician to significant follow-up to ensure recovery from all injuries. In this light, the issue of rehabilitation in chiropractic practice has been gaining greater attention. Rehabilitation is an extremely important part of the care of the geriatric patient. A minor hip, knee, back, or ankle injury can very significantly reduce the ability of a person to perform functional activities of daily living. Prevention of fibrosis and initiation of degenerative changes must be aggressively addressed.

Strategies involve passive range of motion of the joint to stimulate proprioceptive facilitation, stretching to maintain normal motion, exercises to develop normal active motion and proprioception, resistive exercises to retain strength, and extended exercises to develop endurance of the area. An example of exercises that can be used to develop normal motion should be reviewed with the patient in the office.

PROMOTING WELLNESS IN OLDER PERSONS

The principles of exercise, nutrition, minimizing disuse, and rehabilitation may all be employed as indicated in the management of a geriatric patient. In addition, they are principles that must be applied in an effort to achieve the primary goal of geriatric health care—to prevent the development of dependency.

Preventing acute and subacute episodes of physiologic loss

Opportunities to provide counseling for illness and disease prevention abound. The clinician should make available to patients at an early age information about risks and benefits of various methods of care, methods of prevention, and strategies to avoid injury. In addition, the skilled clinician will always be on the lookout for depressive or maladaptive behaviors in patients facing exogenous stress.

Nutrition

As the population ages beyond 60 years, a larger, more heterogeneous group of people interested in preventive medicine is emerging. An area of particular interest is specific nutrient requirements.

Fat is the most caloric-dense nutrient with 9.0 kcal/g. It should represent approximately 30% of caloric intake. Though often touted, the need to reduce cholesterol in older patients has not been shown to relate to any reduced risk of cardiovascular disease. A low-fat diet has been advocated to reduce the risk of certain cancers, most notably cancer of the breast and colon.[26]

Protein has a caloric density of 4.0 kcal/g. Protein intake should account for between 10% to 20% of the total caloric needs. Carbohydrates have a caloric density the same as that of protein. Caloric intake should be between 50% and 60% of the diet and represent the primary source of energy. They should primarily be in the form of starches with fewer calories in the form of simple sugars.[26]

Moreover, carbohydrates represent fiber intake as fiber is that fraction that is not hydrolyzed by digestive enzymes. The average American diet currently contains approximately 20 g of dietary fiber per day. There is a suggestion that increasing fiber intake to approximately 30 g/day may aid in treatment of functional constipation, irritable bowel symptoms, and diverticular disease. High-fiber diets may actually protect against diverticular formation and possibly decrease the risk of colon cancer. Use of high-fiber diets can, however, interfere with micronutrient absorption and result in deficiencies when marginal intake exists.[26]

There remains much to be learned about optimum intake of micronutrients to promote healthy aging. The recommended daily allowance (RDA) guidelines are established as the minimum to prevent deficiency diseases in the absence of stress or malabsorption. There is concern that many older people are at risk for subclinical or marginal deficiencies of vitamin C, vitamin D, pyridoxine, thiamin, folate, riboflavin, and zinc. Contributing factors include marginal intake as documented by diet surveys and age-related changes in absorption and metabolism, alcohol consumption, and drug therapy. Symptoms of marginal vitamin deficiency include fatigue, anorexia, anxiety, and irritability. These symptoms are nonspecific and are often attributed to other chronic diseases.

It is extremely difficult to assess vitamin deficiency based on dietary history alone, and a history often correlates poorly with biochemical measurements. Vitamin requirements may be as heterogeneous as the aging population and depend on physiologic age, disease-related factors, and drug therapy. Routine use of vitamin supplements in well older persons who are consuming a well-balanced diet is often thought to be unwarranted, unless the use of antioxidant nutrients for prevention purposes is recommended.

As noted previously, the geriatric patient is more likely to be taking drugs on a regular basis. Drugs may have an effect on nutrient absorption and metabolism. For example, some antibiotics lead to malabsorption of nutrients and a decrease in appetite. Symptoms involving appetite, weight loss, or gastrointestinal system disturbances should always be investigated. Chronic problems in any of these areas should direct attention to an intensive analysis of the patient's nutritional status.

Preventing chronic gradual loss: Regular exercise

An adequate exercise program is difficult to sustain in older adults. Therefore, recommending changes earlier in life is important. Health care providers can provide counseling, however, counseling alone may not be effective in changing exercise patterns. Because exercise must be sustained for long-term physiologic benefits, program elements associated with continuous involvement in exercise may be far more important than the details of the initial exercise regimen.[25]

All geriatric patients should be involved in some form of exercise program. The most effective form of exercise is walking. Other forms of exercise should be reviewed. Many commercial or nonprofit agencies have exercise programs that need to be evaluated by the clinician for their effectiveness. Criteria to use in reviewing programs include:

- All activities begin at a low level of intensity and build gradually.
- Activities are incorporated that deal with cardiorespiratory fitness, flexibility, and muscular strength, including flexibility and strength exercises for all major muscle groups and joints.
- The total caloric expenditure involved in each session is high enough to contribute to optimal improvement of the body composition.
- Designated activities should be easily scaled to the fitness level and health status of each participant.
- The program is easily adapted for use in a wide range of physical settings.
- The program is organized and presented in a manner that promotes enjoyment and long-term adherence.

Education at an early age is an important hallmark of prevention. It is especially true of exercise, where developing habits is important in establishing lifetime benefits. Persuading an older person to adopt a program of regular exercise may be difficult. It may be helpful to emphasize the psychologic and emotional benefits of exercise. Elements of fun and socialization should be incorporated into an exercise program, especially for the socially isolated patient. Involvement in one of the numerous exercise programs sponsored by community agencies is helpful.

An exercise program should have several components as prerequisites. It should be performed 3 to 5 days per week. The intensity of exercise is also important. The American College of Sports Medicine[27] recommends an intensity between 60% and 90% of the maximum heart rate reserve or between 50% and 85% of the maximum oxygen uptake. However, there is evidence that low-intensity exercise has beneficial effects on fitness, if the duration of exercise is increased.

In order to tailor a program to the patient, a review of the person's current level of fitness needs to be done. Evaluation of the patient in the areas of flexibility, strength, balance, and cardiovascular potential is important.

Exercise to promote range of motion should be an integral part of any wellness plan. The use of stretching programs to decrease the onset of connective tissue stiffness and to help prevent injury during activity is important and should begin early in the adult. Maintaining range of motion in the ankle, knee, hip, lower spine, cervical spine, and shoulder are important to the patient performing activities of daily living and in supporting an exercise program. Range of motion should be assessed functionally during such activities as walking, getting up and down from a chair (preferably from a lower-than-normal chair), reaching for an object overhead, and reaching for something on the floor. If a patient is going to be involved in a walking or jogging program, assessment of hip flexor tightness (Thomas test) and ankle dorsiflexion is important.

Many methods of testing can be employed to assess the strength of the patient. Manual muscle testing, isokinetic testing, gait analysis, functional testing, and hand-held dynamometry may all be employed. Table 4 identifies the types of testing and their relative advantages and disadvantages.

Balance testing can be static or dynamic. Static testing such as performed in Romberg's test, the sharpened Romberg test, the postural stress test, and the reach test have all been found to be reliable and provide the clinician with a general set of information regarding the patient's ability to maintain balance in various positions. While static stress tests are hard to grade, they are useful tools in assessing capacity. Dynamic tests include movement platforms, obstacle courses, and other tests. These tests have norms and have been extensively tested, however, the cost of such procedures may be extremely prohibitive.

Table 4. Methods of strength assessment

Type	Advantage	Disadvantage	Example
Manual muscle testing	Can isolate specific muscle groups, provide insight into specific causes of functional loss	Only can identify weakness when patient has lost 40% to 50%	Rising on toes 10 to 20 times on one leg, Trendelenburg test, prone hip extension through full ROM repeated 10 times
Isokinetic testing	Able to determine movement capability at different speeds and identify point of fatigue	Nonfunctional and difficult form for some patients to learn	Isokinetic muscle testing and exercising units using speeds of up to 300 degrees per second in the upper and lower extremity
Gait evaluation	Can be quickly performed and is function of activity	Nonspecific, examiner requires follow-up testing of another form	Assessing gait in velocity, stride length, stride width, and variability in stride
Functional testing	Identifies ADL items and any need for remediation	Nonspecific, weakness may be obscured by ROM deficits	Getting up and down from a chair, walking up and down curbs, climbing stairs, picking up objects from the floor, removing objects from a cupboard
Hand-held dynamometry	Provides instant information when comparing right and left sides	Some instruments more reliable than others, reflects static strength only	Hand-held dynamometry, or strength testing units that require examiner to resist patient

ROM, range of motion; ADL, activities of daily living.

If the patient is initiating an exercise program some level of tolerance testing should be performed. The two most commonly used are the ergometric bicycle or the treadmill with electrocardiogram.

The two most common methods for determining the proper cardiovascular intensity level are exercising to a target heart rate and measuring the maximal work capacity. Measurement of the maximal work capacity needs to be performed in the laboratory and requires more calculations. It is perhaps more flexible and reliable, and it incorporates the oxygen consumption (MET) and work required across a greater level of activities.

Exercise target heart rate is calculated from the maximum heart rate (MHR) and the resting heart rate (RHR). The MHR may be measured during exercise tolerance testing or estimated by subtracting the individual's age from 220. The exercise target heart rate (ETHR) is derived using the following formula:

$$ETHR = P \times (MHR - RHR) + RHR$$

where P equals the percentage of MHR that is desired (usually 60% to 90%). The patient must be taught how to take a pulse, and any exercise may be used that allows the person to attain the target heart rate.

CONCLUSION

Chiropractic clinicians should have a greater awareness of the amount of prevention that must be initiated with the patient starting around the age of 35. It is during the two decades before one enters the 60-year-old range that the stage for the quantity and quality of life is probably set. Illnesses, injuries, habits, and social behaviors that occur during this time frame can have profound benefits or risks for the remainder of one's life.

Just as the first step for the prevention of osteoporosis truly begins with screening for calcium intake during youth, perhaps the greatest preventive health care in general looks toward the minimization of risk factors, not only for the sake of mortality prevention, but also for the sake of improving the quality of life during one's twilight years. Patients need to be confronted with the reality of the consequences of their behaviors early in life.

Still, the older population will continue to present to chiropractic physicians for the care of many complaints, previously preventable or otherwise, that require attention in the present. An understanding of the unique issues surrounding aging and care of older persons can help DCs both optimize their management of the patients in this age group and provide important insight in contributing to preventive management of their younger patients.

REFERENCES

1. Chappell NS. Aging and social care. In: Binstock RH, George LK, eds. *Handbook of Aging and the Social Sciences*. 3rd ed. San Diego, Calif: Academic Press; 1990.
2. Commonwealth Fund Commission on Elderly People Living Alone. *Aging Alone—Profiles and Projections*. Baltimore, Md: The Commonwealth Fund; 1988.
3. Rowe JW, Kahn RL. Human aging: limitations of the morbidity associated with "normal" aging. In: Hazzard WR, eds. *Principles of Geriatric Medicine and Gerontology*. 2nd ed. New York, NY: McGraw-Hill; 1990.
4. Guralnik JM, et al. Morbidity and disability in older persons in the years prior to death. *Am J Public Health*. 1991;81:443–447.
5. Olshansky SJ, et al. Trading off longer life for worsening health: the expansion of morbidity hypothesis. *J Aging Health*. 1991;3:194–216.
6. National Center for Health Statistics. Current estimates from the National Health Interview Survey, 1988. In: *Vital and Health Statistics Series 10, No. 173*. Washington, DC: Public Health Service; 1989. DHHS Publication No. 89–1501.
7. Harris T, et al. Longitudinal study of physical ability in the oldest-old. *Am J Public Health*. 1989;79:698–702.
8. Wenger NK, Furberg CD, Pitt E. Coronary heart disease in the elderly: working conference on the recognition and management of coronary heart disease in the elderly. New York, NY: Elsevier; 1986.
9. Cadieux RJ. Drug interactions in the elderly: how multiple drug use increases risk exponentially. *Postgrad Med*. 1989;86:179–186.
10. Ciccone CD. Geriatric pharmacology. In: Guccione AA, ed. *Geriatric Physical Therapy*. St. Louis, Mo: Mosby–Year Book; 1993.
11. Halbach JW, Tank RT. The shoulder. In: Gould JA, Davies GJ, eds. *Orthopaedic and Sports Physical Therapy*. St. Louis, Mo: Mosby; 1985.
12. Buskirk ER, Hodgson JL. Age and aerobic power: the rate of change in men and women. *Fed Proc*. 1987;46:1824–1829.
13. Thomas SG, Cunningham DA, Rechnitzer PA, et al. Determinants of the training response in elderly men. *Med Sci Sport Exerc*. 1985;17:667–672.
14. Hagberg JM. Effect of training on the decline of V_{O_2} max with aging. *Fed Proc*. 1987;46:1830–1833.
15. Blair SN, Kohl HW, Paffenbarger RS, et al. Physical fitness and all-cause mortality: a prospective study of healthy men and women. *JAMA*. 1988;262:2395–2401.
16. Shephard RT. *Physical Activity and Aging*. Rockville, Md: Aspen Publishers, Inc; 1987.
17. Makrides L, Heigenhauser GJ, McCartney N, et al. Physical training in young and older healthy subjects. In: Sutton JR, Brock RM, eds. *Sports Medicine for the Mature Athlete*. Indianapolis, Ind: Benchmark Press; 1986.
18. Green HJ. Characteristics of aging human skeletal muscles. In: Sutton JR, Brock RM, eds. *Sports Medicine for the Mature Athlete*. Indianapolis, Ind: Benchmark Press; 1986.
19. Fiatarone MA, Marks EC, Ryan ND, et al. High-intensity strength training in nonagenarians. *JAMA*. 1990;263:3029–3034.
20. Rauterberg J. Age-dependent changes in structure, properties, and biosynthesis of collagen. In: Platt D, ed. *Gerontology, 4th International Symposium*. New York, NY: Springer-Verlag; 1989.
21. Ghosh P. Articular cartilage: what it is, why it fails in osteoarthritis, and what can be done about it. *Arthritis Care Res*. 1988;1:211–221.
22. Bell RD, Hoshizaki TB. Relationship of age and sex with range of motion of seventeen joint action in humans. *Can J Appl Sport Sci*. 1981;6:202–206.
23. Bassey EJ, Morgan K, Dallosso HM, et al. Flexibility of the shoulder joint measured as a range of abduction in a large representative sample of men and women over 65 years. *Euro J Appl Physiol*. 1989;58:353–360.
24. Raab DM, et al. Light resistance and stretching exercise in elderly women: effect upon flexibility. *Arch Phys Med Rehabil*. 1988;69:268–272.
25. Ausman LM, Russell RM. Nutrition and aging. In: Schneider EL, Rowe JW, eds. *Handbook of the Biology of Aging*. San Diego, Calif: Academic Press; 1990.
26. Brown M. The well elderly. In: Guccione AA, ed. *Geriatric Physical Therapy*. St. Louis, Mo: Mosby–Year Book; 1993.
27. American College of Sports Medicine. Position stand on the recommended quantity and quality of exercise for developing and maintaining cardiorespiratory and muscular fitness in adults. *Med Sci Sports Exerc*. 1990;22:265–274.

18
Manipulative Care and Older Persons

Thomas F. Bergmann and Link Larson

The population of the United States is aging rapidly. Currently, 12% are 65 years of age or older.[1]

This rapid growth has led to an increase in the number of older people who experience functional disability. As persons grow older, the goals of maintaining social independence, functional mobility, and cognitive ability become increasingly important and challenging. Functional impairments frequently accompany the aging process and can lead to an inability to meet the demands of daily life. Functional decline is often the initial symptom of illness in an older person and, in some cases, may be the only symptom.[2]

Of concern is that some older patients may not seek professional opinion and help for these problems. Often they consider the problems a part of the normal aging process. However, with organic disease ruled out, functional impairments may considerably affect the quality of life and will have a major influence on all aspects of care. Therefore, it is essential in the care of older patients to determine whether cognitive or functional loss has occurred.[3]

INTRODUCTION

The ability of older persons to perform activities of daily living depends on their capacity to maneuver safely and effectively. Early identification and treatment of those persons with reduced mobility, deconditioning, and risks for injury can help prevent or delay functional problems that jeopardize independence.

Standard neuromuscular examination is insufficient for evaluating mobility. Direct assessment is necessary to identify problems in gait, balance, ability to transfer, and joint function.[4] The ability of older persons to remain independent has a profound influence on the perceived quality of life and the costs incurred for assistance.[5]

Exercise and rehabilitation assist in restoration of function, maintenance of current abilities, and reduction of the risks of falls.[6,7] While the role of activity and exercise in maintaining function in the older person has been evaluated to some degree, there is no current information available supporting the use of manual therapy. Chiropractic principles suggest that manipulative therapy would include appropriate mechanical, soft tissue, and neurologic effects that might have a beneficial change for joint dysfunction in the older patient. Anecdotal information and case reports also exist to support the role of manipulative therapy and chiropractic care in maintaining joint function in the older population.[8–13] If manual therapy can prevent, delay, or reverse functional decline, the independence of older people can be prolonged so that they can remain in an independent living arrangement for a longer period of time. An independent living arrangement usually promotes a higher quality of life and is less costly than an institutional setting such as a nursing home.[5,14]

FORMS OF MANUAL THERAPY

The form of manual therapy emphasized by the chiropractic profession is a specific short lever contact, high-velocity low-amplitude thrust procedure. It is theorized that these procedures are more precise in correcting local subluxation/dysfunction without inducing stress or possible injury to adjacent articula-

The authors acknowledge the work of Kathy Sroga in manuscript preparation and the help of Dr Brian Jongeward in the literature review.

tions. However, a number of chiropractic diagnostic and therapeutic procedures (techniques) have developed empirically in the profession by an individual or association of individuals.[15] These techniques are then commonly assembled as a system incorporating theoretical models of dysfunction with procedures of assessment and treatment.

Chiropractic technique should not be confused with chiropractic therapy or treatment, which includes the application of all the primary and ancillary procedures appropriate in the management of a given health disorder. These are limited by individual state statutes but may include such procedures as joint mobilization, therapeutic muscle stretching, soft tissue manipulation, sustained and intermittent traction, meridian therapy, physical therapeutic modalities, application of heat and cold, dietary and nutritional counseling, therapeutic and rehabilitative exercises, biofeedback, and stress management.

MOBILIZATION

Another form of manual therapy is termed *mobilization*, which is applied within the physiologic passive range of joint motion and is characterized by a nonthrust, passive joint movement. By taking the joint to its barrier and repetitively moving along or beside it, it is thought that the barrier will be encouraged to recede.[16] Characteristics of a mobilization include a general contact on a number of bony structures with a single movement; a specific contact on a single bony structure with a multiple, repetitive movement action; or a general contact on a number of bony structures with a multiple, repetitive movement action. Mobilization procedures help to loosen and break adhesions and fixations, allowing the adjustment to be more effective.

TRACTION

Manual traction is yet another form of manual therapy in which joint surfaces are held in sustained separation for a period of time. Traction may be done solely through contacts made by the clinician, or it may be aided through the use of a mechanized table or other devices. These forces may be applied manually or mechanically. Traction techniques serve to aid adjustments by first allowing physiologic rest to the area, relieving compressive pressure due to weight bearing, applying an imbibing action to the synovial joints and discs, and opening the intervertebral foramen to allow a break in reflex neurologic cycles. Many of these procedures are also quite useful for older patients when a high velocity adjustment may not be indicated.

SOFT TISSUE TECHNIQUE

Manual procedures can also be specifically directed to the soft tissues. Even though all manual techniques, whether adjustment, mobilization, or traction, produce movements of the soft tissues, the justification for a separate classification is to draw attention to the prime importance of including techniques that have the specific purpose of improving the vascularity and extensibility of the soft tissues.[17] If one of the primary goals of manipulative therapy is the restoration of normal painless joint motion, then it is essential that treatment include measures to relax muscle and restore its normal vascularity and extensibility to the soft tissues. Soft tissue manipulations include massage (stroking or effleurage, kneading or petrissage, vibration or tappomont, transverse friction massage), trigger point therapy, connective tissue massage, and body wall reflex techniques (Chapman lymphatic reflexes, Bennett vascular reflexes, acupressure point stimulation), and muscle energy techniques. Soft tissue manipulation will tend to relax hypertonic muscles so that when the adjustment is given equal tensions will be exerted across the joint. Table 1 lists a number of light force and soft tissue manual procedures.

While the use of soft tissue techniques is generally considered to be fairly safe and innocuous, there are some cautions regarding their use with older persons. Patients using nonsteroidal anti-inflammatory drugs (NSAIDs) such as aspirin and ibuprofen will have a tendency to bleed easily. With some of the pressures applied to the soft tissues it is possible to create bruising (hematoma). Bruising is even more of a concern when the patient is on a blood thinner such as heparin or coumadin.

To determine if a given health complaint is manageable with chiropractic care, the physician must first form a clinical impression based on the patient's presentation, findings from the physical examination, and laboratory test results. Once an impression is formed, the physician must decide if

---

Table 1. Light force techniques that can be used with older patients when thrust techniques are not indicated or contraindicated

- Logan basic
- Pelvic blocking (eg, sacro-occipital technique)
- Distractive techniques (eg, Cox distraction table)
- Spondylotherapy (spinal percussion)
- Hand-held mechanical adjusting instruments (eg, Activator)
- Soft tissue procedures
  – Classic massage (effleurage, petrissage, tapotemont, etc)
  – Nimmo receptor tonus technique (trigger point therapy)
  – Connective tissue massage
  – Muscle energy techniques
  – Chapman's lymphatic reflexes
  – Bennett's vascular reflexes
  – Acupressure point stimulation

his or her clinical experience and the current standard of care support chiropractic therapy for this condition. Appropriate treatment decisions are founded on the understanding of the pathophysiology and natural history of the disorder being considered for treatment and on an understanding of the physiologic effects of the considered therapy.

If it is determined that the patient is suffering from a condition appropriately treated by chiropractic care, and other contraindications have been ruled out, then the presence of such conditions provides sufficient justification for a trial of adjustive therapy. If care is initiated, monitoring procedures must be maintained to assess whether the patient's condition is responding as expected. If treatment does not provide results within the expected period of time it should be terminated and other avenues of therapy investigated.[18]

Conditions inducing altered structure and/or function in the somatic structures of the body are the disorders most frequently associated with the application of manual and adjustive therapy. The component of these disorders that is conventionally associated with an indication for adjustive therapy is the identification of joint subluxation/dysfunction. Although the identification of joint subluxation/dysfunction is critical in the determination of whether or not to apply adjustive therapy, it does not terminate the doctor's diagnostic responsibility. The physician must also be able to determine if the dysfunction exists as an independent entity or as a result of other somatic or visceral disease. Joint subluxation/dysfunction may be the product of the disorder rather than the cause, or it may exist as an independent disorder, worthy of treatment, but not be related to the patient's chief complaint.[18]

CLINICAL FINDINGS OF JOINT DYSFUNCTION

Joint subluxation/dysfunction is detected primarily by clinical examination. Where joint subluxation/dysfunction is encountered as the primary lesion, its evaluation and justification for the application of adjustive therapy are complicated by the limited understanding of the pathomechanics and pathophysiology of this disorder.[19] In the early stages of primary joint subluxation/dysfunction functional change or minor structural alteration may be the only measurable events.[20] Evident structural alteration is often not present or not measurable with current technology, and a singular gold standard for detecting primary joint subluxation/dysfunction does not currently exist.

The physical findings usually associated with the detection of joint subluxation/dysfunction and the outcome measures for determining successful treatment include pain, postural alterations, regional range of motion alterations, intersegmental motion abnormalities, tissue texture changes, muscle tone, hyperesthesia/hypesthesia, and functional capacity measures.[19] Although radiographic evaluation is commonly used to identify joint subluxation, it must be incorporated with physical assessment procedures to determine the clinical significance of suspected joint subluxation/dysfunction. Moreover, in geriatric patients the use of radiographic evaluation takes on a different significance. As supported by the Agency for Health Care Policy and Research (AHCPR) guidelines for acute back pain in adults, individuals over the age of 50 with complaints of pain should have plain film radiographs.[21] In addition, Medicare typically requires radiographic evidence of subluxation to justify care for its beneficiaries, the majority of whom are older persons.

At what point specific physical measures are considered abnormal or indicative of joint dysfunction is controversial and a matter of ongoing investigation. The profession has speculated about the structural and functional characteristics of the optimum spine, but it has not reached a consensus on the degree of, or combination of, abnormal findings that is necessary to identify joint dysfunction. However, because of the complexity of the joint systems of the body, no single evaluative tool should be relied on to identify the presence of joint dysfunction. Therefore, structural evaluation of the spinal column should be viewed in terms of a multidimensional index of segmental abnormality.

PARTS

Whether assessing a geriatric patient or a younger individual, the mnemonic PARTS[22] can be used to establish the five diagnostic criteria for spinal dysfunction (subluxation). These criteria are as follows:

1. **P**—Pain/tenderness. The perception of pain and tenderness may be evaluated in terms of location, quality, and intensity. Most primary musculoskeletal disorders manifest primarily by a painful response. The type and location of pain are ascertained by palpating osseous and soft tissues and noting the location and intensity of tenderness as reported by the patient. Pain and tenderness findings are further qualified through observation, percussion, and additional palpation. Furthermore, changes in pain intensity can be objectified using visual analog scales, algometers, pain questionnaires, and so forth.
2. **A**—Asymmetry. Asymmetric qualities on a sectional or segmental level are noted. Such notations would include observation of posture and gait, as well as palpation for misalignment of vertebral segments. Findings of asymmetry are identified through observation (posture and gait analysis), static palpation, and static radiograph evaluation.
3. **R**—Range of motion abnormality. Changes in active, passive, and accessory joint motions are noted. These changes may be an increase or a decrease in mobility. It is thought that a decrease in motion is a common component of joint dysfunction. Range of motion abnor-

malities are identified through the procedures of motion palpation and stress radiographic evaluation.
4. **T**—Tissue tone, texture, temperature abnormality. Changes in the characteristics of contiguous and associated soft tissues including skin, fascia, muscle, and ligament are noted. These changes are identified through the procedures of observation, palpation, instrumentation, and tests for length and strength.
5. **S**—Special tests. Those testing procedures that are specific to a technique system are performed (leg check, arm fossa test, therapy localization, and so forth). In addition, visceral relationships are considered as well as other testing procedures deemed necessary from data previously obtained.

The findings derived from the PARTS evaluation can be used to decide which areas are in need of an adjustment. The clinical decision as to whether an adjustment will be made, how it will be done, and where and when it will be applied can be determined by which area has the most findings from each category. Minimum findings can be established (ie, one from each of the first four categories).

If practitioners were to standardize their evaluation, comparisons of treatment effectiveness and efficiency could be done. Until a professional standard of care is established, each practitioner must use reasonable and conservative clinical judgment in the management of subluxation/dysfunction. The decision to treat must be weighed against the presence or absence of pain and the degree of noted structural or functional deviation.

SPECIFIC CLINICAL PROBLEMS

Pain occurs more frequently in older adults than in younger persons. Often the degenerative diseases that seem to cluster in old age, including arthritis, osteoporosis, and neuromuscular disorders, are responsible.[23] Older patients often have difficulty describing pain and tend to underreport it, possibly because they consider some of their symptoms to be normal consequences of aging.[23]

Immobility can have dire consequences for many older adults. Function must be emphasized so that acute pain is not allowed to progress and cause disability in deconditioning that may be much more difficult to reverse than the pain itself.[23] From 60% to 70% of older adults are sedentary, without routine physical activity.[24] A lack of physical activity may be due to pain, which in turn leads to more pain, and a vicious cycle results. Older adults who maintain high levels of flexibility, strength, and cardiovascular endurance rarely are candidates for dependent long-term care.[24] Regular exercise is an effective nonpharmacologic therapy for stress, sleep disorders, depression, and anxiety, as well as such chronic conditions of aging as hypertension, obesity, diabetes mellitus, coronary artery disease, hyperlipidemia, and constipation.[24] Regular activity is only possible if the amount of pain is minimized.

A reason for institutionalization is the deterioration of function that prevents an individual from carrying out the essential activities of daily living unaided. Muscle strength may be insufficient to lift the body mass from a chair or toilet seat, flexibility at major joints may be inadequate to allow dressing or climbing into a bath, and oxygen transport may no longer be sufficient to meet the needs of the muscles during light aerobic work.[14] Improved physical function allows the older person to maintain personal independence and facilitates a reduction in demands for both acute and chronic medical services.[14]

Disturbances of postural stability and unsteadiness of gait together account for one of the major problems faced by many older people in their everyday lives.[25] Loss of the normal afferent input from the type 1 cervical articular mechanoreceptors for any reason gives rise to clinically significant disturbances of postural sensation (often involving vertigo) and of kinesthesis (upon which precise control of voluntary movements, including walking, depends) even in the presence of a normally functioning vestibular system. Because increasing age is inevitably associated with progressive degenerative loss of mechano-afferent systems related to all tissues of the body, it seems probable that involvement of the cervical spinal articular mechanoreceptor systems in this process may contribute significantly to the impairment of postural and kinesthetic sensation from which most older people suffer to varying degrees.[25] Therefore some consideration should be given to the perceptual and reflexogenic importance of cervical articular mechanoreceptor systems in the design of rehabilitation programs intended to ameliorate postural instability and ataxia in older patients.[25]

Pain, immobility, and decreased muscle strength may result from joint dysfunction and can be complicated by the degeneration process associated with aging. Manual procedures have the ability to restore joint function with the potential of relieving pain, improving mobility, and increasing strength.

With age comes almost a universal tendency, especially in women, for a forward head posture to develop. This posture becomes the primary cause of many cervical, cranial, and shoulder dysfunctions. These dysfunctions can include cervical degenerative joint disease leading to spondylosis and even myelopathy, consequent radiculopathies, shoulder impingement syndromes, subcranial restrictions, headache, and craniomandibular dysfunction. Combined, these conditions can lead to disturbances in balance and gait as well as a cognitive loss of awareness in relation to one's environment.[26]

The postural mechanoreceptors are most numerous in the cervical and upper cervical spines. For a mechanoreceptor to fire, the receptors must be distorted, thus requiring that the capsule in which they reside be stretched. If movement of the facet capsules is restricted due to forward head posture, however, the individual will lack information from these important mechanoreceptors, and postural awareness will be impeded. Clinically, restoring cervical spine movement and improving posture may lead to improvement of self-awareness and the ability to relate to the environment.[26] Postural treatment should follow, not precede, joint and soft tissue manipulation of the upper thoracic and subcranial regions. To attempt postural correction while the patient's joints and myofascia are restricted could create further stress in an already dysfunctional area.[26]

Low back pain is a common complaint in chiropractic offices, and the older patient is no exception. The diagnostic challenge, however, is perhaps greater in older patients. In most older adults with low back pain, no cause is found, and the eventual diagnosis is nonspecific or regional back pain. A search for specific systemic causes is warranted, however, as many have serious consequences. Among older adults, slightly higher percentages are expected for compression fractures and malignancy. Older adults are at somewhat higher risk for some less common causes of low back pain, including osteoporosis-related vertebral compression fractures, lumbar spinal stenosis, and metastatic disease. However, the final diagnosis for most will be nonspecific or regional back pain, although they will almost invariably have degenerative changes on spinal films.[27]

The etiology of regional back pain is unknown. If pain is usually associated with activity, the cause is considered to be mechanical, although a specific inciting event cannot always be identified. Back pain in 5% to 10% of patients will have a radicular component, and muscle spasm and tenderness may be present as well. Management of the geriatric patient with low back pain should be conservative with manipulation a primary consideration. The patient should be advised to restrict activities but avoid prolonged bedrest. Heating pads or cold packs may be prescribed, and soft tissue trigger point therapy can often provide symptomatic relief.[27]

Age-related changes in the shoulder joint can result in impaired range of motion. At least one of every four older persons has shoulder pain.[28] Thoracic kyphosis, degenerative arthritis, occupational trauma, disuse, and cellular collagen and elastin changes in combination reduce shoulder strength, integrity, and mobility.[5] Clinical syndromes include rotator cuff tears or tendonitis, impingement, acromioclavicular arthritis, and the frozen shoulder (adhesive capsulitis). Nevertheless, almost half of the shoulder-related complaints are unreported despite the fact that more than 70% are due to soft tissue lesions responsive to nonsurgical treatments.[29]

SPECIFIC MANUAL AND MANIPULATIVE PROCEDURES FOR OLDER PATIENTS

Osteoarthritis, osteoporosis, and chronic degenerative disc disease are common degenerative spinal conditions with which the doctor of chiropractic must deal on a daily basis when caring for geriatric patients. Because these conditions are permanent and progressive, many chiropractors may choose to use light force adjustments combined with therapeutic adjunctive measures directed toward symptomatic relief. While this approach is understandable, it is most certainly not mandatory. Consideration can be given to the use of specific, high-velocity low-amplitude thrust technique in the care of older patients.

An adjustment is characterized by the application of a specific force or forces to a dysfunctional joint with the purpose of restoring position and/or motion to the joint. The applied force must be sufficient to move the joint against the resistance. Other options such as heat or cold therapy, massage, traction, mobilization, and ultrasound may be useful. Hydrotherapy may be particularly beneficial in improving range of motion in older patients with painful muscles and joints. Nonpharmaceutic options should be considered for initial management.[23]

The mechanical stimulation of the chiropractic vertebral adjustment provides normal cytologic stimulation to the cellular components of the cord neuromeres and may also help augment the vascular and lymphatic exchanges. This action enhances the normal activities of the spinal cord pathways and mediations and helps to obtain an optimal central nervous system conduct. For this reason this type of therapy is thought to help contain or retard central nervous system disease.[30]

Of course, fundamental to the appropriate application of manipulative therapy is reducing the risk of complication. Table 2 indicates the major contraindications to spinal manipulative therapy and suggests modifications that need to be implemented when treating geriatric patients.

The doctor of chiropractic must be able to sufficiently determine the nature and extent of the patient's problems, being able to diagnose the conditions that are applicable to conservative care from those that are not. All treatment is dose related; that is, the type and amount of treatment depend on the problems identified by the evaluation. The anatomic, physiologic, and psychologic condition of the patient, as well as the physician's own skill in the use of a variety of techniques, will serve as the limiting or determining factors in which procedures are or are not applied.

Properly applied, with the right direction and force, high-velocity thrust techniques can be effective for relieving somatic dysfunction.[11] The most significant modification to the established thrust techniques for the older patient would be the use of broader or less specific points of contact. In the thoracic spine, for example, double thenar contacts established over three or four transverse processes may be more appropriate than the focused thrust of pisiform contacts on one transverse process. Table 3 identifies specific modifications to high-velocity thrust techniques that may be considered with the older patient.

Table 2. Geriatric conditions that may contraindicate or require modification to high-velocity, low-amplitude spinal manipulative therapy

Condition	Potential complication of manipulation	Method of detection	Modification of management
Atherosclerosis of major blood vessels	Blood vessel rupture (hemorrhage), dislodged thrombi	Palpation, auscultation, radiographic visualization, Doppler	Soft tissue and mobilizing techniques with light adjustments, refer to vascular surgeon
Aneurysm	Rupture and hemorrhage	Irregular pulse, abdominal palpation, auscultation, radiograph	Refer to vascular surgeon
Tumors	Metastasis to spine, pathologic fracture	Palpation, radiograph, laboratory findings, MRI, CT	Referral*
Fractures	Increased instability, delayed healing	Radiograph, CT	Referral*
Severe sprains	Increased instability	Stress radiograph, motion palpation	If severe, referral; if not, manipulation of area of fixation
Osteoarthritis (late stage)	Neurologic compromise	Radiograph	Mobilization, gentle manipulation
Uncoarthrosis	Vertebral artery compromise	Radiograph	Gentle traction, mobilizing and soft tissue techniques
Clotting disorders	Spinal hematoma	History of anticoagulant therapy, pulse, bruises	Forceful manipulation contraindicated
Osteopenia (osteoporosis)	Pathologic fracture	History of long-standing steroid therapy, postmenopausal females, anticonvulsive medications, malabsorption syndrome, nutritional deficiencies, radiograph	Forceful manipulation contraindicated, use mobilizing technique with light adjustments
Space-occupying lesions	Permanent neurologic compromise	MRI, CT, (myelography)	Referral*
Diabetes (neuropathy)	Unresponsive to pain	Laboratory findings, examination of lower extremity skin and pulses	Referral*
Alzheimer's disease	Inappropriate response or unresponsive to pain and/or treatment	Mental status evaluation	Gentle manipulation, mobilizing and soft tissue techniques

MRI, magnetic resonance imaging; CT, computed tomography.
*While referral for medical treatment of the specific pathologic process is deemed appropriate and necessary, it does not preclude the patient from receiving manipulative therapy to unaffected areas or, in some cases, to the areas of pathology for symptomatic relief.
Adapted with permission from Gatterman MI. *Chiropractic management of spine related disorders.* Baltimore, MD: Lippincott Williams & Wilkins. 1990: 67–68.

The following procedures do not represent an all-inclusive treatise on the use of chiropractic technique for geriatric patients but rather they should be viewed as possible considerations for spinal joint dysfunction and pain.

Atlanto-occipital articulation

Bilateral thenar occiput—prone

This procedure can be used for intractable headaches, posterior atlanto-occipital jamming, decreased movement of the atlanto-occipital articulation, and suboccipital muscle hypertonicity. The patient is placed in the prone position with the headrest lowered slightly to the patient's tolerance and the patient's chin tucked in to induce flexion. The doctor stands at the side of the table, facing headward, in a lunge position. The doctor establishes thenar contacts with both hands at the base of occiput. The doctor's thumbs point toward the vertex of the skull while the fingers fan out laterally. The doctor applies body weight in a cephalad direction. Traction is held 15 to 20 seconds with the pressure released slowly or a very quick and shallow thrust can be applied.

Table 3. Modifications to high-velocity, low-amplitude manipulative procedures that can be considered with the older patient

- Broad contacts taken over large area to disperse thrust
- Multiple lighter (less force) thrusts
- Sustained pressure rather than quick thrust
- Use of specific active or passive motion with specific contacts
- Addition of mechanical assistance (eg, drop piece)

Bilateral thenar occiput—sitting

This procedure is an alternative to the previous technique and may therefore also be used for patients with intractable headaches, posterior atlanto-occipital jamming, decreased movement of the atlanto-occipital articulation, and suboccipital muscle hypertonicity. The patient is placed in the seated position, and the doctor stands behind. The doctor establishes both thenar contacts over the base of the occiput with the thumbs pointing to the vertex of the skull and the fingers fanned out laterally.

Cervical spine

Cervical distraction

This procedure is done to produce distraction of the cervical interbody spaces and to influence the cervical curve. The patient is placed in the supine position, with the headrest lowered when emphasizing cervical extension or raised when emphasizing cervical flexion. The doctor stands at the head of the table and either establishes digital contacts of both hands or places the edge of a rolled towel over the middle cervical segments to induce extension. Alternatively, digital contacts or the edge of a rolled towel is established over the base of the occiput to induce flexion. The doctor then applies cephalad traction, sustaining the force for a few seconds, releasing, and repeating.

Calcaneal cervical break

This procedure is used to induce some rotational movement in the cervical spine with cervical spondylosis and facet arthrosis, where a specific and focused segmental thrust would not be indicated due to the extent of the degenerative condition. The patient is placed in the supine position, with the head turned in the direction of thrust. The doctor establishes a calcaneal contact (heel of the hand) of the ipsilateral hand over multiple cervical artrricular pillars (laminae). The other hand grasps the contralateral aspect of the neck and side of the head to produce some minimal rotational and lateral flexion prestress away from and over the points of contact, respectively. A shallow thrust is applied in the posterior-to-anterior direction.

Cervical compression-translation (stair-stepping)

This procedure provides general mobility to the cervical spine with emphasis on the translational (gliding) quality of segmental motion. The patient is placed in the supine position, and the doctor sits at the head of the table. The doctor establishes contacts with both hands over the lateral aspect of the patient's head and face, straddling the ears with the middle and ring fingers. Keeping the head and face level, compressive force is applied equally through both contacts, footward to the head. This procedure should cause the chin to elevate due to posterior-to-anterior translation of the cervical segments. More compression will translate more segments. In addition, side gliding and slight rotational movements can be induced.

Thoracic spine

Bilateral (double) thenars

This procedure is used to provide mobility to the thoracic spine, especially when an increased or senile kyposis is present. The patient is placed in the prone position, and the doctor stands at the side of the table, facing headward, in a lunge position. The doctor establishes the thenar contacts of both hands over the transverse processes of several thoracic segments. The thumbs point headward while the fingers are directed laterally to ensure no contact is made over the ribs. The patient is instructed to breathe out while the doctor applies body weight through the contacts to prestress the articulations and remove the springiness of the ribs. At the end point, the doctor delivers a quick and shallow impulse thrust in a posterior-to-anterior direction. A slight inferior-to-superior vector can be considered as well, because sometimes it is more comfortable for the patient.

Thoracic rock

This procedure is used to increase mobility of the rib cage and thoracic spine in flexion. The patient is placed in the supine position with hands interlaced behind the head and the elbows together. The doctor stands at the side of the table, facing headward, in a lunge position. The doctor establishes contact over both of the patient's proximal forearms with corresponding hands. The patient is rocked into flexion and then returned to the supine starting position. This procedure may be done once or repeated. If the patient can tolerate it, one hand can be placed under the patient, establishing a flat hand contact over a thoracic spinal segment to induce some specific movement.

Sitting thoracic

This procedure is done to induce rotational and/or lateral flexion movement in the thoracic spine and rib cage. The patient is placed in the sitting position, straddling the table, if able to do so comfortably. The doctor sits behind the patient, also straddling the table. The doctor reaches under the patient's arm to grasp the opposite distal humerus. This procedure will prestress the thoracic cage into rotation. The doctor can then establish a broad contact over several thoracic transverse processes or rib angles to deliver single or multiple thrusts. Alternatively, the prestress can be produced in lateral flexion by applying downward pressure on one shoulder with a broad calcaneal contact established alongside several spinous processes and single or multiple thrusts imparted.

Ilio-costal lift

This procedure is done to induce mobility in the rib cage, to increase thoracic expansion, and to influence intercostal function for such conditions as intercostal neuralgia. The patient is placed in the prone position, with the doctor standing in a square stance to the table on the side of the table opposite to the side to be manipulated. The doctor's cephalad hand is used to establish a thenar contact in the intercostal space below the rib to be manipulated. The caudal hand then establishes digital contacts over the anterior superior iliac spine (ASIS). The caudal hand prestresses the pelvis in an anterior-to-posterior direction while headward and lateral pressure are applied to the rib. At tension, a separating thrust is applied. This procedure can also be done to the lumbar spine by establishing contacts over the mammillary process to mobilize the lumbar segments.

Lumbar spine and pelvis

Lumbosacral stretch

This procedure is done to distract the lumbar segments, especially when there is evidence of hyperlordosis, facet syndrome, or swayback postural changes. It can be done manually or with mechanical assistance. The patient is placed in the prone position with the lumbar and pelvic sections raised on an articulated table or over a roll on a bench-style table. When done manually, the doctor stands at the side of the table, facing footward, in a lunge position. The doctor establishes a broad contact over the sacral base with the inside hand; the other hand reinforces the contact, and traction is applied using the body in a footward direction. The traction may be sustained, or a light thrust may be applied. When done with mechanical assistance, the doctor stands on the side of the table in a lunge position, facing headward. The cephalad hand establishes a contact over the spinous process of a lumbar segment. The caudal hand is used to depress the pelvic section of a distraction table or apply caudal traction on a leg.

Apex contact

This procedure is done for sacroiliac dysfunction and chronic sacroiliac strain. The patient lies in the prone position with the doctor sitting, facing headward, on the side opposite the short leg or posterior innominate. The doctor's caudal hand is used to establish a thumb contact over the sacrotuberous ligament. The other hand usually applies a light stroking action over the lumbar paraspinal muscles. The contact is held, applying about 3 to 5 lb of pressure against the sacrotuberous ligament for up to 3 minutes.

Pelvic blocking

This procedure is done for sacroiliac dysfunction. The patient is placed in the prone position. The doctor identifies the side of short or posterior innominate. The doctor then places padded wedges (blocks) under the acetabulum on the posterior innominate or short-leg side and under the ASIS on the other side. The patient can be left alone in this position for 3 to 6 minutes, letting gravity affect the sacroiliac joints, or the doctor can contact the posterior superior iliac spine (PSIS) and ischial tuberosity on the sides opposite the blocks and apply single or multiple oscillatory thrusts.

Other approaches

Other approaches that could be beneficial and would be appropriate for geriatric musculoskeletal conditions include specific soft tissue manipulative procedures, resisted range of motion procedures (ie, proprioceptive neurologic facilitation [PNF]), mechanical drop section procedures, and mechanical adjusting instruments (eg, Activator).

CONCLUSION

The mere fact that an individual is aging does not mean that spinal manipulative therapy cannot be used or that it must be modified. Indeed, many musculoskeletal conditions affecting older persons can be treated using conservative treatment. Various manual and manipulative procedures can be used provided some precautions are taken and modifications are made when indicated. Adequate assessment procedures to rule out potential complications become especially important with the geriatric patient. Furthermore, the use of broader contacts, attention to proper patient positioning/prestress, and application of the least amount of force necessary to influence joint function are necessary considerations when applying manual therapy to older patients.

There is enough anecdotal evidence to justify further study to evaluate the effectiveness of manual therapy and specifically chiropractic adjustive procedures for improving functional performance in older individuals. Areas of further study include determining the types of older patients who are most likely to benefit from manual therapy, determining the optimal combination of exercises for functional gains, and determining appropriate activities to maintain functional gains once manual therapy has been discontinued. Other areas of study should address psychosocial factors that will improve a subject's motivation and compliance with recommended therapy. Last, a randomized clinical trial is needed to demonstrate the effectiveness of manual therapy for improving gait, balance, and functional performance.

Little evidence exists to validate one form of therapy as being more effective than another for a specific dysfunctional problem. No comparative studies have been done to date. However, full understanding and absolute validation may not be attainable with the technology and knowledge of today. Therefore, in the meantime, clinical success may carry more weight. The notion of clinical success is relative and fragile. It behooves practitioners to make every effort to substantiate the principles and procedures of clinical practice.[31]

REFERENCES

1. Harada N, Chiu V, Fowler E, Lee M, Reuben DB. Physical therapy to improve functioning of older people in residential care facilities. *Phys Ther.* 1995;75:830–839.
2. Pinholt EM, Kroenke K, Hanley JF, Kussman MJ, Twyman PL, Carpenter JL. Functional assessment of the elderly: a comparison of standard instruments with clinical judgment. *Arch Intern Med.* 1987;147:484–488.
3. Applegate WB, Blass JP, Williams TF. Instruments for the functional assessment of older patients. *N Engl J Med.* 1990;322:1207–1214.
4. Tinetti ME, Ginter SF. Identifying mobility dysfunctions in elderly patients: standard neuromuscular examination or direct assessment? *JAMA.* 1988;259:1190–1193.
5. Fleming KC, Evans JM, Weber DC, Chutka DS. Practical functional assessment of elderly persons: a primary care approach. *Mayo Clin Proc.* 1995;70:890–910.
6. Tinetti ME, Baker DI, McAvay G, et al. A multifactorial intervention to reduce the risk of falling among elderly people living in the community. *N Engl J Med.* 1994;331:821–827.
7. Province MA, Hadley EC, Hornbrook MC, et al. The effects of exercise on falls in elderly patients: a preplanned meta-analysis of the FICSIT trials. *JAMA.* 1995;273:1341–1347.
8. Osterbauer P, DeVita T, Fuhr A. Chiropractic treatment of a chronic mechanical low back pain in a geriatric population: a practitioner-scientist protocol. In: *Proceedings of the International Conference on Spinal Manipulation, FCER.* Arlington, Va: FCER; 1991.
9. Cassata DM. An interview with Donald M. Cassata on chiropractic care of the elderly. *J Chiro.* 1991;28:5–9.
10. Winterstein J. Perspectives on clinical practice: practical management of the geriatric patient. *J Aust Chiro Assoc.* 1990;20:62–65.
11. Dodson D. Manipulative therapy for the geriatric patient. *Osteopathic Ann.* 1979;7:114–119.
12. Sandoz R. Chiropractic care of the aged patient. *Ann Swiss Chiro Assoc.* 1985;8:167–191.
13. Clemen M. Adjusting geriatric patients. *Today's Chiro.* 1987;16:77–78.
14. Shephard RJ. Exercise and aging: extending independence in older adults. *Geriatrics.* 1993;48:61–64.
15. Bergmann TF. Various forms of chiropractic technique. *Chiro Tech.* 1993;5:53–55.
16. Bourdillon JF, Day EA. *Spinal Manipulation.* 4th ed. Norwalk, Conn: Appleton & Lange; 1987.
17. Grieve GP. *Common Vertebral Joint Problems.* 2nd ed. Edinburgh, Scotland: Churchill-Livingstone; 1988.
18. Bergmann TK, Peterson DH, Lawrence DJ. *Chiropractic Technique Principles and Procedures.* New York, NY: Churchill-Livingstone; 1993.
19. Triano JJ. The subluxation complex: outcome measure of chiropractic diagnosis and treatment. *J Chiro Tech.* 1990;2:114–120.
20. Kirkaldy-Willis WH, ed. *Managing Low Back Pain.* 2nd ed. New York, NY: Churchill-Livingstone; 1988.
21. Bigos SJ, Boyer OR, Braen GR, et al. *Clinical Practice Guideline Number 14: Acute Low Back Pain in Adults.* Rockville, Md: US Department of Health and Human Services, Public Health Service, Agency for Health Care Policy and Research; 1994.
22. Bergmann TF. The chiropractic spinal examination. In: Ferezy JS, ed. *The Chiropractic Neurological Examination.* Gaithersburg, Md: Aspen Publishers, Inc; 1992.
23. O'Brien JG. Acute pain in the elderly. *Postgrad Med.* August 1992:49–56.
24. Kligman EW, Pepin E. Prescribing physical activity for older patients. *Geriatrics.* 1992;47:33–47.
25. Wyke B. Cervical articular contributions to posture and gait: their relationship to senile disequilibrium. *Age Ageing.* 1979;8:251–257.
26. Paris SV. Cervical symptoms of forward head posture. *Top Geriatr Rehabil.* 1990;5:11–19.
27. Lazaro L, Quinet RJ. Low back pain: how to make the diagnosis in the older patient. *Geriatrics.* 1994;49:48–53.
28. Chakravarty KK, Webley M. Disorders of the shoulder: an often unrecognized cause of disability in elderly people. *Br Med J.* 1990;300:848–849.
29. O'Reilly D, Bernstein RM. Shoulder pain in the elderly. *Br Med J.* 1990;301:503–504. Editorial.
30. Janse JJ. *Principles and Practice of Chiropractic, Gerontology in Chiropractic Practice.* Lombard, Ill: National College of Chiropractic; 1976.
31. Zucker A. Chapman's reflexes: medicine or metaphysics? *J Am Osteopath Assoc.* 1993;93:346–352.

19

Trauma in the Geriatric Patient: A Chiropractic Perspective with a Focus on Prevention

Lisa Zaynab Killinger

I am 38 years old. Over the winter break, I broke my arm in a somewhat bizarre sledding accident involving a plastic sled and an unintentional flight over a large snow ramp. On the same day, a 5-year-old boy I know sustained the same Colles' fracture of the radius and ulna that I did.

The three decades of age difference between us soon became apparent in the way we recovered from our respective traumas. About 5 weeks after fracture, the 5-year-old boy was out of his cast and back on ice skates, flying around like nothing had ever happened. In the meanwhile, my cast had been replaced with an internal/external fixator consisting of three pins, four screws, and a rather space-age device to uncrush my radius. I did 3 months of physical therapy to get my hand to function properly. After the fixator was removed, I did another 2 months of therapy to regain the use of my wrist and arm. Almost 5 months later, my arm still is not completely back to normal.

This incident made me think about how someone three decades older than me would be affected by a similar trauma. In fact, some of the older patients I saw in physical therapy were struggling a year after Colles' fractures to gain enough hand strength to open a can, jar, or package of food. Experience taught me that these older patients were not lazy, but rather were experiencing a longer recovery simply due to their age.

Chiropractors, are caring for an increasingly older population of patients. It is our responsibility to learn about how health care providers, can successfully manage and prevent trauma in our geriatric patients.

OUR AGING WORLD

We live in a world marked by a rapidly aging population. By the year 2030, there will be about 70 million older persons, more than twice the number seen in 1990. Those 65 and older are projected to represent 13% of the population in the year 2000; by the year 2030 they will comprise 20%.[1]

When faced with the statistics on health care and the aging population, we can view the statistics as apocalyptic, or as an opportunity to refine our health care system to better care for those who will use it most. In America, older people accounted for 37% of all hospital stays in 1994.[2] In the late 1980s, older persons represented only 12% of the US population,[1] but accounted for 36% of the total personal health care expenditures. These expenditures totaled $162 billion (an average of $5,360 per person) in contrast with only $1,290 per person per year for younger Americans.[2] The chiropractic profession must recognize that health care is primarily geriatric health care, and it will remain so for quite some time.

TRAUMATIC INJURY OF OLDER PERSONS

Trauma is the fifth leading cause of death in patients over 65 years of age,[3,4] and injuries sustained by this population are much more likely to have a fatal outcome.[5,6] The factors that predispose geriatric patients to injury may be hearing and vision deficits, balance or equilibrium disturbances, or cognitive losses. Musculoskeletal changes such as bone loss and muscle atrophy also may be contributing factors.

In chiropractic practice, we care for many geriatric patients who may experience traumatic injury. It is our respon-

---

Adapted from *Top Clin Chiro* 1998; 5(3): 10–15
© 1998 Aspen Publishers, Inc.

Ryan Kain assisted in obtaining research for the preparation of this chapter.

sibility to understand the types of traumatic injuries to which older patients are prone, to offer preventive services, to provide comprehensive patient care to injured patients, and to offer or facilitate rehabilitative services.

GOALS FOR GERIATRIC TRAUMA PATIENTS

The basic principle that guides geriatric health care is its emphasis on function.[7] Therefore our care of geriatric trauma patients should be focused on the restoration of function. In this way, we can maximize our geriatric patient's ability to perform activities of daily living and subsequently promote his or her independence. This concept of independence, although important to all patients, is critical to the self-esteem and will to survive in older patients.

COMMON GERIATRIC TRAUMATIC INJURIES

Trauma in older patients can be classified into three major categories: fall-related injuries, motor vehicle accidents, and pedestrian injuries. Nearly 80% of traumas in patients over 65 are due to these three mechanisms of injury. Moreover, falls alone account for nearly half of all trauma in older patients.[8] These findings contrast to the mechanisms of injury in younger persons. Violence (such as beatings, stabbings or gunshot wounds) is responsible for over 25% of injuries in younger patients, and automobile accidents are responsible for nearly 33%.[3,8]

Fractures and falls

Castillo and Pousada[4] report that older patients have a seven times greater rate of fall-related injuries than younger patients (under 55 years old). This figure is based on emergency department (ED) data. The data also indicate that fractures comprise 23% to 37% of ED diagnoses in older patients.[4] The most common fractures involve the hip, proximal humerus, wrist, and spine (compression fractures).[9]

Motor vehicle accidents

Approximately 28% of all injuries to older persons are due to motor vehicle accidents. Poor vision, hearing deficits, and slower reaction times may all contribute to this statistic. In addition, a lower rate of seat belt use in older drivers could be a contributing factor. A more complete discussion of these issues can be found later in this article.

EFFECTS OF AGE ON RECOVERY FROM TRAUMATIC INJURY

The ways in which an older body responds to injury are unique. Health professionals, including chiropractors, are just beginning to understand and appreciate the distinctions in the diagnoses and prognoses of older versus younger patients. Although patients 65 and older are less likely to be injured than other age groups, injuries in this age group are, unfortunately, more likely to have a fatal outcome.[5] More specifically, trauma to the central nervous system (ie, brain or spinal cord injury) has a mortality rate of nearly 90% in geriatric patients.[10,11]

Why do older patients die from trauma that would be survived by younger patients? Although it was once thought that chronic diseases were responsible for poorer outcomes in geriatric trauma patients, research does not support this theory.[5,9,11] The reasons for this disparity are complex, and both physiologic and psychosocial concerns play a role.

RECOVERY GOALS OF OLDER TRAUMA PATIENTS: ARE THEY DIFFERENT FROM THE DOCTOR'S GOALS?

The goals for which the physician strives may differ quite markedly from the goals of the geriatric patient. Whereas the provider must be desirous of facilitating the patient's progress in improved scores on outcome assessments and return to normal ranges of motion, the patient's goal may be much more straightforward—independence.

Perhaps the most profound impact that traumatic injury can have on the geriatric patient is a decrease in the patient's ability to care for himself or herself. If this concept is hard to visualize, try to imagine having to ask for help every time you need to open a package, envelope, jar, can, or container (all tasks requiring two functional hands). Or imagine suddenly requiring assistance in getting dressed. These tasks are simple for the able-bodied individual but quite impossible for an older trauma victim. This inability to perform daily tasks may have a huge impact on the individual's self-esteem, pride, and will to survive. The "will to live" is crucial to the health status of all patients, but particularly so in older patients.

With older patients, it is particularly important, to talk about what activities they are limited in performing due to their injury. The doctor may not understand the injury's full impact on the patient's daily life. The doctor should work with the older patient to develop a strategy to regain abilities that the patient perceives as most important for the activities he or she pursues. Depression can be a serious concomitant factor in the recovery from traumatic injury. Patients must not feel alone in their struggle to return to independent living.

THE ROLE OF CHIROPRACTIC IN THE MANAGEMENT OF OLDER TRAUMA PATIENTS

Acute phase

Typically, a chiropractor may not be the only health care provider involved in the management of traumatic injury in the older patient. The most common cause of injuries in older patients is falling, with the most common injuries being fractures of the hip, wrist, or spine. These injuries will first be managed in an emergency department, followed by an orthopaedic surgeon's office. The traditional strategies used for management of fractures may include casting, splinting, metal pins and screws, or prosthetic devices.

Ambulatory phase

The chiropractor may gain his or her first access to the trauma patient once the patient is ambulatory. The alteration of normal gait (in immobilized lower extremity injuries) or in arm and shoulder girdle use (in arm or wrist fractures) will almost certainly affect the larger musculoskeletal picture of every patient. With chiropractic's focus on joint and spinal mechanics, chiropractors are a suitable choice for the care of the injured patient, particularly in the non-emergency phase of treatment.

When co-management occurs, it is in the patient's best interest for providers to have regular communication on management issues. A co-managed patient is much more likely to share important information if he or she knows that the providers are also communicating with each other. Providers may also be able to enhance the appropriateness and relevance of their care if they are aware of other providers' management plans.[12] Frequently chiropractic care is only a part of a larger team of essential providers in the care of a serious traumatic injury. Although most chiropractors are comfortable with leaving orthopaedic surgery to the surgeons, their role relative to other providers (eg, physical therapists, neurologists, home care specialists, case managers) can be clouded. Through open communication and discussion, the role of the chiropractor in caring for the complex musculoskeletal and neurologic intricacies of a trauma patient can be made clear to the patient and to the other providers.

The chiropractor's contribution to the team

Chiropractic attention to the spine may be appropriate in any traumatic injury to the limbs, back, head, or chest. Although it is beyond the scope of this article to examine in-depth biomechanical relationships of the spine with general trauma, the obvious kinetic linkage of muscular attachments and articular relationships between the extremities and the axial skeleton suggests that stresses and compensations in the periphery may influence spinal function. The sheer weight of casts and the effects of long-term joint immobilization can have a devastating impact on a patient's functional status. The chiropractor can help a patient regain the ability to perform the activities of daily living important to the patient. Some chiropractic adjustive procedures and other mechanical strategies may require modification in older patients. Excellent discussions of chiropractic techniques appropriate for older patients are offered by Bergmann and Larson[13] and McCarthy.[14]

Extremity adjustment also may play an important role in enhancing and maintaining extremity joint function. The chiropractor's contribution is often enhanced once any orthopaedic immobilizing devices have been removed and the rehabilitation phase of the injury is begun. For example, a wrist that has been immobilized due to a fractured radius may benefit greatly from gentle, specific adjustment, when indicated. The return to mobility after months in a cast or splint is a joyous, albeit painful, event for a trauma patient, and gentle passive movements typical of some manipulative and adjustive interventions help speed return of function.

Other members of the trauma management team

Athletic trainers, physical therapists, and occupational therapists (to name a few) are important members of the health care team for a trauma patient. In fact, their expertise in the muscular component of injury is complementary to chiropractic and orthopaedic care. The rehabilitation of a patient is a time-consuming, long-range process, one that may best be facilitated by experts in rehabilitation.[3,7] These experts may be the professionals listed above, or they may be chiropractors with specialized training (eg, a diplomate in rehabilitation).

The rehabilitation of a geriatric trauma patient may involve tasks that are not routine for most chiropractors (eg, applying and changing bandages and dressings). Nursing professionals or rehabilitation staff with training in wound and postoperative care might be more appropriate choices to manage these patient care tasks. Again, communication between providers on the rehabilitation team is crucial to the management of the geriatric trauma patient.

It is important to recognize the potential advantages of a team approach to trauma management. Chiropractors can be essential elements of the trauma care team, and both patients and providers will gain much from a treatment plan that is collaboratively developed and executed.

STRATEGIES FOR PREVENTION

Chiropractors often emphasize prevention and strive to improve balance and proprioception through appropriate care. Balance and proprioception are important factors in the prevention of falls, which account for most traumatic injuries to older patients.

Although chiropractic adjustments are important to patients, chiropractors and their office staff can assume a more active role in counseling patients in the prevention of traumatic injuries. This counseling might address motor vehicle use, safety in the home, exercise and nutrition, osteoporosis, and hormone replacement therapy. Algorithm 1 identifies trauma prevention strategies.

Automobile safety

Older patients did not grow up wearing seat belts, nor was any emphasis placed on teaching this segment of the population the importance of their use. Encouraging seat belt use is every doctor's responsibility. In fact counseling on the importance of seat belt use, along with periodic vision and hearing screening to identify deficits, is a recommended preventive strategy for health care providers.[15] Chiropractic offices may choose to offer incentive programs for patients participating in such "wellness activities." Seat belt use is a good habit worthy of reminders.

Driving: Is it time to turn over the keys?

Many older people continue to drive long after they have lost the ability to do so safely. As physicians we may be able to offer a professional opinion on a patient's driving status. A patient who demonstrates vision or hearing losses or impaired reaction times should be counseled on the advisability of continued driving. The physician's opinion may be the deciding factor, which could save the patient severe injury or death.

Perhaps the biggest challenge in this area is the direct conflict such a decision presents with the older person's most desired goal of independence. Therefore, the chiropractor must identify community resources, as well as enlist family and friends, to aid in this transition.

Safety in the home

Many simple steps can be taken to reduce the risk of injury and falls at home (eg, removing throw rugs or rugs with curled edges, repairing loose banisters, installing rails or banisters on porches and steps, and installing non-slip strips on stairs). In fact, several environmental or fall hazards checklists exist that allow patients and their families to identify conditions in the home that may precipitate a fall or other injury. Any patient experiencing gait or balance deficits, or anyone over the age of 50, should complete such a checklist.

Other simple and relatively inexpensive home modifications may offer significant help and facilitate independence. Representative examples include installing different shape knobs on drawers, using lever-style door handles, installing support bars in tubs or showers, and locating stools and seats in areas where tasks are routinely performed.

Patients of all ages appreciate a doctor who cares about them as a whole person. Taking an active role in keeping patients healthy at home is a worthwhile use of time.

Exercise, nutrition, and prevention

The patient can play an active role in preventing traumatic injury through appropriate nutrition and exercise. Soundness of muscular function and heightened fitness levels can help prevent falls and pedestrian accidents—two of the three leading causes of trauma to older patients.[16] Often injury results because the patient lacks the muscular strength to catch himself or herself after tripping or slipping. Chiropractors can and should encourage patients to be physically active in order to maintain and promote muscular coordination and fitness. Chiropractors also should be vigilant in observing the patient's weight patterns for evidence of poor or inadequate nutrition. A patient weakened by poor nutrition is at greater risk for falls and injury. Nutritional neglect may be the result of difficulty with meal preparation, problems with opening packaging, or lack of access to fresh foods. Advice on proper nutrition may require the doctor to explore issues regarding access to foods and their preparation. Specific questions regarding how often a patient gets to the store, how much time and difficulty are involved in cooking and eating, and other similar questions will provide insight.

Osteoporosis

Osteoporosis, the most common skeletal disorder in the world, is the second most common cause of disability in older persons.[17] Osteoporosis is the main reason why falls that do not jeopardize a younger patient's health can be quite serious in older individuals. Statistics reveal there are 1.3 million osteoporotic fractures sustained annually.[18]

Osteoporosis may be first discovered in the chiropractor's office through radiography. Because 30% to 50% of skeletal calcium may be lost before osteoporosis is detected on a plain film radiograph, any level of osteoporosis should be reported to the patient and the patient's other health care providers. Further radiographic studies designed to quantify bone density may be needed if osteoporosis is apparent on plain films.[19-21]

A diagnosis of osteoporosis may influence the chiropractor's selection of chiropractic adjusting techniques. In some cases, it may preclude the use of forceful adjusting techniques to prevent iatrogenic fractures. Specific adjustment techniques may require modification as discussed by Bergmann and Larson.[13]

It is important for the chiropractor to be aware of the geriatric patient's bone density status and to counsel the patient who is at risk for osteoporosis-related fractures. Chiropractors can, in most states, advise patients on dietary and exercise programs that can prevent osteoporosis or arrest its progression. This type of patient education is appropriate for patients of all ages, because this disease manifests itself slowly over several decades. Osteoporosis can take years to reverse.

Hormone replacement therapy: A sensitive issue

An older patient's medical physician may suggest hormone replacement therapy (HRT) for osteoporosis. This topic remains controversial within the medical and pharmaceutical fields.[17,18,22,23] Any advice on drug therapy lies outside the chiropractic scope of practice,[24] however, patients and family members may seek information on this topic from many health care providers, and they may appreciate receiving current literature on this topic. Two concise overviews of the literature can be found elsewhere.[22,23] Furthermore, patients with osteoporosis should be counseled on home safety due to their increased risk for fractures.

CONCLUSION

Most articles on trauma in geriatric patients are found outside the chiropractic literature.[3–11,15–23] Existing chiropractic literature on geriatrics does not focus on traumatic injury specifically.[13,14,25–31] Opportunities for research and case studies on the chiropractic management of the geriatric trauma patient are immense and relevant, given that chiropractic is the most widely used alternative/complementary health care profession.[28,31]

Of particular importance is the growth of the geriatric patient population. As chiropractic use patterns and the older patient population increase, a greater need will exist to provide health and information services to geriatric patients. Quality-of-life issues are sure to increase and, as more and more older people remain active longer, the prevalence of traumatic injury is destined to rise. All health professionals must address techniques for the management of geriatric patients,[32] particularly those with traumatic injuries.

In addition to the treatment of trauma, the prevention of trauma should be a focus in chiropractic training. The chiropractic profession is well suited to take on a leadership role in prevention services, given our philosophical emphasis on wellness and our training in conservative musculoskeletal patient care strategies.[30] The shift of some of our nation's vast health resources toward prevention may result in a decreased need for emergency and rehabilitative geriatric health services and a healthier older population. Healthy, functional, independent older patients is an important goal for all health care providers.

REFERENCES

1. Bureau of the Census. *Statistical Abstracts of the United States, 1996.*
2. US Department of Health and Human Services. *A Profile of Older Americans: 1996.* Administration on Aging and the Program Resources Dept. American Association of Retired Persons.
3. Champion HR, Copes WS, Buyer D, et al. Major trauma in geriatric patients. *Am J Public Health.* 1989;79:1278–1282.
4. Castillo PA, Pousada L. Emergency services use by elderly individuals. *Clin Geriatr Med.* 1993;9(3):491–497.
5. Horst HM, Obeid FN, Soren VJ, et al. Factors influencing survival of elderly trauma patients. *Crit Care Med.* 1986;14:681–684.
6. Broos TL, Stappers KH, Rommens PM. Polytrauma in patients sixty five and over: injury patterns and outcome. *Int Surg.* 1998;73:119–122.
7. Mosqueda LA. Assessment of rehabilitation potential. *Clin Geriatr Med.* 1993;9(4):689–699.
8. Baker SP, Harvey AM. Fall injuries in the elderly. *Clin Geriatr Med.* 1985;1:501–512.
9. Levy DB, Hanlon DP, Townsend RN. Geriatric trauma. *Clin Geriatr Med.* 1993;9(3):601–620.
10. Miller JD, Butterworth JF, Grundeman SK, et al. Further experience in the management of severe head injury. *J Neurosurg.* 1981;54:289–299.
11. Oreskovich MR, Howard JD, Copass MK, et al. Geriatric trauma: injury pattern and outcome. *J Trauma.* 1984;24:565–572.
12. Hawk C, Nyiendo J, Lawrence D, Killinger L. The role of chiropractors in the delivery of interdisciplinary health care in rural areas. *J Manipulative Physiol Ther.* 1996;19(2):82–91.
13. Bergmann TF, Larson L. Manipulative care and older persons. *Top Clin Chiro.* 1996;3(2):56–65.
14. McCarthy KA. Management considerations in the geriatric patient. *Top Clin Chiro.* 1996;3(2):66–75.
15. Rubenstein LZ. Update on preventive medicine for older people. *Generations.* 1996–1997;4:47–53.
16. Schwab CW, Kauder DR. Trauma in the geriatric patient. *Arch Surg.* 1992;127:701–704.
17. Holbrook TL, et al. The frequency, occurrence, impact, and cost of musculoskeletal conditions in the United States. In: *Proceedings: American Academy of Orthopedic Surgeons.* Chicago; 1985.
18. Cummings SR, et al. Epidemiology of osteoporosis and osteoporotic fractures. *Epidemiol Rev.* 1985;7:178–208.
19. Taylor JAM, Hoffman LE. The geriatric patient: diagnostic imaging of common musculoskeletal disorders. *Top Clin Chiro.* 1996;3(2):23–45.
20. Genant HK, Boyd D. Quantitative bone mineral analysis using dual-energy computed tomography. *Invest Radiol.* 1977;12:545–551.
21. Sartoris DJ, Sommer FG, Marcus R, Maadvig P. Bone mineral density in the femoral neck: quantitative analysis using dual energy projection radiography. *Am J Roentgenol.* 1985;144:605–611.
22. Yaffe K, et al. Estrogen therapy in postmenopausal women. *JAMA.* 1998;279(9):688–695.
23. Petrovich H, et al. Pros and cons of postmenopausal hormone replacement therapy. *Clin Care Update.* Winter 1996–1997:7–12.
24. Lamm LC, Wegner E, Collord D. Chiropractic scope of practice: what the law allows–update 1993. *J Manipulative Physiol Ther.* 1995;18(1):16–20.
25. Kohler A. Balancing act: changes in equilibrium trip up elderly. *ACA J Chiro.* 1991;28(10):34–36.
26. Kovar MG, Feinleib M. Older Americans present a double challenge: preventing disability and providing care. *ACA J Chiro.* 1991;28(10):28–30.
27. Souza T, Soliman S. Back to basics: normal aging. *Top Clin Chiro.* 1996;3(2):1–9.
28. Coulter ID, Hurwitz EL, Aronow HU, Cassata DM, Beck JC. Chiropractic patients in a comprehensive home-based geriatric assessment, follow-up and health promotion program. *Top Clin Chiro.* 1996;3(2):46–55.

29. Bowers LJ. Clinical assessment of geriatric patients: unique challenges. *Top Clin Chiro*. 1996;3(2):10–22.
30. Hawk C, Killinger LZ, Zapotocky B, Azad A. Chiropractic training in care of the geriatric patient: an assessment. *J Neuromusculoskel Sys*. 1997;5(1):15–25.
31. Hurwitz EL, et al. Use of chiropractic services from 1985 through 1991 in the United States and Canada. *Am J Public Health*. 1998;88(5):771–777.
32. *Shortage of Health Professions Caring for the Elderly: Recommendations for Change. A report by the chairman of the select committee on aging; House of Representatives*. Washington, DC: Government Printing Office; 1993. Com. publication 102–915.

Algorithm 1

Trauma prevention strategies in older patients

Killinger L. Trauma in the geriatric patient:
A chiropractic perspective with a focus on prevention.
Topics in Clinical Chiropractic 1998; 5(3).
Seed Algorithm by Linda J. Bowers, DC

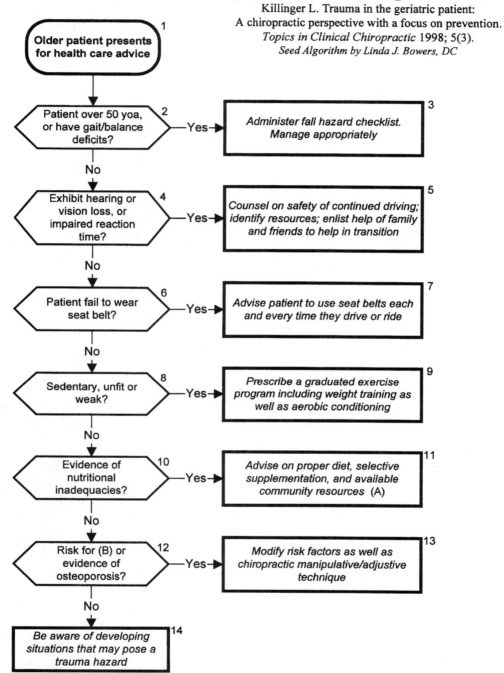

Annotations:
(A) e.g., Meals-on-Wheels, food stamps, grocery delivery services
(B) e.g., over age 60, thin, sedentary, Caucasian/Asian, family history, female, postmenopausal, cigarette smoking, excessive alcohol, fiber, caffeine consumption, inadequate dietary calcium or vitamin D intake

APPENDIX III–A

Internet Sites for Seniors

General Information:

Administration on Aging	pr.aoa.dhhs.gov/
American Association of Retired Persons	www.aarp.org
American Physical Therapy Association Section on Geriatrics	geriatricspt.org
Elderhelp	www.elderhelp.com
Merck Manual of Geriatrics	www.merck.com/pub/mm_geriatrics/
National Council on Aging	www.ncoa.org/
National Council of Senior Citizens	www.ncscinc.org
Senior.Com	www.senior.com
Spry Foundation	www.spry.org/
Third Age	www.thirdage.com

Cancer Information:

American Cancer Society	www.cancer.org/
Cancer Care, Inc.	www.cancercareinc.org/
CANCERLIT Topic Searches	cancernet.nci.nih.gov/canlit/canlit.htm
CancerNet	cancernet.nci.nih.gov
Cansearch	www.access.digex.net/~mkragen/index.html
NCI Cancer Information Service	cancernet.nci.nih.gov/occdocs/cis/cis.html
The National Cancer Institute Cancer Centers Program	cancernet.nci.nih.gov/global/glo_pt.htm#nci-designated
PDQ	cancernet.nci.nih.gov/pdq.htm
OncoLink	oncolink.upenn.edu/

Index

A

Activities of daily living index, geriatric patient, 176
Acute lymphocytic leukemia, 57–59
    clinical algorithm, 58
    laboratory tests and studies, 58
    prognosis, 59
    signs and symptoms, 58
    treatment, 58–59
Adolescent
    back pain, 70–71
    on-line and text health resources, 85
    periodic health examination, ages 13-18, 83–84
    subluxation, pathology, 70–71
Adverse drug reaction, geriatric patient, 186
Aging, 159–166
    bladder, 166
    bone, 164
    cardiovascular system
        clinical features, 164–165, 165
        response to exercise, 165
    categories, 159
    central nervous system
        anatomy, 160
        morphology, 160
        motor, 162
        neurophysiologic changes, 160
        normal, 160–163
        sensory, 160–162
        sleep, 162–163
        structure, 160
    characteristics, 159
    connective tissue, 164
    consequences, 161–162
    demographics, 204
    effects, 160
    exercise, 186–189
    gastrointestinal tract, 166
    hematologic alterations, 165
    joint, 164
    kidney, 165–166
    musculoskeletal system, 163–164
        fat pad syndrome, 163
        muscle cramp, 164
        spontaneous muscular fasciculation, 163–164
    pulmonary system, 166
    spine, 164
    temporomandibular joint, 164
    theories, 159–160
    vs. disuse or misuse, 159
AIDS, resources, 154
Algorithm by consensus, xviii
Anabolic therapy, osteoporosis, 107
Analgesic, otitis media, 37
Antihistamine, otitis media, 37
Anti-inflammatory drug, otitis media, 37
Apex contact, geriatric patient, 202
Atherosclerosis, 6
Atlanto-occipital articulation, geriatric patient, 200–201
Autism, 46–48
    case study, 47–48
    informational resources, 47
    signs, 46
    treatment, 46–47

B

Back pain, 199
    adolescent, 70–71
    child, 70–71
Bilateral (double) thenars, geriatric patient, 201
Bilateral thenar occiput, geriatric patient
    prone, 200
    sitting, 200
Bladder, aging, 166
Body composition, child, 27
Bone, aging, 164
Bone mass density, 100
Bone tumor, child, 60–61
    laboratory tests, 61
    prognosis, 61
    signs and symptoms, 60–61
    treatment, 61
Brain tumor, child, 59–60
    risk factors, 59
    signs and symptoms, 60
    treatment, 60
Breast cancer, 124–134
    causation theories, 127–128
    classification, 129–130
    clinical algorithm
        clinical breast examination, 134
        diagnostic mammography, 133
    diagnosis, 131
    epidemiology, 124–125
    laboratory markers, 130–131
    prevention, 128–129
    primary prevention, 128

resources, 154
risk factors, 125–127
secondary prevention, 129
signs and symptoms, 130
staging, 130
tertiary prevention, 129
traditional therapies, 131
unconventional therapies, 131

C

Calcaneal cervical break, geriatric patient, 201
Calcitonin, osteoporosis, 106
Calcium, osteoporosis, 104–105
Cancer
   child, 56
      bone tumor, 60–61
      brain tumor, 59–60
      chiropractor's role, 64, 66
      comparison of adult cancer, 57
      epidemiology, 56–57
      life after, 65–66
      nutritional aspects, 66
      psychosocial aspects, 66
      red flags, 57
      risk factors, 57
   resources, 155
Cardiorespiratory fitness, child, 27
Cardiovascular system
   aging
      clinical features, 164–165, 165
      response to exercise, 165
   health resources, 155
Care pathway, xv, xvii
Central nervous system, aging
   anatomy, 160
   morphology, 160
   motor, 162
   neurophysiologic changes, 160
   normal, 160–163
   sensory, 160–162
   sleep, 162–163
   structure, 160
Cerebral palsy, 44–46
   case study, 45–46
   categories, 44, 45
   etiology, 44
   problems associated with, 44, 45
   treatment, 44–45
Cervical compression-translation, geriatric patient, 201
Cervical distraction, geriatric patient, 201
Cervical manipulation, otitis media, 35
Cervical spine, rotational adjustments, 77–78
Child, xiii. *See also* Special needs child
   back pain, 70–71
   behavioral choices, 19
   body composition, 27
   bone tumor, 60–61
      laboratory tests, 61
      prognosis, 61
      signs and symptoms, 60–61
      treatment, 61
   brain tumor, 59–60
      risk factors, 59
      signs and symptoms, 60
      treatment, 60
   cancer, 56
      chiropractor's role, 64, 66
      comparison of adult cancer, 57
      epidemiology, 56–57
      life after, 65–66
      psychosocial aspects, 66
      red flags, 57
      risk factors, 57
   cardiorespiratory fitness, 27
   clinical assessment, 3–15
   diagnostic imaging, 25, 26
   dietary behavior, 17–18
   endurance, 27–28
   flexibility, 27
   health history, 22–23
      elements, 22
   health promotion, 16–19
   Hodgkin's lymphoma, 62–63
      laboratory tests, 63
      prognosis, 63
      signs and symptoms, 63
   injury prevention counseling, 28
   internet health sites, 86
   musculoskeletal examination, 24–25
   nervous system examination, 24–25
   neuroblastoma, 61–62
      laboratory tests, 62
      prognosis, 62
      signs and symptoms, 61–62
   non-Hodgkin's lymphoma, 63–65
      laboratory tests, 64
      prognosis, 65
      signs and symptoms, 64
   nutrition assessment, 26–27
   periodic health examination, 21–28
      ages 2-6, 81
      ages 7-12, 82
      birth to 18 months, 80
   physical examination, 23–25
   practice guidelines, 8
   sexual behavior, 18–19
   social drug use, 16–17
   spinal adjustment, 69–78
      adjusting apparatus, 72–74, 75, 76
      adjustive technique modifications, 71–76
      age-related changes, 71–72
      positioning options, 72–74, 75, 76
      specificity of contact points, 72, 73
      thrust characteristics, 73–76
   strength, 27–28
   subluxation, 69
      pathology, 70–71
   vertebrobasilar stroke, 76–78
      cervical spine rotational adjustments, 77–78
      incidence, 76–77
      mechanism of injury, 76–77
Chiropractic research, research policies, xiii
Cholesterol, 6, 92–93
Clinical algorithm, xv
   action box, xx, xxi
   acute lymphocytic leukemia, 58
   breast cancer
      clinical breast examination, 134
      diagnostic mammography, 133
   caveat, xv
   clinical state box, xx, xxi
   critiquing, xxiii
   decision box, xx, xxi
   defined, xvii
   development, xviii, xxvi
   diagnostic sequences, xx
   endpoints of therapeutic cycles, xx
   end-users, xix
   geriatric patient
      clinical assessment, 181–182
      mental status assessment, 183
      trauma prevention strategies, 210
   heart disease, women's risk factors, 98
   history, xvi
   hypercholesterolemia, 15
   implementation, xviii
   improving, xxiii
   infantile colic, 55

lead toxicity, 4
leukemia, 58
link box, xx, xxi
osteoporosis, prevention, 112
otitis media, 12, 13
partner abuse, identifying victim, 152–153
premenstrual syndrome, management, 122–123
relevance, xv
sudden infant death syndrome, 11
terminology, xvi
testing, xxiii
titling, xx, xxii
use of annotations, xx, xxii
writing, xix
Clinical guideline, xvii
Colic. *See* Infantile colic
Comprehensive geriatric assessment, 168
Connective tissue, aging, 164

D

Denver Developmental Screening Test, 23
Diagnostic imaging
    child, 25, 26
    infant, 25, 26
Diet, premenstrual syndrome, 118
Dietary behavior, child, 17–18
Disphosphate, osteoporosis, 107
Domestic abuse. *See* Partner abuse
Down syndrome, 48–49
    characteristics, 48
Dual-energy X-ray absorptiometry, 102
Dual-photon absorptiometry, 102

E

Eating disorder, resources, 155
Elderly client, xiv
Endometriosis, resources, 155
Endurance, child, 27–28
Estrogen, 113
    osteoporosis, 106–107
Ewing's sarcoma, 60–61
Exercise
    aging, 186–189
    cool-down exercises, 188
    defined, 26–27

geriatric patient, 186–189
    preventing chronic gradual loss, 192–193
premenstrual syndrome, 118
warm-up exercises, 188

F

Falling
    geriatric patient, 169–170
        risk factors, 170
    osteoporosis, 100
        risk factors, 100
Family planning, resources, 155
Fat pad syndrome, 163
Fertility, resources, 155
Flexibility
    child, 27
    women, 136–137
Fluoride, osteoporosis, 107
Forward head posture, 198–199
Functional assessment, geriatric patient, 175–176

G

Gait, 198
Gait disturbance, 7
Gastrointestinal tract, aging, 166
Geriatric patient, 170–171
    activities of daily living index, 176
    activity inhibitors, 190–191
    adverse drug reaction, 186
    apex contact, 202
    atlanto-occipital articulation, 200–201
    atypical presentations, 185–186
    bilateral (double) thenars, 201
    bilateral thenar occiput
        prone, 200
        sitting, 200
    calcaneal cervical break, 201
    cervical compression-translation, 201
    cervical distraction, 201
    changes in health care strategies, 185
    clinical algorithm
        clinical assessment, 181–182
        mental status assessment, 183
        trauma prevention strategies, 210
    clinical assessment, 168–183

connective tissue, 189–190
degeneration, 189–190
diagnostic testing, 177–179
exercise, 186–189
    preventing chronic gradual loss, 192–193
falling, 169–170
    risk factors, 170
family relationships, 184
frail health
    causes, 190–191
    preventing, 190
functional assessment, 175–176
health history, 169–171
ilio-costal lift, 202
immunization, 170
incontinence, 170
instrumental activities of daily living scale, 176
Internet sites, 211
lack of knowledge about exercise, 190
lifestyle factors, 170–171
living arrangements, 184
lumbar spine, 202
lumbosacral stretch, 202
management, 184–193
manipulative care, 195–203
    clinical findings of joint dysfunction, 197
    forms of manual therapy, 195–196
    mnemonic PARTS, 197–198
    mobilization, 196
    procedures, 199–203
    soft tissue technique, 196–197
    traction, 196
mental health status assessment, 172–175
morbidity
    functional disability, 184–185
    health disability, 184–185
multiple pathologies, 185
nutrition, 191–192
nutritional assessment, 176–177
pelvic blocking, 202
pelvis, 202
physical examination, 171–172, 173–174
preventing acute and subacute episodes of physiologic loss, 191
promoting wellness, 191–192
response to therapy, 186
rest dogma, 190

screening test, 170–171
sitting thoracic, 201–202
stair-stepping, 201
stiffness, 189–190
techniques for geriatric interviewing, 171, 172
thoracic rock, 201
trauma, 204–210
  automobile safety, 207
  common injuries, 205
  driving, 207
  effects of age on recovery, 205
  epidemiology, 204–205
  exercise, 207
  falls, 205
  fractures, 205
  goals, 205
  home safety, 207
  hormone replacement therapy, 207–208
  motor vehicle accidents, 205
  nutrition, 207
  osteoporosis, 207
  prevention, 206–208
  role of chiropractice in management, 205–206
unique aspects of geriatric health care, 185–186
vision and hearing tests, 172
vital signs, 171–172
Growing pains, 6–7
Gynecological care, resources, 155

H

Health history
  child, 22–23
    elements, 22
  infant, 22–23
    elements, 22
Health promotion, child, 16–19
Heart disease, women, 89–98
  characteristics, 89–90
  cholesterol, 92–93
  hypertension, 90–91
  management, 95
  menopause, 93
  obesity, 93–94
  pathogenesis, 90
  plasma homocysteine, 95
  risk factors, clinical algorithm, 98
  smoking, 94
  thrombogenic risk factors, 94–95

Hodgkin's lymphoma, child, 62–63
  laboratory tests, 63
  prognosis, 63
  signs and symptoms, 63
Hormone replacement therapy, 207–208
Hypercholesterolemia, 6
  clinical algorithm, 15
Hypertension, 90–91
Hysterectomy, resources, 155

I

Ilio-costal lift, geriatric patient, 202
Immobility, 198
Immunization, 170
Incontinence, geriatric patient, 170
Infant
  clinical assessment, 3–15
  diagnostic imaging, 25, 26
  health history, 22–23
    elements, 22
  musculoskeletal examination, 24–25
  nervous system examination, 24–25
  neuroblastoma, 61–62
    laboratory tests, 62
    prognosis, 62
    signs and symptoms, 61–62
  nutrition assessment, 25–26
  periodic health examination, 21–28
Infantile colic, 50–55
  biomedical causes, 50–51
  clinical algorithm, 55
  clinical manifestations, 51
  definition, 50
  epidemiology, 51
  etiology, 50–51
  incidence, 51
  management, 51–53
  psychological and social causes, 51
Injury prevention counseling, child, 28
Instrumental activities of daily living scale, geriatric patient, 176

J

Joint, aging, 164

K

Kidney, aging, 165–166

L

Lead toxicity, 5–6
  clinical algorithm, 4
Leg length inequality, 135, 136
Leukemia, 57–59
  clinical algorithm, 58
  laboratory tests and studies, 58
  signs and symptoms, 58
  treatment, 58
Local heat, otitis media, 36–37
Low back pain, 199
Lumbar spine, geriatric patient, 202
Lumbosacral stretch, geriatric patient, 202

M

Manipulation
  geriatric patient, 195–203
    clinical findings of joint dysfunction, 197
    forms of manual therapy, 195–196
    mnemonic PARTS, 197–198
    mobilization, 196
    procedures, 199–203
    soft tissue technique, 196–197
    traction, 196
    terminology, 136
Menopause, 93
  resources, 155
Menstrual cycle, 113–114
Mental health, resources, 156
Mental health status assessment, geriatric patient, 172–175
Morbidity, geriatric patient
  functional disability, 184–185
  health disability, 184–185
Muscle cramp, 164
Muscle strength, 198
Musculoskeletal conditions, 6–8
Musculoskeletal examination
  child, 24–25
  infant, 24–25
  newborn, 23–24
Musculoskeletal system, aging, 163–164
  fat pad syndrome, 163
  muscle cramp, 164
  spontaneous muscular fasciculation, 163–164

N

Nasal decongestant, otitis media, 37
National Institutes of Health, research policies, xiii
Nervous system examination
  child, 24–25
  infant, 24–25
  newborn, 23–24
Neuroblastoma
  child, 61–62
    laboratory tests, 62
    prognosis, 62
    signs and symptoms, 61–62
  infant, 61–62
    laboratory tests, 62
    prognosis, 62
    signs and symptoms, 61–62
Neurolymphatic stimulation, premenstrual syndrome, 119
Newborn
  musculoskeletal examination, 23–24
  nervous system examination, 23–24
Non-Hodgkin's lymphoma, child, 63–65
  laboratory tests, 64
  prognosis, 65
  signs and symptoms, 64
Nutrition
  geriatric patient, 191–192
  resources, 156
Nutrition assessment
  child, 26–27
  geriatric patient, 176–177
  infant, 25–26
Nutritional supplementation, premenstrual syndrome, 118

O

Obesity, 93–94
Osteopenia, 99
Osteoporosis, 99–112
  adjustment, 137–138
  advanced diagnostic testing, 102–103
  anabolic therapy, 107
  calcitonin, 106
  calcium, 104–105
  characterized, 99
  clinical algorithm, prevention, 112
  clinical examination, 101–102
  conventional radiography, 102
  defined, 99
  disphosphate, 107
  dual-energy X-ray absorptiometry, 102
  dual-photon absorptiometry, 102
  estrogen, 106–107
  falling, 100
  fluoride, 107
  fracture treatment, 107–108
  management, 103–104
  pathogenesis, 100–101
  preventive measures, 104
  quantitative computed tomography, 102
  rate of fracture occurrence, 99
  resources, 156
  risk, 99
  risk factors, 101
  single-photon absorptiometry, 102
  vitamin, 106
  vitamin D, 105–106
Osteosarcoma, 60–61
Otitis media, 3–4
  analgesic, 37
  ancillary studies, 33–34
  antihistamine, 37
  anti-inflammatory drug, 37
  auricular adjusting, 35–36
  cervical manipulation, 35
  clinical algorithm, 12, 13
  conservative treatment options, 34–35
  diagnosis, 30
  endonasal technique, 36
  epidemiology, 31
  etiology, 30
  evaluation strategy, 31–34
  external ear, 32
  history, 31
  inspection of head, neck and ears for symmetry and signs of infection, 32
  local heat, 36–37
  management protocol, 34–38
  manual therapy, 35–36
  middle ear, 32
  nasal decongestant, 37
  natural history, 31
  neck biomechanics, 33
  over-the-counter medication, 37
  physiotherapeutic modalities, 36–37
  recurrent, 37–38
    acute otitis media, 37–38
    dietary and nutritional considerations, 37–38
    management, 37–38
    prevention, 37–38
    serous otitis media, 37–38
  referral or consult, 37
  reviewing conservative treatment strategies, 34
  risk factors, 31, 32
  self-care advice, 37
  signs of infection, 31
  soft tissue manipulation, 36
  sources of referred pain, 33
  symptoms and signs, 32–33
  therapeutic objectives, 34
  tympanic ventilation, 36
  vital signs, 32
  warm oil, 36
Over-the-counter medication, otitis media, 37

P

Pain, 198
Partner abuse, 145–153
  clinical algorithm, identifying victim, 152–153
  clinician's legal responsibilities, 150
  cycles of family violence, 146
    honeymoon phase, 146
    tension-building phase, 146
    violent phase, 146
  exit plan, 149–150
  identifying victim, 146–147
  intervention, 148–150
  patient history, 147
  physical examination, 147–148
  safety plan, 149
  scope of problem, 145, 146
Patient history, special needs child, 41–42, 43
Pelvic blocking, geriatric patient, 202
Pelvis, geriatric patient, 202
Periodic health examination
  adolescent, ages 13-18, 83–84
  child, 21–28
    ages 2-6, 81
    ages 7-12, 82
    birth to 18 months, 80
  infant, 21–28
Physical activity, defined, 26–27

Physical examination
  child, 23–25
  infant, 23–25
  special needs child, 42, 43
Physical fitness
  assessment, 26–28
  defined, 26–27
  resources, 156
Plasma homocysteine, 95
Postural stability, 198
Practice guidelines
  child, 8
  infant, 8
Practice parameter, xvii
Pregnancy
  adjustment, 138–143
  biomechanical changes, 138–139
Premenstrual dysphoric disorder, 114
  criteria, 114
Premenstrual syndrome, 113–123
  blood sugar levels, 115
  characterized, 113
  clinical algorithm, management, 122–123
  coping mechanisms, 118
  decreased serotonergic activity, 114
  deficient cofactors, 115
  diagnostic criteria, 115–116
  diet, 118
  estrogen excess, 114
  etiology, 114–115
  exercise, 118
  lifestyle modifications, 116
  management, 116–120
  menstrual cycle, 113–114
  neurolymphatic stimulation, 119
  nutritional supplementation, 118
  patient daily self-assessment form, 117
  pharmacologic agents, 119–120
  prevalence, 114
  progesterone deficiency, 114
  prostaglandin, 115
  psychologic factors, 115
  psychoneuroendocrine mechanisms, 115
  psychosocial interventions, 116
  reflexology, 119
  relaxation response, 116
  spinal manipulation, 119
  surgery, 120
  symptoms, 114
  thyroid function, 114–115
Prepuberty, 17–18
Prostaglandin, 115
Pulmonary system, aging, 166

Q

Quantitative computed tomography, 102

R

Reflexology, premenstrual syndrome, 119
Relaxation response, premenstrual syndrome, 116

S

Scoliosis, 7–8
Screening test, geriatric patient, 170–171
Seed algorithm, xvii
  development, xviii
  graphic programs, xxii
  testing, xxi
Seed guideline, xvii
  development, xviii
  graphic programs, xxii
  testing, xxi
Seed pathway, xvii
  development, xviii
  graphic programs, xxii
  testing, xxi
Self-help, resources, 156
Sexual behavior, child, 18–19
Sexual health, resources, 156
Shoulder joint, 199
Single-photon absorptiometry, 102
Sitting thoracic, geriatric patient, 201–202
Sleep, 162–163
Smoking, 94
Social drug use, child, 16–17
Soft tissue manipulation, otitis media, 36
Special needs child, 41–49
  patient history, 41–42, 43

Spinal adjustment
  child, 69–78
    adjusting apparatus, 72–74, 75, 76
    adjustive technique modifications, 71–76
    age-related changes, 71–72
    positioning options, 72–74, 75, 76
    specificity of contact points, 72, 73
    thrust characteristics, 73–76
  osteoporosis, 137–138
  pregnancy, 138–143
  terminology, 136
Spinal cord injury without radiographic abnormality, 69
Spinal manipulation, premenstrual syndrome, 119
Spine, aging, 164
Spontaneous muscular fasciculation, 163–164
Stair-stepping, geriatric patient, 201
Standards of care, xvii
Strength, child, 27–28
Subluxation
  adolescent, pathology, 70–71
  child, 69
  pathology, 70–71
Substance abuse, resources, 156
Sudden infant death syndrome, 3
  clinical algorithm, 11

T

Temporomandibular joint, aging, 164
Thoracic rock, geriatric patient, 201
Trauma, geriatric patient, 204–210
  automobile safety, 207
  common injuries, 205
  driving, 207
  effects of age on recovery, 205
  epidemiology, 204–205
  exercise, 207
  falls, 205
  fractures, 205
  goals, 205
  home safety, 207
  hormone replacement therapy, 207–208
  motor vehicle accidents, 205
  nutrition, 207

osteoporosis, 207
prevention, 206–208
role of chiropractice in management, 205–206

V

Vertebrobasilar stroke, child, 76–78
    cervical spine rotational adjustments, 77–78
    incidence, 76–77
    mechanism of injury, 76–77

Vitamin, osteoporosis, 106
Vitamin D, osteoporosis, 105–106

W

Warm oil, otitis media, 36
Women, xiii
    anatomic differences, 135
    chiropractic clinical considerations in women's care, 135–143
    initial evaluation, 136

    flexibility, 136–137
    health resources guide, 154–156
    heart disease, 89–98
        characteristics, 89–90
        cholesterol, 92–93
        hypertension, 90–91
        management, 95
        menopause, 93
        obesity, 93–94
        pathogenesis, 90
        plasma homocysteine, 95
        smoking, 94
        thrombogenic risk factors, 94–95